Breast Cancer Recurrence and Advanced Disease

Breast Cancer Recurrence and Advanced Disease

Comprehensive Expert Guidance

Barbara L. Gordon, PhD

Heather S. Shaw, MD

David J. Kroll, PhD

Brooke R. Daniel, MD

Duke University Press
Durham and London 2010

© 2010 Duke University Press
All rights reserved
Printed in the United States of America
on acid-free paper ∞
Designed by Amy Ruth Buchanan
Typeset in Chaparral Pro and Officina Sans
by Tseng Information Systems, Inc.
Library of Congress Cataloging-in-Publication
Data appear on the last printed page of this book.

DISCLAIMER

The information provided in this book is based on
research and experience and believed to be correct
when written; however, it is provided without guarantee or warranty, whether expressed or implied,
as to its accuracy, completeness, usefulness, time-
lessness, suitability, or reliability. Any mention, or
Internet link, leading to other texts, images, organizations, facilities, or persons is not an endorsement of these sources of information or care. These
sources are independent entities. No information
offered in this book is to be relied upon as a substitute for consulting directly with experts for advice
and care. Neither Duke University Press, its employees, nor its authors are responsible or liable for any
direct, indirect, special, incidental, or consequential
damages, or any other damages, however caused,
arising out of the use of any information offered in
this book.

Dedicated to those
who commit themselves
to alleviating the suffering
of others

Contents

Chapter 8. Emotional and Spiritual Well-Being 263

Reflections on Death 293

List of Online Resources

Preface

I was diagnosed with Stage II infiltrating ductal breast cancer when I was forty-two. Not long before I had wondered whether or not something was wrong with my right breast since, as unscientific as this may be, I felt a periodic tingle in the spot where the tumor was eventually found. In fact, the tingle motivated me to get a mammogram a year preceding the discovery of my cancer. The resultant radiology report stating that nothing was abnormal had given me a false assurance. Later I learned that mammograms are not particularly effective in detecting cancer in dense breast tissue, the firm tissue many women have before menopause. I also now realize that I did not press down hard enough when I examined my breasts. A year later, when my gynecologist guided my hand to the suspicious lump, at my fingertips was something different from any lump I had felt before, unmistakably foreign, like a marble suspended in my flesh.

It took me weeks to come to terms with the hard reality of that lump and its consequences. My incredulity about the possibility of having a serious disease—indeed my arrogance in believing I could be in anything other than good health—in retrospect is a bit embarrassing. At the time my lump was discovered, I was heading to Italy for the first time to encounter my heritage and prepare for bringing students abroad in the future. All the arrangements had been set and of course, investigating this lump was, at a minimum, inconvenient. With the encouragement of a friend, I did what was sensible and made a follow-up appointment for an ultrasound and new mammogram. When the radiologist at the follow-up called me into a dark room with my scans in his hands and a bit nervously told me I should see a surgeon, my eyes welled with tears. Regardless, I thought seriously about flying away to Italy, unwilling to exchange Tuscany for an operating table. But in the end, I met with the surgeon who advised me to have the lump removed sooner rather than later. Shortly after the surgery, as I heard what the surgeon said when she called with the biopsy results, I felt ushered into an alternate reality. I slunk down onto the beige carpet that hot June afternoon and sobbed while my cats, unperturbed, purred and rubbed their heads against my legs. Still not fully accepting I had breast cancer, I went to the surgeon's office a few days later and questioned whether my results had gotten mixed up with someone else's. When it was clear they had not, the diagnosis became true and fixed.

I gathered all the external and internal resources I could muster in an effort to deal with my diagnosis. I am a teacher and one groundbreaking study from my graduate school days came back to me. The researchers found that students were more likely to succeed in school if they could exercise some control in their learning environment. I never forgot this, and as a patient it took on new meaning. Though we do not have control over everything in life, we can make choices that can significantly shape outcomes. I wanted to be sure to the best of my ability that I made decisions about my cancer that would enhance my well-being. Others offered help. A woman from the American Cancer Society who a year earlier had been diagnosed with my stage and type of cancer came to speak with me about her surgery and treatment. Two women at my workplace who had cancer shared what they had been through and gave me reading material. I embarked on a crash course to educate myself on both traditional and alternative therapies.

Before I learned that I had breast cancer, with the exception of gynecological checkups, I shied away from traditional Western medicine. My misgivings stemmed mostly from traditional medicine's often narrow focus, aiming care at the disease, sometimes neglecting the rest of the person. Also, when I was diagnosed with cancer, the traditional medical world offered mostly harsh treatments (surgery, radiation, and chemotherapy). On the other hand, my confidence in alternative therapy was eroding. I was overwhelmed by the variety of options and appalled by some literature insinuating that I had caused my illness or had fallen out of cosmic good graces. I also thought it criminal that some alternative literature advocated rejecting standard medical treatment on the basis of conspiracy theories and anecdotal evidence.

My dreams revealed my confusion over these two types of therapies. In one I found myself standing on an airport runway, two large planes heading straight at me, full speed. Just as they began lifting off a short distance from me, they swerved into one another, colliding. I fell to my knees covering my head with my arms as the debris barreled toward me. Over time, I realized that therapies do not always pose an either/ or choice. Alternative treatment can be a misnomer since it sometimes can be integrated with traditional treatment. Both kinds of care share the same objectives—to prevent, alleviate, or eradicate pain and illness. I am heartened that well-intentioned health practitioners, rather than being threatened by methods of healing different from their own, sometimes join forces for the benefit of those in their care. I have become more cautious of all medicines. I track down the evidence-based information, consider my tolerance for risk, and listen to my intuition.

Over the ensuing months of treatment I felt at times as though the debris from the planes' collision was pelting me. I was sore from probings and pricks, sick of being sick to my stomach, and weary of appointments and decisions, but I was shielded and guided through the onslaught. A particularly loyal friend was at my side for nearly every hurdle. I had in my hands *Dr. Susan Love's Breast Book*, the only book on the market at that time that imparted medical information about breast cancer to lay readers. Because of what I learned in those pages, I was informed when I went to my appointments. I could move to the "next" questions. I asked my surgeon if he could spare certain nerves when conducting the lymph node dissection. When I learned the size of my tumor and the lymph node involvement, I was able to stage my cancer and anticipate my treatment regimen, which gave me time to investigate statistical information on chemotherapies to decide if I was willing to submit myself to certain harsh medicines. I learned it was possible to build up a tolerance to some chemotherapies, which led me not to enroll in a clinical trial, thinking that later on I may need the drug being tested if I were to have a recurrence. Before being told that my chemotherapy regimen would likely induce menopause, I already knew this would be a consequence, allowing me to mourn the loss of my reproductive years in private and remain clearer headed as I listened to what my oncologist had to say about what was ahead. Information enabled me to feel more in control, better able to have intelligent conversations with doctors and participate in my care. This feeling of empowerment kept immobilization and depression from taking hold. I developed a curiosity about my disease that led me to appreciate my physicians' expertise and develop confidence in my own choices.

So I felt particularly disempowered when two years after my initial treatment, believing my breast cancer had spread to my lungs, I could not find authoritative, detailed medical information for late-stage breast cancer. For many months I believed that my cancer had metastasized. My lungs felt heavy. I had a constant cough, intermittent sharp pains on both sides of my chest and in my back, and an overall feeling of malaise. At my regular cancer checkup a chest x-ray was ordered. Within a few days, while I was sweeping my kitchen floor, the sun streaming in, I got the bad news over the phone. Something abnormal was spotted on my chest X-ray. It confirmed my suspicion. As with my earlier diagnosis, this news came at an inconvenient time. (When doesn't it?) I had been cleaning in anticipation of a visit from my mother and stepfather, who would house-sit while I headed to a writing workshop; in response to the news, I simply told the cancer clinic that I would make a follow-up appointment in about two weeks. But two days later, as I drove from my home in the middle of North Carolina to the workshop in Wilmington on the coast, the reality of my situation became more pressing with each mile marker. In the quiet hum of the long interstate drive, I could no longer compartmentalize what I knew.

Halfway to the coast I got out of my car at a rest stop, gathered myself, and used a pay phone to call the Morris Cancer Clinic at Duke University Hospital to see if I could be squeezed into the appointment schedule. I did not have enough change to remain on hold, so I said I would call back. I drove on, still heading toward the ocean, then stopped at the next rest stop to call the head of the workshop, explaining my circumstances, asking if I could simply forfeit my deposit and cancel, which the workshop leader kindly allowed. A bit further down the road I stopped yet a third time to call Duke again. I could get in the next day. As soon as I saw a spot for a U-turn, I swung the car around and headed back, realizing the hardest part was next: sharing the news with my unsuspecting mother. Within moments of opening the door and seeing her surprised look, I told her why I had returned. Her first words were, "Whatever happens, we will go through it together." We headed to a local bookstore, where I assumed there would be that next book about breast cancer, the one written by an oncologist about procedures and treatment for metastatic breast cancer. I figured my local bookstore just did not stock it, but after thorough library searches, I finally conceded that it did not exist.

Without that book I was plunged into darkness, stumbling forward, not knowing what came next. Thinking my X-ray had confirmed my me-tastasis, I was surprised when I was sent for a CT scan at my next appointment. Shortly afterward my oncologist brought me into a room with lit images displayed in a row above us. He said something close to, "Unfortunately, it looks as though the cancer has spread to every quadrant, but we have ways we can keep it at bay for two or three years." I could see in the images what looked like spotted cotton candy floating in my lungs. He turned from those and gave me a good hard look, as though he was trying to reconcile some difference between the body before him and what he saw on film. Then he asked if I was all right. I was impassive; it was what I had expected. I was ready to discuss a treatment regimen, but I was surprised to learn I needed another test—a bronchoscopy, something that I could not pronounce and sounded unfriendly. This was how I learned the degree to which oncologists must be certain someone has had a recurrence and what kind it is, before prescribing treatment. Again I lamented that I had no outside medical resource to which to turn, to empower me with information as I had had during my initial cancer diagnosis. I wanted to know if this was the normal course of diagnosing a metastasis. I wanted to know about the procedure. I wanted to know if treatment would be much different from before. And, I was thinking about the big questions: How long might I live? How functional would I be and for how long? What do I need to do to prepare for death? I wanted to take care of business and be free to live as fully as possible in whatever time I had left.

Late Friday night, a day or two after the bronchoscopy, my oncologist called to say that so far the results did not show metastasized cancer. As incongruous as it sounds, that too seemed predictable. Perhaps it was the curious look he gave me at the office when showing me the images, or perhaps I was numb. On Monday, another call was less hopeful. A gathering of doctors felt the CT scan and bronchoscopy were inconclusive, and they recommended exploratory lung surgery. It was when I awoke from that surgery, in the moments I was coming to consciousness, that this book was born. I had a foggy memory of nurses remarking that I did not have breast cancer in my lungs, and on a second slightly more lucid awakening, the pulmonary surgeon was beside me, repeating that news, saying I had an autoimmune disease called sarcoidosis.

Though I was not yet able to see where I was, I was able to eke out a wheezy, "How sure are you?" In a flood of statistics, my kindly doctor handed me back my life, assuring me that no more testing was needed. I laughed, or attempted to. Having the objective world of science directed at me in this most extraordinary moment seemed incongruous. And, perhaps I was laughing at the vagaries of life and was in need of an emotional release. Rather than laughter, what emerged were sputtering coughs. Directly following that outburst, gratitude welled in me and out toward others—those who take care of patients, researchers, and particularly advocates, who, like me, have breast cancer but who, unlike me, have devoted themselves to bettering the lives of fellow cancer patients. I knew to my core that I was a recipient of their efforts. I had donated money to breast cancer organizations but felt compelled to do more. Before I could fully open my eyes from that operation, I made a vow to do so.

By the time I left the hospital, it was clear to me what my contribution could be. Using my background in writing, interest and coursework in science and statistics, and experience as a breast cancer patient, I was determined to find an oncologist with whom I could collaborate to write that nonexistent book I had longed for and could not find. Thus began a long process that included more than seven years of researching, writing, and managing this undertaking. Many people contributed to this effort — clinicians, researchers, social workers, and fellow writers, whose names you will see in the acknowledgments — and I am honored that three co-authors with specialized backgrounds, good humor, and bountiful altruism signed on. Without their expertise, this book would not have come into existence.

I did not have to look far beyond my own experience to know that the information in this book could help others. While I was working on the manuscript, sadly, my mother was diagnosed with breast cancer; a woman I regard as my stepsister died of it; two of my close friends lost their cousins to the disease; and a colleague at my workplace passed away from inflammatory breast cancer. Over this period I was reminded repeatedly that my own cancer could spread. A polyp was removed from my uterus. An ultrasound revealed a growth on my ovary. A colonoscopy led to an MRI that showed a growth was pressing on my lower intestine. And, a CT scan was ordered to investigate a lump that appeared above my left collarbone. In each case, I was fortunate that the growths were benign.

In addition to these reminders of breast cancer's prevalence and possible reemergence, immersing myself in information about advanced breast cancer was alternately frightening, comforting, and fascinating. In learning the symptoms of recurrence I could dismiss certain aches and pains as likely something other than cancer. I was comforted when I saw a graph that showed the chances of a recurrence sharply decline a few years out from an initial diagnosis. But, I also became aware of how unpredictable breast cancer can be and how elusive a cure is. As researchers plumb the depths of the workings of cancer, its complexity provokes new challenges for treatment. No matter how much is discovered, certain aspects of what is life prolonging and what initiates our deaths remain mysterious.

In working on this book, I heard and read heart-wrenching and heart-warming accounts of others' experiences with late-stage breast cancer. I have come ever more to appreciate everyone's unique journey and means of grappling with serious illness and death. When death was close at hand in my life, it became clear that contributing to easing the suffering of others is life's task. I hope this book accomplishes that end. To those of you who have come to hold this book in your hands, my co-authors and I trust you find empowerment and comfort in the pages ahead. We offer you knowledge and wish you strength, hope, courage, and peace.

—**Barbara L. Gordon, PhD**

Acknowledgments

Many people generously and graciously lent their expertise to this book. First and foremost I want to thank Heather Stuart Shaw, MD, David J. Kroll, PhD, and Brooke Ratliff Daniel, MD, who without hesitation joined in this effort to bring needed information to people with breast cancer and those who care for them. I also want to single out Edward K. Lobenhofer, PhD, who initiated me into the world of breast cancer research and lent his keen eye to the scientific chapters. Without Ed's guidance at the inception of this project, I could not have gone forward with it. Special thanks to Renea M. Valea, head of Duke Hospital's Oncology Team of Licensed Clinical Social Workers, who arranged for a meeting with colleagues Evelyn M. Reed, Roberta D. Calhoun-Eagan, Sandra A. Scott, Amy E. Powell, Gregory J. Bankoski, and Debra J. Huntoon that resulted in the addition of essential information in the chapter on practical matters. Mary Honeycutt, volunteer coordinator of the University of North Carolina Hospice, and her colleagues Elizabeth Hart, RN, CHPN, Andrea Tuttle, MSW, and Tanya Thompson, MSW, LCSW, were also very helpful in responding to sections of this book related to end-of-life concerns. Robert James, Associate Director of Access Services in the Duke University Medical Center Library, was always quick to respond with needed information, as was Shaunta Alvarez, collection development librarian of Belk Library at Elon University.

I am appreciative of the sabbatical awarded by Elon University that allowed me to complete the first draft of this book and am appreciative of many in my workplace who gave their time to this endeavor, including Robert Springer, Director of Institutional Research, and Kirsten Doehler, Assistant Professor of Mathematics, who offered clear explanations in answer to numerous statistical questions; Shaun Adkins, Elite Program Consultant, who spent many hours helping me scan and resize images; and Pat Jones, program assistant to the English and Human Services Departments, who good-heartedly and deftly helped prepare the final manuscript more than once.

A thousand bows of gratitude to Cassie Kircher, Janet Myers, and Janet Warman, my writing group and the midwives of this book. Nearly every page passed under their eyes for their insightful responses. From beginning to end they provided steadfast support. I am grateful to other dear friends who not only frequently inquired about the book's progress, but who also were able to proofread and respond to chapters in a pinch, including Denise L. David, Teitaku Gardiner, Jo Grimley, Constance (Zo) Tanzo, Sandy Stewart, and G. Douglas Meyers.

From this book's beginning—a promise to myself on a hospital gurney to do more for others with breast cancer—to its publication has been a long, arduous journey. My parents, James and Lee Gordon, and my brother, Jim Gordon, did everything possible to make that journey a smooth one, and no one I know is more pleased than they are to see that promise fulfilled. Along the way, loved ones enabled me to scale obstacles by lending their ears and their wisdom, particularly G. Douglas Meyers and Sandy Stewart. Many others provided encouragement and inspiration, including Rita Pollard, Mary Pudaloff, Sheila Arnold, Annie and Ken Hassell, Betsy and Ronald DePersis, Eve Weingarten, Jeffery Levine, Bobbi Chaville, and Gregory Maunz. I am indebted to all those whose names are listed here, along with some whose names are not. In varying and significant ways all of them added their shoulders to turn the wheel that brought this book into being.

—Barbara L. Gordon, PhD

....

I would like to thank my fellow authors, without whom this book would not exist. I have special thanks for Brooke Daniel, MD, who got the medical expert parts of the manuscript moving on the right track at the same time that she kept me on track in clinic. Of course thanks go to my dear family members for their help (David Kroll) and patience (Phoebe Kroll) in this endeavor. Thanks must also go to my many colleagues and mentors in breast cancer research and treatment. Without the wonderful mentorship of Eric Winer, MD, Linda Sutton, MD, James Vredenburgh, MD, J. Dirk Iglehart, MD, and Jeffrey Marks, PhD, I would not have become a breast cancer clinician and researcher. I could not have become such a well-rounded clinician without my wonderful colleagues at Duke University, who taught me about multidisciplinary care of breast cancer patients on a daily basis: in Breast Imaging, Jay Baker, MD, Mary Scott Soo, MD, and

Ruth Walsh, MD; in Pathology, Rex Bentley, MD, and Alan Proia, MD; in Radiation Oncology, Ellen Jones, MD, PhD, Larry Marks, MD, and Leonard Prosnitz, MD; in Surgical Oncology, Bryan Clary, MD, Thomas D'Amico, MD, George Leight, MD, John Olson, MD, PhD, Scott Pruitt, MD, PhD, and Lee Wilke, MD. My colleagues in Medical Oncology always served as wonderful supports, sounding boards, and collaborators: Kimberly Blackwell, MD, Gretchen Kimmick, MD, and P. Kelly Marcom, MD. Finally and most important, thank you to all of the amazing women with breast cancer who have allowed me the privilege of caring for them.

—Heather S. Shaw, MD

I wish to thank my friend and co-author, Barbara Gordon, PhD, for the invitation to join in this effort. It is a rare privilege for a basic scientist to have the opportunity to directly address cancer patients and their needs. I am honored to have the chance to share in this project.

I am eternally grateful to my wife and co-author, Heather S. Shaw, MD, for her dedication to the care and education of hundreds of breast cancer patients like those who will read this book. Beyond being an incredible life partner, she has patiently spent many hours of discussion with me on the aspects of basic science that are most important in cancer care. Her selfless devotion to her patients and her unending quest to provide them with compassionate and cutting-edge care is an inspiration to all of us. I am indebted to our daughter, Phoebe Talbot Kroll, for understanding that Mommy and Daddy often had to take time away from her to complete this project. Phoebe is fortunate to have her mother as a role model, and I hope that she can look back on this book with pride and an appreciation of how important it is for her mom to serve her patients.

I also wish to acknowledge my own mother, Barbara Kroll Holzapfel, RN, whose diagnosis with breast cancer and subsequent twenty-three years free of the disease catalyzed my interest in pursuing a cancer research career. I am thankful for her unwavering support of my education and career path, even though I never became a "real" doctor. Her example of personal strength through breast cancer and the nearly quarter-century of extended life she has enjoyed serve as a continual reminder not only of the progress cancer research has made for some, but also the need for us to continue our fight to offer the benefits of such progress to others.

I could not have gained a level of scientific stature consistent with being selected to contribute to this book without the support of my scientific and journalism mentors over the years: my PhD mentor, Thomas C. Rowe, PhD; my postdoctoral mentors, Arthur Gutierrez-Hartmann, MD, and James P. Hoefler, PhD; my academic departmental chairmen, V. Gene Erwin, PhD, and David Ross, PhD; my natural products research colleagues, Nicholas H. Oberlies, PhD, and Ara DerMarderosian, PhD, as well as Mansukh C. Wani, PhD, the late Monroe E. Wall, PhD, co-discoverers of Taxol and camptothecin; Joe Graedon, MS, and Terry Graedon, PhD, of *The People's Pharmacy*; and Tom Linden, MD, of the medical journalism program at the University of North Carolina, Chapel Hill.

Finally, I wish to thank you, the reader, for your confidence in our expertise to pick up and read this book. I hope that we have been able to serve as a source of comfort and objective, understandable information in your journey through cancer.

—**David J. Kroll, PhD**

I would like to thank Barbara Gordon for giving me the opportunity to contribute in this book. I would like to thank Heather Shaw for her mentorship and friendship. She taught me my foundations in breast oncology. I would like to thank my husband, Davey Daniel, for his love and patience. I would also like to thank my patients, whose wisdom and insight continue to motivate me.

—**Brooke R. Daniel, MD**

Introduction

Worldwide, breast cancer is the most commonly diagnosed cancer in women; an estimated 1.3 million people (mostly women) were diagnosed with the disease in 2007 (1).* Fortunately, the majority of people who learn they have breast cancer are in early stages of the disease. They go on to comprise the largest group of those living with breast cancer, and most do not have their lives cut short by the disease. Still, nearly all whose lives have been touched by cancer are haunted, to some degree, with the specter of their cancer recurring. You may be among them. After your initial treatment ended, you may have been seeking information about recurrence, information that is less readily available than the information you sought when you first were diagnosed. This book can address many of your concerns. We offer explanations about types of recurrence and discuss their symptoms. We discuss pathological factors that predict chances of a recurrence and present information about testing, prescriptions, and lifestyle choices that may minimize that likelihood.

You may, however, be among a different group of the millions living with breast cancer: those who were diagnosed initially with late-stage cancer or those who have had a recurrence in which the cancer has invaded an organ, referred to as metastatic cancer. In this book we provide you with information about the diagnostic tests, potential surgeries, and treatment options that may be prescribed to help manage your disease. We suggest means for getting the best care, ways to evaluate complementary therapies, and avenues for alleviating physical pain and depression. We address sensitive questions that people are often reluctant to discuss, including when treatment should stop, what one might experience as the disease progresses, and what it might be like to die of the disease.

Though this book is written primarily for those with breast cancer, the subjects covered can be useful to nearly everyone whose cancer is in a late stage. People with potentially incurable cancers need to know what

---

* Numbers in parentheses correspond to texts listed in the reference section of this book.

hospice provides, what legal documents should be prepared, how to plan memorial services, and how others have dealt with the psychological and spiritual challenges of facing death. This book can also be helpful to you if you are among those who take care of, or advocate for, those with cancer since we offer information to enable you to talk more knowledgeably with doctors, to advocate for patients' medical rights, and to comfort someone when death approaches. If you are a cancer health-care professional, sections of this book can complement your area of expertise so that you can direct your patients to resources and more comprehensively address their concerns.

We recommend that in using this book, you peruse the contents and index so that you can pinpoint the section that best suits your needs. The topics were chosen to address what readers most want to know, and embedded throughout chapters you will find resource boxes with in-depth and updated information for you to access. The Web links within these resource boxes lead to authoritative sites that Internet searches do not readily display, including sites such as the National Institutes of Health (NIH) Fact Sheets on Supplements, the Physician Data Query (PDQ) of the National Cancer Institute (NCI), Web casts from the San Antonio Breast Cancer Symposium, and sites with information on legislation related to patients' rights.

Considerations in Reading This Book

Be aware that this is a time of unprecedented progress in cancer health care, with new drugs emerging every few months and clinical trial results regularly altering treatment guidelines. The dynamic nature of cancer medicine and health-care legislation makes it difficult for any book or Web site to be as entirely current or thorough as a professional's knowledge. Therefore, use this book as an aid and an adjunct when speaking with professionals. Breast oncologists, attorneys who study medical law, hospice nurses, and local social service counselors are uniquely informed in the intricacies of their areas. While the pages that follow can assist you in making choices in your best interests, the material contained in them is not a substitute for the expert opinion of those most knowledgeable about your particular case and the laws and resources in your locality.

In selecting information for this text, we aimed to fill the gap between the brief, sometimes commercial, material found in pamphlets and on

Web sites and the lengthy, complex expert material found in medical journals known to professionals. Striking this middle ground is challenging
and can exclude audiences for whom some material presupposes background knowledge. However, in making this expert information accessible to many more people, we anticipate that it will be disseminated more
widely through breast cancer networks and through those who interrelate
with patients, including nurses, physicians' assistants, hospice personnel,
breast cancer advocates, social workers, and physicians.

Given our backgrounds, this book reflects breast cancer care in the
United States. Readers in other countries may have access to different
treatments and may not have access to some of the treatments that are
mentioned here. A 2007 study in *Annals of Oncology* noted that the use
of new cancer drugs is most rapidly implemented in the United States,
Austria, France, and Switzerland and more slowly in the United Kingdom,
New Zealand, South Africa, Poland, and the Czech Republic (2). Conversely,
treatments considered unconventional in the United States may be more
acceptable in other countries. Philosophies vary as well. Oncologists in the
United States may be more likely than their international counterparts to
employ aggressive treatments and less likely to discontinue therapy.

The culture of oncology is influenced by each country's medical training
of its professionals and the respective national system of health care. You
will see that we have included a section in this book about medical rights
and ways to cover medical bills, a particular concern in the United States.
Access to treatment, however, is a concern in much of the world. For this
reason a portion of the proceeds from this book are being donated to Partners In Health, a non-profit organization whose mission is to help the
world's poor obtain good health care. Though cancer is thought to be more
a disease of the developed world, men in developing countries have close
to the same cancer mortality rate as their counterparts in the developed
world, and women in developing countries have a higher mortality rate in
comparison with women in developed countries (3).

The word choice in this book reflects its primary readership—women.
Since the vast majority of individuals with breast cancer are women, we
use "she" to refer to those with breast cancer when a singular pronoun
is called for. We regret the off-putting nature of that choice for the approximately two thousand men diagnosed annually with breast cancer in
the United States (approximately 1 percent of all cases) and for the many
other men worldwide (4). We generally use feminine singular pronouns
as well when referring to oncologists in an effort to break down gender

stereotypes and to recognize the dramatic increase of women oncologists. However, we want to acknowledge in this introduction the great number of dedicated male oncologists caring for those who have cancer.

As authors we each bring a unique perspective and background in contributing to the content in this book. With diverse knowledge and experience — from patient to pharmacology researcher to oncologists — we have worked together to offer a comprehensive collection of expert information. We hope this serves you well and that you find much in the pages that follow that will aid, empower, and enliven you.

CHAPTER 1

Local and Distant Recurrence

Do not be anxious about tomorrow;
tomorrow will look after itself.
—Matthew 6:34

Even cowards can endure hardship;
only the brave can endure suspense.
—Mignon McLaughlin, *A Woman's Notebook*

Over millennia the word "cancer" has inspired concern. Humankind has wrestled with its nature, seeking to define, understand, and overcome it. Physicians thousands of years ago in ancient Greece recognized the disease, calling abnormal growths *oncos*, the origin for our word "oncology." The word "cancer" comes from what the Greeks called solid growths, *karkinos*, meaning crab, a derivative of the Indo-European word for hard.

You probably know personally how frightening a diagnosis of cancer can be since you are reading this book. You may be among the many millions of people worldwide living with cancer or among the many who care for them. In the United States alone, almost 2.45 million women were living with a diagnosis of breast cancer in 2005, the latest year for which data were available at this writing (1). This number will likely increase as newer treatments extend lives. Though the disease has not significantly altered since it was first identified, our ability to manage it has greatly improved. Increasingly we know more about its workings, and increasingly people have access to advancements in treatment and good care. This book is a part of that care. We bring to you and your loved ones expert information about recurrence and advanced breast cancer. In conjunction with your health-care professionals, what you learn in these pages can empower you to make knowledgeable decisions for your complete well-being—body, mind, and spirit.

In this chapter on recurrence, we introduce important concepts in the diagnosis and treatment of breast cancer. The common questions that are posed in the following section form the basic outline of topics in this chapter. For those of you who have metastases at the time of diagnosis, some of the material on recurrence may be less helpful. However, the discussion of the diagnosis of cancer will give you a good working knowledge of breast cancer to aid in reading your medical reports and in understanding the therapeutic options available to you.

Common Questions about Recurrence

What Is a Recurrence?

Nearly everyone who has been treated for breast cancer worries about cancer returning or, in other words, worries about having a recurrence. Many do not realize that a breast cancer recurrence refers to a number of different conditions. Though any recurrence is scary, some are far less life threatening than others. Recurrences are of various types and differ significantly in terms of treatment and prognosis. A recurrence can be *local*, meaning that cancer has reappeared in the same breast or scar area; *regional*, meaning that cancer has reappeared in nearby lymph nodes, such as those under the collarbone or in the chest wall; or *distant*, meaning that cancer has reappeared in an organ in the body such as in a bone, a lung, the liver, or the brain.

Recurrences are usually caused by a return of cancer cells from the original tumor, cells that remained despite prior surgery, chemotherapy, and radiation. Most often a local recurrence occurs in the mastectomy or lumpectomy scar. Following the original surgery, the breast cancer cells at the edges (margins) of the removed areas of the breast may have been too few or too far apart to be seen by a pathologist looking at tissue through a microscope. These cells can lie dormant, and though radiation, chemotherapy, and hormonal therapies may have been used to destroy them, occasionally some survive and reappear. It is also possible, though less likely, that a local recurrence is the result of the original cancer circulating in the body and reappearing in the breast; this is a more serious condition. Cancer that recurs or is discovered in a distant site is called metastatic cancer.

What Is My Chance for Recurrence?

Your oncologist may use a number of sources of information to determine your risk of cancer recurrence. A computer program called Adjuvant! Online can give general estimates of chances of recurrence based on the size, grade, and estrogen-receptor status of your tumor, in combination with the number of lymph nodes with metastases. These factors are discussed under "Predictors of Recurrence." The estimate calculated with Adjuvant! Online is not highly specific; it does not distinguish between distant and local recurrences, nor does it currently take HER2—an important indicator of a tumor's response to certain drugs as well as its potential aggressiveness—status into account. Newer tests that look at a gene signature may soon more accurately predict the risk of distant recurrence.

How Can I Prevent a Recurrence?

Depending on your specific cancer, chemotherapy, hormonal therapy, and/or radiation may be, or may have been, recommended to reduce the chances of a recurrence. Exercise and a healthy diet appear to prevent recurrences, and specific recommendations are discussed below under "Reducing Chances of Recurrence."

How Is a Recurrence Detected?

Some recurrences are easy to see, such as those that occur in the skin. These can be diagnosed with a simple skin punch sample or biopsy. Recurrences in the lymph nodes, such as those in the armpit (axilla) or around the collarbone (clavicle), are usually found as hard lumps that can be sampled with a needle to confirm a recurrence. Recurrences in other sites, such as the lung, liver, or bone, are detected with scans such as a CT scan or bone scan. Areas of concern must also be sampled with a needle to confirm a recurrence. This is further discussed in "Detecting a Local or Regional Recurrence" and "Detecting and Confirming a Metastatic Recurrence."

How Can Recurrence Be Treated?

Depending on the site and type of recurrence, combinations of hormonal therapy, chemotherapy, immunotherapy, radiation therapy, and surgery can be used. Further discussion of local and regional recurrence can be found in this chapter under "Treatment of Local or Regional Recurrence," and a more extended discussion of treatments, particularly for distant (metastatic) recurrence, can be found in chapter 3.

What Does It Mean to Have a Distant Recurrence?

A distant recurrence is the reappearance of cancer in an organ away from the site of the original cancer, such as the bone or lung. A distant recurrence signals that initial treatment did not destroy all the malignant cells. At the time of this writing, no treatment can guarantee the eradication of all cancer cells.

If the Cancer Comes Back in My Bone/Lung/Liver, Is It Bone/ Lung/Liver Cancer or Breast Cancer?

If the original cancer reappears in your bone or in another organ, it is not bone or another type of cancer, but breast cancer that has spread (metastasized) to the bone or that organ. Regardless of the organ to which breast cancer has metastasized, it is still breast cancer and keeps the features of breast cancer.

Does It Matter How Quickly a Recurrence Is Detected? Why Doesn't My Doctor Get Scans on Me Routinely?

It improves chances of survival to detect a local or regional recurrence as early as possible. This fact guides the recommendation for monthly breast self-examination; annual mammograms; and regular follow-up appointments with a physician after diagnosis. (See "Conducting a Breast Self-Exam" resource box in this chapter.) Unfortunately, detecting a distant recurrence early, such as seeing cancer on a CT or bone scan, does not significantly improve chances of survival. Once a tumor has spread outside the local or regional area, it is no longer curable. It is, however, treatable, as will be discussed. Many women with metastatic breast cancer have a good quality of life and live many years.

Current surveillance guidelines from major cancer organizations do not include routine scans other than mammography or other breast imaging on an annual basis. The American Society of Clinical Oncology (ASCO) recommends physical examinations every three to six months for the first three years after diagnosis, every six to twelve months for years four and five, and annually thereafter. Yearly mammographic evaluation should also be performed. The National Comprehensive Cancer Network (NCCN) recommends annual mammograms and physical examinations every four to six months for the first five years after diagnosis and annual exams after five years. Neither ASCO nor NCCN recommends tumor markers or other blood tests as part of surveillance.

Is the Diagnosis of Recurrence Going to Affect How Long I Will Live?

If your cancer has spread locally, then your risk for distant metastases increases. If you have distant metastases, then most likely breast cancer will shorten your life. Where the metastases are; how well your cancer responds to therapy (chemotherapy, hormonal therapy, radiation therapy, and/or immunotherapy); your age; and your underlying health will all affect how long you will live. Women with metastatic breast cancer are now living longer than ever with new treatments. This is further discussed in this chapter under "Prognosis of Distant Metastasis."

Predictors of Recurrence

Oncologists and pathologists can estimate the risk of your cancer returning in various ways. In general, your type of cancer is compared to similar types of cancer. The number of times out of one hundred that type of cancer was seen to have returned in the past is estimated as your chance of recurrence. Estimates can be made based on the size and spread of the cancer (stage of cancer), the way the cancer looks under the microscope (pathologic type), the types of proteins present on the cancer, and (most recently) a specific gene "signature." Estimates of recurrence will likely continue to become more personalized such that risk will be determined for each individual's specific tumor, not simply her tumor type.

Cancer Staging

Cancer staging is a means of indicating the amount of cancer present in the body when the disease is first diagnosed. It is also the best means at this time for predicting your risk of recurrence, although this is changing as newer molecular tests are being developed. The system most often used to describe the extent of breast cancer is the TNM staging system of the American Joint Commission on Cancer (AJCC). In TNM staging, information about the tumor (T), spread to nearby lymph nodes (N), and distant metastases (M) is combined, and a stage is assigned to specific TNM groupings. The TNM stage groupings are described using Roman numerals from 0 to IV.

The *clinical stage* is determined by what the doctor learns from the physical examination and imaging tests. The *pathologic stage* includes the findings of the pathologist after surgery. Most of the time, the pathologic stage is the most important since involvement of the lymph nodes can be accurately determined only by examining them under a microscope.

TNM Staging System of the American Joint Commission on Cancer (AJCC) — Categories of TNM

T Categories: T categories are based on the size of the breast cancer and whether it has spread to nearby tissue.

> **Tis:** T is used only for carcinoma *in situ* (noninvasive breast cancer), such as ductal carcinoma *in situ* (DCIS) or lobular carcinoma *in situ* (LCIS).
>
> **T1:** The cancer is less than or equal to 2 cm in diameter (about ¾ inch).
>
> **T2:** The cancer is more than 2 cm but not more than 5 cm in diameter.
>
> **T3:** The cancer is more than 5 cm in diameter.
>
> **T4:** The cancer is any size and has spread to the chest wall, skin, or both. This category includes inflammatory breast cancer. To learn more about inflammatory breast cancer, see "Inflammatory Breast Cancer" at the end of this section.

N Categories: The N category is based on which of the lymph nodes near the breast, if any, are affected by the cancer.

> **N0 Clinical:** The cancer has not spread to lymph nodes, based on clinical exam.
>
> **N0 Pathological:** The cancer has not spread to lymph nodes, based on examining them under the microscope.
>
> **N1 Clinical:** The cancer has spread to lymph nodes under the arm on the same side as the breast cancer. Lymph nodes are not attached to one another or to the surrounding tissue.

N1 Pathological: The cancer is found in 1–3 lymph nodes under the arm.

N1 Clinical: The cancer has spread to lymph nodes under the arm on the same side as the breast cancer, and lymph nodes have attached to one another or to the surrounding tissue. Alternatively, the cancer can be seen to have spread to the internal mammary lymph nodes (next to the breastbone) but not to the lymph nodes under the arm.

N2 Pathological: The cancer has spread to 4–9 lymph nodes under the arm or to the internal mammary lymph nodes.

N3 Clinical: The cancer has spread to lymph nodes above (supraclavicular) or just below (infraclavicular) the collarbone on the same side as the breast cancer and may or may not have spread to lymph nodes under the arm. Alternatively, the cancer has spread to the internal mammary lymph nodes or the superclaviclular and axillary lymph nodes under the arm, both on the same side as the cancer.

N3 Pathological: The cancer has spread to ten or more lymph nodes under the arm or also involves lymph nodes in other areas around the breast.

M Categories: The M category depends on whether the cancer has spread to any distant tissues and organs.

M0: No distant cancer spread.

M1: Cancer has spread to distant organs.

Once the T, N, and M categories have been assigned, the information is combined to assign an overall stage of 0, I, II, III, or IV. The stages identify tumor types that have a similar outlook and thus are treated in a similar way. For a further look at staging, use the link in the following resource box.

BREAST CANCER STAGING

- American Cancer Society, Breast Cancer Staging: Provides information on breast cancer staging.

    http://www.cancer.org/docroot/CRI/content/CRI_2_4_3X_How_is_
    breast_cancer_staged_5.asp?sitearea

resources

Inflammatory Breast Cancer

Inflammatory breast cancer is a special type of breast cancer that is given its own T designation, T4d. A breast involved with inflammatory breast cancer is red, swollen, and warm, and the condition can be easily confused with an infection of the breast. These symptoms do not go away with antibiotic treatment, unlike in an infected breast. Often the skin of the breast resembles the peel of an orange, called "peau d'orange." Frequently these skin changes are found without a lump that can be felt (a palpable mass), and a mammogram may show only skin thickening. A skin biopsy performed on an affected area shows tumor cells in the lymph channels of the skin, the dermal lymphatics. These cancers are particularly aggressive, and spread to the local lymph nodes is common. Distant disease is present at initial diagnosis more often than in other types of cancer, and a CT scan and a bone scan are usually performed soon after diagnosis. With newer presurgical (neoadjuvant) chemotherapy and targeted treatment for HER2 overexpressing tumors, long-term survival from this cancer has significantly improved.

resources

INFLAMMATORY BREAST CANCER

- Inflammatory Breast Cancer Research Foundation: Provides information on symptoms and where to receive special care.
  PO Box 90117
  Anchorage, AK 99509
  877-786-7422
  http://www.ibcreasearch.org
  E-mail: librarian@ibresearch.org

- National Institute Fact Sheet on Inflammatory Breast Cancer
  http://www.cancer.gov/cancertopics/factsheet/Sites-Types/IBC

- Inflammatory Breast Cancer Association: Includes treatment information and forums.
  http://www.ibchelp.org

Pathology Reports for Diagnosis and Prognosis

The staging of a cancer relies heavily on a pathology report. In addition to noting physical evidence, such as the size of a tumor and the amount of lymph node involvement, pathology reports note the histological type of cancer (how the cancer cells look under the microscope), the aggressiveness of the cancer in terms of how rapidly the cells appear to be dividing, and the extent cancer cells have invaded surrounding tissue. Last, pathology reports include biomarkers, special features of a tumor that can reveal what may have contributed to the growth of a particular cancer. These pathology indicators help physicians determine the treatment to which a cancer may respond and predict both the chances of a recurrence and the chances of a normal life span.

The process of assigning labels and numbers to some pathology indicators is an art—an interpretive science—that depends on the ability and diligence of the pathologist. Often more than one pathologist reviews and interprets the slides of a person's cancer cells. They determine the type of breast cancer by looking at the shape and size of the cells under a microscope. The degree of cell abnormality is a relative measure and is generally a way of describing how similar the abnormal cells appear to be to normal ductal or lobular breast cells. Thus, a grade 1 tumor is well differentiated—that is, it looks nearly like a normal breast cell. A grade 3 tumor, in contrast, is called poorly differentiated and looks least like a normal breast cell. Grade 2 tumors are in between these two.

Histologic Types of Breast Cancers

Figure 1 shows the locations of the two primary types of cells from which cancer can develop in the breast, the cells of the ducts and, less frequently, the lobules. The two photos in the figure show the appearance of invasive lobular carcinoma and invasive ductal carcinoma under the microscope.

The brief explanations of the following terms used frequently on pathology reports will enable you to better understand your report and the nature of your cancer.

Invasive Ductal Carcinoma: Invasive (or infiltrating) ductal carcinoma is the most common type of invasive breast cancer, accounting for 80–85 percent of all diagnoses. Under the microscope, one can see that invasive ductal carcinoma cells start in the duct and invade through the walls into

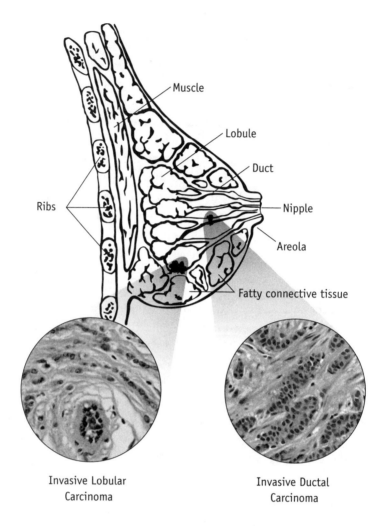

Invasive Lobular
Carcinoma

Invasive Ductal
Carcinoma

1. Anatomy of the breast showing invasive lobular and ductal carcinoma.

the rest of the breast. These cells generally grow in nests of cells, as seen in figure 1.

Invasive Lobular Carcinoma: This is the second most common type of invasive breast cancer, accounting for about 15 percent of diagnoses. Under the microscope one can see that lobular carcinoma cells start in the lobules, where breast milk is formed. The cells tend to spread into the surrounding tissue in single-file strands, as seen in figure 1, resulting in greater difficulty in detection by mammography.

Mixed Invasive Carcinoma: This type of cancer has features of both lobular and ductal carcinoma.

Rare Subtypes of Ductal Breast Cancer:

—*Tubular*: Tubular breast cancer is a rare subtype of ductal carcinoma that forms tubules. This type of cancer rarely spreads throughout the body and rarely causes death.

—*Mucinous or Colloid*: Mucinous or colloid carcinoma is another rare subtype of ductal carcinoma in which the cancer cells are surrounded by pools of mucin, a component of mucus. This type of cancer rarely spreads but can grow to be very large.

—*Medullary*: Medullary carcinoma is a rare subtype of ductal carcinoma that generally contains a large number of white blood cells and a specific growth structure. These tumors are generally estrogen- and progesterone-receptor-positive and have a better prognosis than typical ductal carcinoma.

There are also types of *in situ* (noninvasive) cancers. While not considered invasive cancers, they do increase the risk of one's developing an invasive cancer.

—*Ductal Carcinoma in Situ (DCIS)*: DCIS is the most common type of noninvasive breast cancer. These breast cancer cells are confined within the walls (basement membrane) of the duct and have not spread into the rest of the breast tissue. The duct is a small area, and the rapidly growing cancer cells can cause irritation and cell damage, leading to the formation of suspicious calcifications that are often detected on mammograms. In some women, the cancerous cells will eventually spread outside the duct and become invasive; for others, the cells will remain confined. Because it is not yet possible to determine whose DCIS cells will spread outside of the duct, all cases are treated as if they will. This typically means surgery to remove the area of DCIS, then a discussion of radiation therapy with a radiation oncologist if a lumpectomy was performed and a discussion of hormonal therapy with a medical oncologist if the cells are estrogen-receptor-positive.

—*Lobular Carcinoma in Situ (LCIS)*: LCIS is the lobular form of *in situ* carcinoma. Generally this histologic type has not been considered a cancer, but rather an accumulation of atypical cells in the lobules that signifies an increased risk of developing cancer in either breast, even in the nonaffected breast. Unlike DCIS, in which the area must be removed, LCIS is not thought to require surgery, although this assumption has recently been called into question. People with LCIS need to be vigilant in examining their breasts and in having regular mammograms. They may benefit from breast cancer prevention with an agent such as tamoxifen or raloxifene.

Additional Indicators of Pathology

Histologic Grade: The histologic grade is a score given to a breast cancer to identify it as a more favorable (less aggressive) cancer or an unfavorable (more aggressive) cancer. The most commonly used scoring system is the Nottingham Combined Histologic Grade. This scoring system evaluates three variables: the tubule formation, or the way cells form ducts; nuclear grade, or the shape and size of the central part (nucleus) of the cells; and mitotic count, or the number of cells that are actively dividing in a tumor. The tumor is assigned a score from one to three, with one being the most favorable, least aggressive breast cancer.

Gross Size of Tumor: This is the size of the mass that was surgically removed as it is seen by the naked eye. It can contain both invasive cancer and precancerous cells, as well as benign tissue.

Size of Invasive Component: This is the size of the invasive breast cancer as seen under the microscope. The stage of your cancer will be based in part on this size (the "T" part of TNM).

Vascular or Lymphatic Invasion: This is how pathologists communicate whether they see any evidence of the breast cancer invading blood or lymphatic vessels. If invasion is present, it increases the chances of the tumor spreading through the blood supply or lymphatic system respectively; however, it does not automatically mean that you have, or will develop, a distant metastasis.

Surgical Margin Status: A surgeon tries to remove breast tissue until the margins are clear, meaning that pathologists no longer find cancer cells under a microscope when they look at the edges of the tissue surrounding the cancer. The more locally invasive the cancer has been, the wider a surgeon has to cut to reach a clear margin.

Axillary Lymph Node Status: If lymph nodes were removed during surgery, pathologists will analyze them to determine how many, if any, contained breast cancer cells. The size and number of metastases present in the lymph nodes are used in assigning a stage to the cancer. Breast cancer that has spread to the axillary nodes (nodes in the armpit) is referred to as "metastatic to the lymph nodes," but this is very different from Stage IV cancer, in which cancer has invaded an organ.

Biomarkers

In addition to one laboratory providing tumor descriptions based on pathologists' visual examinations, a different laboratory will test for some, or all, of the biomarkers below. A biomarker is a measurable characteristic of a disease or condition; for example, pathologists often look for greater quantities than normal of a particular substance in a cell; such an indicator is a clue to what may be causing the cell to grow out of control. The numbers assigned to biomarkers are the results of molecular tests. Some biomarkers have been so recently discovered that it is difficult to know their full potential for prognostic or treatment purposes. At a minimum, all breast cancers should have estrogen receptor (ER), progesterone receptor (PR), and HER2/neu levels measured.

Estrogen Receptors (ER): Estrogen receptors are proteins found inside the cancer cell that bind with circulating estrogen. Once triggered by estrogen, the receptor signals the cell's nucleus to grow and divide. ER presence can be reported as a percentage of cells positive, the number of femtomoles per milligram of protein, or an Allred score. A positive result, or overexpression of estrogen receptors, means the breast cancer cells are sensitive to estrogen and will likely respond to hormonal therapies. About 80 percent of tumors in postmenopausal women are estrogen receptor and/or progesterone receptor (see below) positive, as are 30–50 percent of tumors in premenopausal women.

Progesterone Receptors (PR): Progesterone receptors are proteins that bind to progesterone and interact with the estrogen receptor. PR presence can be reported as a percentage of cells positive, the number of femtomoles per milligram of protein, or an Allred score. A positive result means, again, that the cells are likely sensitive to hormonal therapies. Some tumors will be estrogen receptor negative and progesterone receptor positive. Hormonal therapies are also options in these cases.

HER2/Neu Overexpression: HER2/neu (also called ErbB2) is a receptor on the cell's surface that responds to certain growth factors that make cells divide more quickly. In about 25 percent of breast cancers, HER2 is overexpressed, meaning that larger than normal quantities of HER2 are found. HER2 is generally reported on a scale of 0–3+, with 3+ being strongly expressed. Cancers that moderately overexpress HER2 (2+) are usually tested for the actual number of HER2 genes per cell (normal is 2). A result greater than 6 copies per cell, or a ratio greater than 2.2, is considered amplified. In general, HER2 is thought to be an adverse prognostic indicator. Its presence does, however, mean your cancer may respond to certain biologic treatment—such as Herceptin (trastuzumab) or Tykerb (lapatinib)—and may respond better to certain chemotherapies or hormonal therapies.

Epidermal Growth Factor Receptor (EGFR): EGFR is related to HER2 and likewise can be overexpressed, resulting in more rapid cell growth. It is particularly of interest in a subclassification of breast tumors that are negative for ER, PR, and HER2—so-called triple-negative or basal-type carcinomas (discussed below). As more targeted therapies are developed against EGFR, your cancer may respond to them.

Ki-67: The Ki-67 antigen is a protein expressed only in the nuclei of cells that are proliferating, or growing. A high Ki-67 is associated with a more aggressive, or more rapidly dividing, cancer.

S-Phase: S-phase is the time in a cell's life in which DNA is being made or synthesized. A high S-phase fraction indicates your cancer is dividing quickly and is more aggressive. The range of S-phase fraction is established by each testing laboratory.

Triple-Negative or Basal-Type Carcinoma:
A Special Subtype of Breast Cancer

Some tumors do not express ER, PR, or HER2 by pathology examination. These tumors are called "triple-negative" tumors. Researchers believe that many of these tumors arise from basal cells in the ducts. Triple-negative tumors do not respond to hormonal therapy and likewise do not respond to drugs that bind to HER2, such as Herceptin. These tumors appear to respond readily to chemotherapy but tend to be more aggressive than similar tumors with receptor expression. Often these tumors overexpress EGFR, which may be a target for therapy in the future. Treatment of these tumors prior to surgery (neoadjuvant treatment) is favored as response to treatment can be monitored. Additionally, a pathological complete response—absence of tumor cells under the microscope when the site of cancer is removed by surgery—appears to predict a better overall survival (2).

Prognostic Gene Signature Tests

Gene tests that have emerged in the last few years are now in limited use for helping tailor treatment by determining the likelihood a cancer will metastasize, primarily in people with breast cancer that has not spread and with negative nodes and ER-positive tumors. These tests, such as OncotypeDX™ and MammaPrint®, examine the levels of expression of key genes in the primary tumor and appear to predict more accurately than other tests the chance for distant recurrence. As mentioned above, tests such as these will likely become standard in the near future.

OncotypeDX

OncotypeDX is a gene test that measures the expression of twenty-one different genes, then separates people into high, intermediate, and low risk for distant (not local or regional) recurrence. High-risk patients are recommended to undergo additional chemotherapy, while low-risk patients are not. It is unclear what the best treatment is for intermediate-risk patients. Currently a worldwide trial called TAILORx is being undertaken to determine the best treatment for these patients. OncotypeDX has been validated only in women with ER-positive, node-negative, HER2-negative tumors (3).

MammaPrint

MammaPrint is a gene test for levels of seventy different genes that separates patients into good and poor risk, with patients falling into the poor-risk group having five times the risk of distant recurrence. MammaPrint has been validated only in women younger than sixty-one years old, with tumors smaller than 5 cm and negative nodes (4). A clinical trial, MIND-ACT, is ongoing in Europe to assess treatment in patients who have conflicting results based on gene testing by MammaPrint and traditional risk-assessment measurements.

PREDICTING RECURRENCE

- Adjuvant! Online: Provides a means for medical professionals to assess the risk of recurrence for those with Stage I through Stage III breast cancer.
  http://www.adjuvantonline.com/index.jsp

PATHOLOGY REPORTS
- Imaginis: Offers explanations of terms on pathology reports.
  http://imaginis.com/breasthealth/histologic_grades.asp

- breastcancer.org: Offers online and downloadable basic information about pathology reports.
  http://www.breastcancer.org/pathology_intro.html

GENE SIGNATURE TESTS
- OncotypeDX™
  http://www.genomichealth.com/oncotype/default.aspx?c1=
      google&source=contentkw=breast_cancer_radiation_

- MammaPrint®
  http://usa.agendia.com/index.php?option=com_content&task=
      view&id=27&Itemid=271

Recurrence Statistics

An individual's chance for having a recurrence cannot be known with certainty. Instead, groups of people who have similar cancer characteristics are studied. Statisticians look for the number of people in a group with similar characteristics who had a recurrence over a specific number of years, and this is expressed in terms of a percentage, or how many times out of one hundred someone in this group had a recurrence. The chance that a tumor will come back is also called "risk of recurrence."

An example of percentages (or risk) of cancer recurrence that are gener-

Table 1. Example of Adjuvant! Online estimates for recurrence based on stage at diagnosis. For these estimates, we assumed a fifty-five-year-old woman with an ER-positive grade 3 tumor. (Calculated using www.adjuvantonline.com/breastnew.jsp.)

Initial disease stage	Risk of recurrence over ten years without further therapy
Stage I	21–31%
Stage IIA	45–54%
Stage IIB	59–68%
Stage IIIA	75–92%
Stage IIIB	80–92%
Stage IIIC	89–99%

ated by Adjuvant! Online can be seen in table 1. This table shows the range of estimates of recurrence based on stage at diagnosis in a fifty-five-year-old woman with an ER-positive histologic grade 3 tumor. For example, if her cancer was discovered in Stage I, and if following her surgery to remove the tumor no follow-up treatment was given, her chances over ten years of having either a local, regional, or distant recurrence would be 21–31 percent. The estimates of recurrence are based on age, ER status, tumor grade, and change over time using historical data from the National Cancer Institute's Surveillance Epidemiology and End Results (SEER) database. Estimates of the likelihood a cancer will respond to hormonal therapy and chemotherapy can also be obtained using Adjuvant! Online.

Prognostic tables and graphs sometimes can be alarming. Be aware that numbers represent generalized information about groups, not information about an individual. These statistics are estimates, only a "best guess" about your possible outcome. Do not assume they represent your particular prognosis. Below are some reasons why.

1. The staging system for cancer is subject to change, and that in turn changes the statistical outcomes. The revision of breast cancer stages in the 2003 *American Joint Committee on Cancer Staging Manual* is a case in point. The manual is updated every five years. Prior to 2003 women with ten or more positive lymph nodes were classified as Stage II, but in 2003 these women were classified as Stage III. If you look at prognostic tables and charts that use the 2003 staging guidelines, you will see improved sur-

vival outcomes for Stage II disease since the women with ten or more lymph nodes were removed from that stage. The women with ten lymph nodes would now see worse outcomes since they are classified as Stage III. Though the actual condition of individual women with ten positive lymph nodes did not change, their statistical prognosis did. Lumping people together in categories distorts the likely outcomes for individuals on the fringes of each category.

2. The percentages in prognostic tables and charts represent the effects of treatments from previous years. The percentages in a table showing disease-free survival five years out from diagnosis are based on treatments used at least five years before the date the table was created. A newer treatment you may have had would not be reflected in these data, and such a treatment may positively affect your prognosis.

3. Your prognosis is changing statistically each year out from your initial diagnosis. If you are many years out from your first diagnosis, your chance of having a recurrence is going down and your potential for a normal life span is increasing. Typically tables present your prognosis based only on your time of diagnosis and do not reflect how your prognosis alters over time.

4. Your prognosis is dependent on your body. Your individual response to a treatment may differ from other people's. Each person's and each tumor's chemistry varies to some extent. A treatment may be more or less effective for you than it was for others in your stage cancer.

5. Most prognostic tables and charts are based on the most powerful predictors for survival and disease-free intervals, usually the number of lymph nodes that were found to have metastases and the size and grade of tumors. A great deal more is becoming known about the characteristics of various types of breast cancer. It may be that an individual who is classified in Stage I has a more aggressive cancer than someone in Stage II, but the prognostic tables are just beginning to account for finer predictive characteristics like receptor status and other biomarkers. Though standard estimates may not as yet take these characteristics into account, doctors often do when discussing prognoses with patients.

CANCER STATISTICS

- National Cancer Institute's SEER Data: Site for the U.S. government's statistics on cancer incidence and survival.
  http://seer.cancer.gov

- Steven Dunn's Cancer Guide: Provides information to help understand cancer statistics, including a copy of Stephen Jay Gould's helpful essay "The Median Is the Message."
  http://cancerguide.org/stats_home.html

No one diagnosed with early-stage breast cancer can be certain that she will not have a recurrence, though in reality an individual's chance for a recurrence may be very small to nonexistent. Most recurrences appear in the first two years following surgery, with the risk of recurrence decreasing significantly two to five years out from surgery and tapering very slowly thereafter (5). In general, hormone receptor-negative tumors are likely to recur earlier than hormone receptor-positive tumors, though a small number of positive receptor tumors are known to occur many years out. Overall, very few people have a recurrence of breast cancer more than twenty years out from their initial diagnosis. The longer you live with no evidence of disease, the more likely it is that your cancer has responded to treatment and that you will live a normal lifespan.

Currently there is no definitive "marker" for breast cancer—in other words, there is no way to detect with certainty through a blood test or other quick measure whether cancer is active in your body, although such tests may be on the horizon (see chapter 4.) Also, there is no definitive time out from your initial diagnosis when a doctor can say with absolute certainty that you are cured. You may be, but not enough is known yet to say with complete assurance that your chance of having breast cancer again is the same as anyone else's in the population; this, in the strictest sense, is the medical definition of "cure." If you live as long as is normal for someone in your generation who does not have breast cancer and you ultimately die from some other cause, most physicians would consider that you were cured. The fact is that sometimes breast cancer is eradicated, sometimes it goes into remission, perhaps for good, and sometimes it is a slow-growing disease that reappears many years later.

Reducing Chances of Recurrence

After a diagnosis of nonmetastatic breast cancer, your doctor likely discussed with you treatments that could reduce the risk of your cancer coming back. These may have included hormonal therapy, biological therapy, chemotherapy, and radiation therapy. Lifestyle changes can also reduce the risk of recurrence for a number of people. It can help you decide if you are willing to engage in some means of reducing your chances of recurrence if you understand the terms *absolute risk* or *relative risk* of reduction. Research results often will distinguish between these terms, and the difference is especially relevant when you are weighing the possibility of taking a medicine that has adverse long-term side effects. To understand the difference, see appendix A. Where possible, we describe results of studies in terms of absolute and relative risk.

We begin this section by mentioning lifestyle changes that are known to reduce the risk of recurrence and conclude with medications that do so as well. In breast cancer groups many substances and activities are suggested as ways to reduce recurrence. In addition to the known ways below, you will find many of these other means covered in more detail in chapter 5, where you can learn which are promising and which have not been shown to be beneficial.

Maintain a Healthy Weight

Being overweight is a risk factor for recurrence, especially in postmenopausal women. Do not gain more than eleven pounds (five kilograms) beyond what you weighed in your early twenties; if you have, it is not too late to reap the benefits of losing weight. Once through menopause, women's ovaries stop making estrogen, but body fat still produces a low amount of estrogen that is implicated in causing some recurrences. A review of thirty-nine studies in an article in the *Journal of Clinical Oncology* shows that your risk of recurrence could increase as much as 30 percent if you are overweight with a body mass index (BMI) of 25 or greater. A normal BMI falls between 18.5 and 24.9 (6). You can calculate your BMI using the links in the next resource box.

Maintain a Regular Exercise Regimen

Though results have been mixed, the large, long-range Nurses Health Study showed that women with breast cancer who exercised the equivalent of walking about 2.5 mph three to five hours per week had longer survival times compared with women who exercised little or not at all. Even walking one hour a week appeared to lower the risk of breast cancer death (7). Physical activity can aid in keeping a woman's weight down as well, which can help prevent recurrence a number of years out from diagnosis (8). Exercising regularly will undoubtedly contribute to your overall health in a number of ways, enabling you to partake in the widest variety of cancer treatments, strengthening your bones and muscles, and reducing stress.

Eat Five or More Servings of Fruits and Vegetables a Day

The Women's Healthy Eating and Living (WHEL) study evaluated the benefit of very high vegetable intake on breast cancer recurrence in over three thousand women diagnosed with early-stage breast cancer. While the consumption of more than seven servings of fruits and vegetables a day added no benefit, evaluation of the comparison group showed that the combination of consuming five or more daily servings of vegetables and fruits and exercise equivalent to walking thirty minutes six days a week was associated with a significant survival advantage. The approximate 50 percent relative reduction in risk associated with these healthy lifestyle behaviors was observed in both obese and non-obese women (9).

Reduce Your Fat Intake

The Women's Intervention Nutrition Study (WINS) randomized women diagnosed with early-stage breast cancer to normal care or a dietary intervention aimed at lowering fat intake. In the control group, women maintained a fat intake of about 50 grams per day, getting about 30 percent of their calories from fat. In contrast, the intervention group lowered fat intake to about 30 grams per day, getting about 20 percent of calories from fat. Women in the low-fat group lowered their chance of recurrence by 24 percent, with a greater benefit seen in women with hormone receptor-negative cancers. Especially if you have a hormone receptor-negative disease, try reducing your fat intake to 30 grams per day, with a concurrent decrease in calories so that you get no more than 20 percent of your calories from fat (10). You can learn more about specific dietary recommendations in appendix B and by using the resource box below.

resources

REDUCING RECURRENCE: DIET AND EXERCISE

- National Institutes of Health Body Mass Index (BMI) Calculator: A tool for maintaining a healthy weight.
  http://www.nhlbisupport.com/bmi

- American Institute for Cancer Research: Provides research results on diet and cancer prevention.
  800-843-8114
  http://www.aicr.org

- breastcancer.org: Provides current information on breast cancer and nutrition.
  http://www.breastcancer.org/tips/nutrition

- Fruits and veggies: Provides serving sizes for fruits and vegetables for eating healthfully.
  http://www.fruitsandveggiesmorematters.org/?page_id=58

- "Nutrition and Physical Activity during and after Cancer Treatment: An American Cancer Society Guide for Informed Choices": A downloadable, well-referenced report of recommendations.
  http://caonline.amcancersoc.org/cgi/content/full/56/6/323

Avoid Medications and Supplements Containing Estrogen or Progesterone, Especially If Your Tumor Is Hormone-Sensitive

Discuss the use of any hormone replacement therapy (HRT) or estrogen replacement therapy (ERT) or hormonal birth control with your oncologist. Such therapies include the brand name drugs Premarin, Estrace, Estratest, PremPro, DepoProvera, and Nuvaring. Two randomized clinical trials in the 1990s indicated that using HRT put women with breast cancer at greater risk for recurrence (11, 12). Occasionally topical medications will be prescribed for the treatment of vaginal dryness or shrinkage (atrophic vaginitis), which may result from a lack of estrogen. A small amount of estrogen can be absorbed into the blood stream via the vaginal lining with these medications, although some forms (such as Estring vaginal ring) have lower systemic absorption than others. Discuss these topical forms of estrogen with your oncologist if you are considering using one. Some herbal supplements also contain certain phytoestrogens (plant estrogens) that can potentially increase your risk of recurrence; the most common phytoestrogen-containing supplements are soy, red clover, and flaxseed. The use of these supplements is discussed further in chapter 5.

Consult with Your Oncologist about Medicines That Block or Reduce Estrogen

Estrogen-blocking and estrogen-reducing drugs have been shown to cut recurrence rates in those who have estrogen and/or progesterone receptor positive breast cancer. Whether these drugs would be a good choice for you depends on a number of factors, such as your type and stage of cancer, your menopausal status, and bone and heart health.

Estrogen-Blocking Drugs: SERMs—tamoxifen (Nolvadex), raloxifene (Evista), toremifene (Fareston)

Starting in the 1970s through the early 2000s, tamoxifen has been standard treatment for reducing recurrence in women with estrogen-receptor-positive tumors. Five years of taking tamoxifen can reduce the relative risk of breast cancer recurrence by up to 50 percent. Tamoxifen is a "selective estrogen-receptor modulator," or SERM, that can block the body's own estrogen from locking onto estrogen receptors in cells. The body's estrogen, which is called estradiol, can trigger cell division in breast cancer cells. Tamoxifen acts similarly to estradiol in some tissues, such as the bone and lining of the uterus (endometrium). In other tissues, such as the breast, it acts as an anti-estrogen. A small percentage of women develops uterine cancer or blood clots as a result of taking this drug. After five years, tamoxifen appears to lose its effectiveness, perhaps because of changes in the shape of the estrogen receptor in breast cancer cells.

Raloxifene is another SERM, similar to tamoxifen, though it is not standard treatment for reducing the risk of recurrence; rather, it is used for breast cancer prevention. In a clinical trial known as STAR, raloxifene was studied in comparison to tamoxifen for its effectiveness in reducing the risk of a first breast cancer in postmenopausal women at high risk of developing the disease. Results from the STAR trial, published in 2006, showed that raloxifene was equivalent to tamoxifen in reducing first invasive breast cancers and had a lower risk than tamoxifen for thromboembolic events (blood clots in the leg and lungs) and cataracts. It did not reduce the number of cases of noninvasive breast cancer or ductal carcinoma *in situ* (DCIS) (13).

Estrogen-Reducing Drugs: Aromatase Inhibitors: letrozole (Femara), anastrozole (Arimidex), exemestane (Aromasin)

In postmenopausal women, whose ovaries are shut down, estrogen continues being produced at low levels by the conversion of testosterone to estrogen in tissues such as fat cells, adrenal glands, and muscle. Aromatase is the enzyme necessary for this conversion. By taking advantage of this finding, researchers developed a new class of drugs that inhibits aromatase, thereby blocking the cell's ability to create estrogen. Aromatase inhibitors are effective in women only after menopause because before this point the ovaries are the primary source of estrogen in the body. Ongoing studies are underway evaluating the effectiveness of chemical ovarian shutdown in combination with aromatase inhibitors in premenopausal women as aromatase inhibitors do not effectively reduce estrogen produced by the ovaries.

Large-scale studies show that aromatase inhibitors are better at reducing the risk of recurrence than tamoxifen in women who are past menopause with estrogen-receptor-positive breast cancer. Aromatase inhibitors have not yet consistently shown gains in lengthening life; this may be in part because these drugs are so new. Their long-term benefits and risks are just emerging. The optimal length of time to take an aromatase inhibitor is not known as of this writing; studies are currently addressing this issue. Many women tolerate the side effects well, but in some, aromatase inhibitors appear to raise the risk of osteoporosis and bone fractures. Many women also experience joint aches and pain as side effects; these are typically mild but can be severe in some women. The joint aches resolve after discontinuation of the drug.

In 2002, the initial results of the Arimidex, Tamoxifen, Alone or in Combination (ATAC) study, involving over nine thousand women, showed that an aromatase inhibitor, anastrozole (Arimidex), taken for five years was approximately 20 percent more effective than tamoxifen taken for five years in reducing recurrence. Overall survival was not evaluated at this analysis (14). This initial report radically changed the adjuvant hormonal management of postmenopausal breast cancer, opening up a new option for thousands of postmenopausal women taking tamoxifen. An update was published confirming the approximately 20 percent improvement in disease-free survival with anastrozole and noting, as yet, no difference in overall survival (15).

In 2003, an article in the *New England Journal of Medicine* reported on the ability of another aromatase inhibitor, letrozole, to reduce recurrence in postmenopausal women who had previously taken tamoxifen for five years. In this study, over five thousand women took either five years of letrozole or five years of placebo (a sugar pill) following four and a half to six years of tamoxifen. There appeared to be a 40 percent relative reduction in the risk of recurrence for those taking letrozole compared to those taking the sugar pill, but there was no difference in overall survival (16). A follow-up report of this study affirmed the 40 percent reduction in recurrence and found a 40 percent relative improvement in survival in women with node-positive disease (17). There was no difference in survival in women with node-negative disease.

In 2004, a study was published describing over four thousand women who were randomized to either switch to exemestane, another aromatase inhibitor, after two to three years of tamoxifen or remain on tamoxifen for a total of five years. The women who switched to exemestane for two to three years had a 32 percent relative reduction in risk of recurrence in comparison to the group that did not switch. No difference in overall survival was found (18).

Since the publication of these early reports, other studies have been published confirming the superiority of aromatase inhibitors taken in a sequential fashion (19) and as a single drug (20) over the former standard of tamoxifen for five years. ASCO and the NCCN Practice Guidelines both recommend that all postmenopausal women with hormone receptor-positive tumor who do not have contraindications to therapy with an aromatase inhibitor receive an aromatase inhibitor for some part of their adjuvant hormonal therapy.

Though aromatase inhibitors have shown good results, their use must be carefully considered for those who have advanced osteoporosis or those who experience severe bone pain. A number of issues are still unclear regarding their use, including the timing of therapy, duration of therapy, and type of aromatase inhibitor used. Some data suggest that in women with ER-positive, PR-negative tumors, anastrozole is significantly better than tamoxifen. Trials are ongoing to determine whether there is any difference between the three approved aromatase inhibitors in terms of freedom from recurrence. Additionally, other trials are being conducted to learn whether taking tamoxifen and then an aromatase inhibitor is better than taking an aromatase inhibitor and then tamoxifen. Still other trials are focusing on determining the optimal duration of aromatase inhibitor therapy. The results of recent studies can be found by using the links in the "Keeping Up to Date with Breast Cancer Developments" resource box in chapter 2.

Consult with Your Medical Oncologist about Whether Chemotherapy Is Indicated for You

Chemotherapy (discussed in depth in chapter 3) may be used before surgery (neoadjuvant) or after surgery (adjuvant) to reduce the chances that your cancer will come back. Whether or not chemotherapy will be helpful depends on the stage, grade, and pathologic type of your tumor. Gene signature tests such as OncotypeDX may be helpful in determining the benefit from chemotherapy if your tumor is ER-positive. Your age is also an indicator of how beneficial chemotherapy will be for you, with women younger than forty years old obtaining the greatest benefit. Few studies of adjuvant chemotherapy have been performed in women over the age of seventy, so there is less information about how helpful treatments are in older women. Chemotherapy is the only systemic therapy that provides beneficial results for women with triple-negative tumors. If you have a tumor that overexpresses HER2, you may benefit from Herceptin therapy.

resources

REDUCING RECURRENCE: MEDICATIONS

- Estrogen receptors/SERMs: The National Cancer Institute offers detailed explanations and updates on these drugs.
    http://www.cancer.gov/cancertopics/understandingcancer/
      estrogenreceptors

- Aromatase inhibitors: The National Cancer Institute provides current updates on these drugs.
    http://www.cancer.gov/cancertopics/aromatase-inhibitors

(Resources, continued)

- Bisphosphonate drugs (see following section): An important clinical trial on these drugs and recurrence is being conducted.
  http://www.cancer.gov/clinicaltrials/ft-SWOG-S0307

Consult with Your Medical Oncologist about Whether Bone-Building (Bisphosphonate) Therapy Is Right for You

A recent study published in the *New England Journal of Medicine* showed a decrease in breast cancer recurrence when zoledronic acid (Zometa) was given at 4 mg intravenously every six months. The study enrolled 1,800 premenopausal women with ER-positive disease who were randomized to receive Zometa or not during endocrine therapy of their early-stage breast cancer. Women who received the Zometa had an absolute reduction of 3.2 percent and a relative reduction of 36 percent in the risk of disease progression (21).

Consult with Your Radiation Oncologist about Whether Radiation Therapy Is Indicated for You

Radiation therapy is recommended to reduce local recurrence if you have had a lumpectomy. Radiation is usually recommended if you have positive lymph nodes or if your tumor was larger than 5 cm (about 2 inches), even if you have had a mastectomy. Some studies suggest that radiation therapy may not only reduce the risk of recurrence, but also improve overall survival.

Uncertain Territory

Though the recommendations listed above are clearly tied to reducing recurrence risk, you may want consider the following suggestions, which have less clear but possible ties to reducing breast cancer risk.

Limit Alcohol Consumption

More than one study has linked alcohol with breast cancer (22–24). Some studies have even associated the consumption of one alcoholic drink per day with an increased relative risk of breast cancer by as much 21 percent as compared with nondrinkers (22). But to keep perspective, the authors of a review in the *Journal of the American Medical Association* suggest, "For those considered sporadic or occasional social drinkers (less than one drink per day), alcohol consumption is unlikely to significantly affect breast cancer risk" (25).

Do Not Smoke

In addition to increasing the risk of heart disease and lung cancer, smoking is implicated in increasing the risk of developing breast cancer (26). There is no evidence as to whether continuing to smoke increases your risk of recurrence, but it is certainly bad for many other aspects of your health.

Make Sure You Have Adequate Vitamin D

Higher blood levels of vitamin D (in the form of 25-hydroxyvitamin D) have been linked to a lower risk of breast cancer (27). While not demonstrated yet in breast cancer, higher vitamin D levels have correlated with increased survival and decreased recurrence in colon cancer patients. In general, vitamin D can be obtained through sun exposure and dietary sources (such as vitamin D–fortified milk). (Further discussion of vitamin D supplementation can be found in chapter 5.) Experts on vitamin D recommend taking a vitamin D supplement of 2,000 iu a day to attain the levels correlated with cancer protection. Vitamin D supplementation is safe as long as you do not have any risk factors for elevated calcium levels (such as bone metastases or granulomatous disease such as sarcoidosis). Ask your doctor to test your 25-hydroxyvitamin D level to ensure you are not deficient.

Rest and Sleep Regularly

Animal and human studies have shown that sleep deprivation has a harmful effect on the immune system. Evidence points to chronic short-term sleep loss as being more detrimental on the immune system than staying awake more than twenty-four hours on rare occasions (28). Additionally, shift workers (those exposed to bright lights at night) are more likely to be diagnosed with breast cancer, perhaps as a result of a disruption of melatonin secretion.

Avoid Potential Carcinogens

There is no scientific evidence that exposure to, or avoidance of, chemical carcinogens following a diagnosis of breast cancer changes recurrence rate or survival. Since cancer can take many years to develop, avoidance of carcinogens may be more important for younger people. If you are concerned, however, about carcinogen exposure, limit working around pesticides in the garden or house and use appropriate protective wear, such as gloves, eyewear, and specially designed face masks. Limit your intake of grilled or charred meats as the high-heat method of cooking produces polycyclic aromatic hydrocarbons (PAHs).

Recently a class of chemicals called endocrine disruptors has been associated with increased breast cancer risk. These chemicals are not classic carcinogens; they appear to cause effects by simulating hormones made in the body. Phthalates, parabens, and bisphenol A are of particular interest. Phthalates can leach into food from plastic containers when heated (29), so one way to avoid exposure is to limit the use of plastics when microwaving food.

Parabens, short for "para-benzoic acid," may be found in many beauty care products such as cosmetics, lotions, sunscreens, and shampoos. Read the labels for methylparaben, propylparben, ethylparben, isobutylparaben, and alkyl parahydroxybenzoate (30). As parabens are absorbed through the skin, they may not be problematic in products that are washed off immediately, such as shampoo. Older women may have no cause for concern, but young girls and adolescents may want to limit exposure to lotions that contain parabens until more is known.

Some substances and activities that were thought to be possible factors in the development of breast cancer appear not to be. According to the breastcancer.org Web site, the current summation of studies has not shown that any of the following increase the risk of getting breast cancer: deodorant/antiperspirant, hair relaxers, hair dye, birth control pills, and natural or induced abortion. A recent epidemiological study (31) has also concluded that there is no increase in breast cancer risk from exposure to electromagnetic fields (EMF). You can learn more about the studies leading to these conclusions using the link in following resource box (32).

REDUCING RECURRENCE: ENVIRONMENT AND LIFESTYLE

- breastcancer.org: Offers research updates on potential environmental carcinogens and lifestyle choices in the prevention of breast cancer and for breast cancer survival.

    http://www.breastcancer.org

- United States Department of Health and Human Services Household Products Database: Provides a health rating for commonly used household products.

    http://householdproducts.nlm.nih.gov/index.htm

It is possible that other measures, in addition to those mentioned above, *could* reduce the risk of a recurrence, but these are more speculative. These measures, which include diet variations, herbal supplements, and mind/body practices, are discussed in chapter 5. Many lifestyle changes and new medicines are being studied to determine what might extend the survival time without a recurrence (disease-free survival) of those who have had a breast cancer diagnosis. We highly recommend that you periodically review the current findings about breast cancer, particularly if your diagnosis is recent. You will find sites that regularly report breast cancer developments and organizations that send periodic updates on the latest breast cancer news in chapter 2 in the "Keeping Up to Date with Breast Cancer Developments" resource box.

Local and Regional Recurrence

You most likely have been checked for a local recurrence by your surgeon or medical oncologist and/or radiation oncologist following your initial breast cancer diagnosis. Typically you will have a checkup every four to six months, and after five years appointments will be annual. These checkups include yearly mammograms along with a physical examination, including palpation (feeling with the fingertips) of the breasts, chest wall, and nearby lymph nodes for any suspicious lumps. Your doctor has likely advised you of the importance of monthly self-examinations between these visits. If you note any changes in your breasts during these exams, such as the development of a lump or swelling, skin irritation or dimpling, nipple pain or retraction (turning inward), redness or scaliness of the nipple or breast skin, or a discharge other than breast milk, contact your doctor right away. Whether you have had a mastectomy or lumpectomy, the scar area is where cancer is most likely to reappear. You can learn to give yourself a thorough breast exam using the link in the following resource box.

CONDUCTING A BREAST SELF-EXAM

- Susan G. Komen for the Cure: More than a series of instructions, this site is a teaching tool that visually shows how to check for changes in your breast.

    http://ww5.komen.org/BreastCancer/BreastSelfExam.html

resources

Detecting a Local or Regional Recurrence

In addition to a woman's feeling and looking for breast abnormalities, the recommended way to check for cancer remains mammography. Digital mammography has been shown to be more effective than standard mammography in certain groups of women. Annual magnetic resonance imaging (MRI) screening has been recommended as well for certain groups of women, as discussed below.

Breast reconstructions usually do not obscure recurrences. Recurrences generally occur in front of an implant. With reconstructive flaps, recurrences generally occur on the margins of the reconstruction, where the original breast tissue and skin remain, not in the flap, which contains transplanted back or abdominal flesh. Tissue in a reconstructed breast is not breast tissue so it does not need to be x-rayed in a mammogram. However, x-rays may be useful if there is any suspicion that breast cancer may recur in the remaining underlying tissues.

Mammography

Mammography can often detect tumors before they can be felt. Tumors are more easily detected in nonfibrous, less firm breast tissue. Mammograms are often better at revealing a tumor after menopause because the tissue becomes less dense. The accuracy of mammography depends on the equipment, procedures, clinic personnel, and radiologist. It is best to go to a radiology clinic that has up-to-date mammography imaging equipment, a radiologist on site (in case follow-up films are needed), and more than one experienced radiologist to read the images.

Check whether the clinic to which you go is accredited by the American College of Radiology. This organization accredits not only radiologists, but also technicians and equipment. It may be advantageous if the clinic has digital mammography available. Digital images can be manipulated to enlarge and change views, can be read by a computer-aided diagnostic program, and can preserve and transfer a good image to another doctor or clinic. One large study has shown that digital mammography is more accurate in women under fifty years old, women with radiographically dense breasts, and premenopausal or perimenopausal women (33).

MAMMOGRAPHY

- American College of Radiology: To learn of an approved site near you.
  800-227-5463
  http://www.acr.org/accreditation/AccreditedFacilitySearch.aspx

- American College of Radiology: To learn more about mammography.
  http://www.radiologyinfo.org/content/mammogram.htm

Ultrasound

Ultrasound is a complementary diagnostic tool used with mammography to further investigate suspicious areas seen on a mammogram or felt during a physical examination. It is not used alone since mammography is more reliable. An ultrasound test is painless, noninvasive, and safe. A cool conducting liquid is placed on an area of your breast, and then a small wand is placed on the fluid and moved around as benign high-frequency sound waves travel through the area being examined to create images. When the area contains solid tissue, white images are transmitted since the waves do not pass through solids easily. If the waves pass through the area, the area is more fluid. A solid area can be suspicious and may need to be biopsied.

Magnetic Resonance Imaging (MRI)

MRI is an additional diagnostic tool to complement mammography. Magnetic resonance images are created by magnetic fields that align hydrogen atoms in the body while radio waves are aimed at those atoms. When the radio waves stop, the hydrogen atoms return to their natural alignment, releasing energy that is picked up and turned into an image. No radiation is used, and as long as metal objects are kept out of the range of the machine's powerful magnets, the procedure is considered safe and painless. Gadolinium is often injected into a vein to enhance contrast in order to improve the quality of the image. If the MRI is done using a breast coil, which allows you to lie on a table face down with your breasts resting in two holes, you will not experience the claustrophobia that occasionally accompanies this procedure when a person is inserted bodily into the cocoon-like MRI machine. Currently the coil for breast imaging is used at large medical centers but is not as widely available as regular MRI machines.

MRI is many times more expensive than mammography. It can be better than mammography in detecting tumors in the scar tissue from a lumpectomy or mastectomy, in detecting whether tumors are in more than one spot in the breast, and in detecting whether a tumor has invaded the chest wall. When such conditions are suspected, an MRI may be ordered. Additionally, there are increasing data that MRI is more effective at screening women at high risk for breast cancer, such as those with a known genetic mutation. MRI images offer views of the breast in any geometric plane, from any angle, allowing for clearer, deeper pictures into dense breast tissue. Unfortunately, it can be difficult for radiologists to distinguish cancerous from noncancerous abnormalities when looking at the images. It also can be difficult to use MRI imagery to guide a needle to a suspicious spot to perform a biopsy, though the abnormality may not be visible with mammography. MRI is recommended in addition to mammography for women who have, have had, or carry the following:

A BRCA 1 or 2 mutation;

A first-degree relative with a BRCA 1 or 2 mutation and are untested;

A first-degree relative who carries a genetic mutation in the TP53 or PTEN genes (Li-Fraumeni syndrome and Cowden and Bannayan-Riley-Ruvalcaba syndromes);

A lifetime risk of breast cancer of 20–25 percent or more using standard risk assessment models;

Radiation treatment to the chest between ages ten and thirty, such as for Hodgkin Disease.

Women with a personal history of breast cancer, carcinoma *in situ*, atypical hyperplasia, or extremely dense breasts may benefit from annual MRI screening; however, the data are not clear enough to make a definite recommendation for or against MRI screening in these cases (34).

ULTRASOUND AND MRI

- Imaginis: Use the search engine to see photos of the machines and review procedures for mammography, ultrasound, and MRI.
  http://imaginis.com/breasthealth

- breastcancer.org: Offers explanations and comparisons of types of screenings, including mammography, ultrasound, and MRI.
  http://www.breastcancer.org/testing_images.html

Confirming a Local or Regional Recurrence: Breast and Lymph Node Biopsies

Biopsies are used to confirm whether or not a suspicious area contains cancerous cells. The greater the amount of suspicious tissue that is removed during a biopsy, the more likely that if there is cancer, it will be discovered. Most doctors begin with the least invasive procedure if the chances are not high that the area to be biopsied is cancerous. The pathology report from a biopsy provides information about the type of cancer and about biomarkers to aid in treatment decisions. (See the preceding section on pathology reports.) A biopsy report that indicates a recurrence can offer different information as compared with an original biopsy report. For instance, receptor status can change over time. In one study, 36 percent of patients whose initial pathology report showed estrogen receptor positive receptors had tumors with negative estrogen receptor status when tested at the time of a recurrence (35).

Types of Biopsies

Fine Needle Aspirate: In this procedure a long, thin, hollow needle is used to extract cells for examination. Usually this can be done in a doctor's office with local anesthetic on suspicious areas. This technique is used most often for recurrences rather than evaluation of a primary tumor.

Core Needle Biopsy: In this procedure a long, thin needle, slightly larger than that used for a fine aspirate, is used to extract more than one piece of tissue from a suspicious area. A surgeon or radiologist usually performs the biopsy with local anesthetic in the doctor's office. Suspicious areas that are not palpable masses will be biopsied with the aid of either ultrasound or mammogram (also called a stereotactic biopsy). Some facilities may also perform biopsies with CT or MRI guidance.

Incisional Biopsy: In this procedure a section of a suspicious mass is removed surgically, usually under mild anesthesia in a clinic or hospital on an outpatient basis.

Excisional Biopsy: In this procedure the entire suspicious mass is removed surgically. It is usually done with mild anesthesia in a hospital on an outpatient basis unless it is part of a larger surgery to remove lymph nodes.

BIOPSIES

- Ultrasound-Guided Breast Biopsy
  http://www.radiologyinfo.org/content/interventional/breast_biopsy_us.htm
- X-Ray–Guided Breast Biopsy
  http://www.radiologyinfo.org/content/interventional/breast_biopsy_xr.htm

resources

Treatment for Local and Regional Recurrence

Treatment varies for local and regional recurrence depending upon a number of factors, including where the cancer has recurred, whether or not it appears to be a return of the previous breast cancer, how soon after the first occurrence of cancer the recurrence took place, and what the previous treatment was.

Recurrence in the Same Breast

If you had a lumpectomy and your cancer recurs in the same breast, you likely will be advised to have a mastectomy. It is generally not possible to radiate a previously irradiated breast as an alternative to mastectomy since the tissue damage to the surrounding muscle, bone, and nerves would be too great. Some clinical trials are testing the suitability of re-irradiation of small portions of the breast; however, this is not yet common practice. After a mastectomy, you can have a flap reconstruction, a procedure where tissue and skin from your back or belly are used to create a breast, but you may not be able to have an implant since the radiated skin is often not pliable enough to be stretched over an implant. You will need to discuss your specific situation with a plastic surgeon. A small percentage of individuals at this point have metastases or locally extensive disease, which generally rules out having a mastectomy since the disease needs to be treated systemically—in other words, with treatment that reaches the whole body.

Cancer in the Opposite Breast

If you develop cancer in the previously unaffected breast, pathologists can compare the cancer cells in this breast with cells from the earlier cancer, if they are available, to try to determine if the new tumor is indeed a recurrence of the original breast cancer or a new cancer. Local (in breast) recurrences versus completely new breast cancers (primary cancers) may also be distinguished by the location of the new tumor. Recurrences after a short time (zero to three years) tend to be in the same quadrant, while those more than seven to ten years out tend to be anywhere in the breast, suggesting a different time course for local recurrences versus new primary cancers. If the tumor is a new cancer, the treatment options are similar to an initial diagnosis—mastectomy or lumpectomy/radiation and lymph node testing. Depending on the stage of the new cancer and your previous treatment, you may be advised to have systemic (whole body) treatment such as hormone therapy and/or chemotherapy.

If the cancer in your previously unaffected breast turns out to be a recurrence of your original cancer, it will likely be treated similarly to a new breast cancer as well, with surgery, a mastectomy or lumpectomy, followed with radiation. The optimal treatment for recurrences is currently unknown, and a large clinical trial—NSABP B-37 (IBCSG 27-02)—is evaluating adjuvant chemotherapy compared to no chemotherapy after locoregional recurrence (in breast, axillary or internal mammary lymph nodes). A recurrence in the other breast, especially within a year or two of an initial diagnosis, signals an aggressive cancer that may lead to distant metastases, so you will be checked for cancer spread and will likely be prescribed systemic treatment.

Recurrence in Regional Lymph Nodes

If you have a regional recurrence — meaning that your original breast cancer has reappeared in nearby lymph nodes around the collarbone (supraclavicular or infraclavicular nodes) or armpit (axillary nodes) — you may have surgery to remove the cancerous lymph nodes, assuming that this can be done safely and without causing you more harm than good. If it can be done safely, your doctors will likely recommend radiation to the involved nodal areas (after surgery, if a resection was performed), often in combination with a sensitizing chemotherapy that makes the cancer cells respond more easily to radiation.

Recurrence in the Chest Wall

If your cancer recurred in the chest wall, surgery is often recommended to remove a portion of tissue and possibly some muscle and bone surrounding the site of recurrence. Depending on the extent of what is removed, a flap reconstruction is possible after this surgery. You will be treated with systemic therapies and may receive radiation therapy as well. Extensive chest wall recurrences may be treated with radiation in combination with local heat, called *hyperthermia*. Only a few centers in the United States have the ability to deliver hyperthermia treatments. Another option for persistently recurring chest wall disease is *photodynamic therapy*. In photodynamic therapy, a light-sensitizing drug such as Photofrin is injected into the vein, and the area of cancer is treated with specialized laser light therapy. In one trial, as many as 89 percent of patients had resolution of disease in the treated areas (36).

More so than with a recurrence in the breast, a regional or chest wall recurrence increases the chances of discovering distant metastases. Tests for distant metastasis, such as a CT and/or bone scan, will likely be ordered, and the possibility of distant spread is why you are likely to be advised to have radiation and systemic treatment, depending on what treatment you had initially.

Distant Recurrence/Metastatic Cancer

When cancer metastasizes to an organ—in other words, when breast cancer cells move through the blood or lymph and start to grow in a distant site away from the breast and nearby lymph nodes—this is termed metastatic cancer. Though breast cancer can spread to almost any tissue in the body, the most common metastasis is to the bone, particularly to the pelvis, hip, shoulder joints, ribs, and spine, the bones that doctors call the "axial skeleton." The second most common site of metastasis is to the lung, third most is the liver, and fourth most are areas of distant lymph nodes. Brain metastases are infrequent as the first area of metastasis, but incidence appears to be increasing in women with HER2-positive disease who receive adjuvant Herceptin (37). Often metastases are found in more than one organ. In one study involving approximately one thousand women, one-third of the women had tumors in more than one site at the time their metastatic cancer was diagnosed (38). As the disease progresses, it typically appears in more organs. Table 2 shows sites of recurrence in a number of women evaluated between 1989 and 2002.

Detecting and Confirming Distant Metastases

Most breast cancer metastases are uncovered when a patient reports symptoms to her doctor. Depending upon the symptoms, specific scans or tests may be ordered. Frequent scans and tests may detect a metastasis a few months earlier than reported symptoms; however, early detection does not appear to confer survival advantage. No matter how early a metastasis is discovered, the disease has already progressed. A few months' lead time does not prolong someone's life. The one possible exception—and this is not certain—is in less common cases, such as one localized tumor in a surgically removable area like the lung, liver, or brain. Patients who present with only one site of metastatic disease probably have a slower-growing cancer than those who present with multiple sites of disease.

Since evidence suggests that finding a metastasis early does not make any difference in length of survival, scans are not recommended unless you have symptoms that indicate possible distant disease. Scans that are performed without accompanying symptoms often uncover noncancerous abnormalities, causing significant worry and further unnecessary testing that can tax your time, finances, and peace of mind. The more tests someone undergoes, the more likely medically insignificant abnormalities will

Table 2. Sites of recurrence in 456 women with breast cancer evaluated from 1989 to 2002. Adapted from Elder et al., "Patterns of Breast Cancer Relapse," *European Journal of Surgical Oncology* 32, no. 9 (2006): 922–27.

Site of recurrence	Percentage of women
Bone	27.4
Local	27.2
Lung	16.0
Liver	12.5
Supraclavicular fossa	5.5
Axilla	3.1
Brain	1.5
Other	5.7
Unknown	1.1
Total	*100*

be discovered; for example, nearly all women have uterine fibroids, and many people have liver cysts.

The fact that a few months' difference in detecting a distant recurrence does not prolong your life does not mean that treatment is of no benefit for advanced cancer. Treatment can enhance and prolong your life, but at this time no evidence clearly indicates that starting treatment earlier is better. Treatments have the same effect on extending your life and/or ameliorating unpleasant symptoms whether started early in the process or later.

Symptoms of Metastatic Disease

Often there are no signs that cancer is growing in an organ until that organ becomes dysfunctional or until the tumor presses against a nerve or blood supply source, causing discomfort or pain. Most aches and pains are not indicative of cancer. It may help you to know some of the common symptoms associated with different metastases to allay your fears or to signal that you should contact your oncologist. These are intended as a guide but should not substitute for the advice of your doctor. Contact your oncologist if you have any questions about your health.

Bone Metastases: Possible symptoms include bone pain, particularly in the hips, legs, arms, or spine. The bones below the elbow and knee are rarely affected. Pain from bone metastases is usually persistent — that is, it does not come and go. It usually begins as a dull pain and over weeks or months increases in intensity. The pain will remain even at night and will sometimes be more pronounced if weight is put on the affected bone. Occasionally a fracture can develop in a site of metastatic disease, and it can cause a sudden onset of pain that does not go away. If bone pain appears only at a certain time of day or comes and goes under certain circumstances such as weather or activity, it is more likely caused by other conditions, such as arthritis or bursitis. Pain relieved by rest is also rarely cancer. If you have steady pain that persists for more than two weeks, contact your doctor.

Lung Metastases: Possible symptoms include shortness of breath or chronic dry cough that over time become more troublesome. Breast cancer in the lungs rarely causes pain. Occasionally a tumor can form that blocks off one of the internal airways, causing pneumonia.

Pleural (Lung-Lining) Metastases: Possible symptoms include pain, particularly with breathing, in contrast to lung metastases. They may also include shortness of breath and difficulty with lying down, due to an accumulation of fluid (a *pleural effusion*) around the lung.

Liver Metastases: Possible symptoms include weight loss and loss of appetite or pain in the upper-right area of the abdomen, felt under the right side of the ribs. Occasionally people will develop jaundice, a yellowing of the skin.

Brain Metastases: Possible symptoms include seizures, loss of coordination and weakness when walking, changes in vision, paralysis, numbness in an area of the body, an inability to speak, nausea, or persistent headaches. A headache caused by a tumor usually is present when you first wake up, improves during the day, and returns at night. Rarely will a person with initial brain metastases display mental or behavioral abnormalities.

Metastases to the Meninges (Lining of the Brain): Possible symptoms include headaches and stiff neck. These can gradually become more severe over days or weeks and can include visual disturbance, drowsiness, and nausea. Sometimes focal areas of weakness or numbness can occur.

Spine Metastases: Possible symptoms may include an increasingly worse continuous aching pain in a specific spot along the spine and possibly pain going down one or both legs (sciatica) when you cough or sneeze or a pain in your shoulder or back. Those with compression of the spinal cord will likely have weakness in their leg muscles and experience numbness in the legs. Other symptoms of spinal cord compression include an inability to urinate and constipation. Let your doctor know immediately if you have leg weakness and/or numbness, particularly if it is accompanied by problems with urination or constipation. If you develop a sudden onset of numbness, weakness, difficulty speaking, and/or facial drooping, these are signs of a stroke—call 911. THIS IS AN EMERGENCY!

Imaging and Tests for Distant Metastasis

It is necessary to know definitively that your breast cancer has spread before treatment can begin. X-rays, bone scans, CTs, MRIs, and Position Emission Tomography (PET) scans are noninvasive ways of investigating possible cancer spread, but they do not confirm it. If scans do reveal a suspicious area, a biopsy is usually performed to determine whether the area is cancerous. Biopsies can confirm if a tumor is malignant; further, the resulting pathology report will determine what treatment may be useful. Under a few circumstances biopsies are not conducted, such as when it is difficult to reach the suspicious area or when other cancerous areas leave little doubt that a new area is also malignant. If a biopsy is performed, it is recommended that estrogen and HER2 testing be redone since these are known to change in 5–20 percent of cases. Below are likely routes for confirming distant metastases for particular organs.

Bone Metastases: A bone metastasis is usually diagnosed by a bone scan. Healthy bone is comprised of two kinds of cells: osteoblasts, which help build up bone, and osteoclasts, which break down bone and help with remodeling. When breast cancer cells metastasize to the bone, they can stimulate overactivity of the osteoclasts, causing bone fractures and lesions. On an X-ray, cancer may appear like a hole in the bone or like a fracture. Bone scans are more sensitive than X-rays in detecting bone metastases. With X-rays at least 30 percent of the bone mineralization must be gone for a lesion to be apparent. A bone scan will pick up approximately 80–90 percent of bone metastases (39). A bone scan gives an idea of the general location of a bone metastasis. If radiation therapy is planned, X-ray imaging, CT scans, or MRIs may be used to better define the area.

Lung Metastases: Lung metastases usually appear as nodules or as a mass on a chest X-ray. Sometimes there will be a pleural effusion around the lung. To investigate further, a chest CT scan is usually ordered. If your radiologists and oncologists believe the films indicate possible lung metastases, you may be advised to have a bronchoscopy, or a CT-guided lung biopsy, to further investigate.

Liver Metastases: Liver metastases can cause loss of appetite, weight loss, fever, and abdominal pain. Usually a tumor must be quite big before any of these symptoms appear. Blood tests such as AST, ALT, alkaline phosphatase, and total bilirubin are used to gauge liver function, but they are not sensitive enough to be certain indicators of a metastasis. CT scans, MRIs, or ultrasound of the liver can be used to evaluate the liver for evidence of metastases. A radiologist with the aid of CT or ultrasound imaging can perform a liver biopsy as an outpatient procedure to confirm cancer.

Brain, Spinal Cord, and Meningeal Metastases: CT scans and MRIs with contrast can be used to detect a tumor in the brain, spinal cord, or meninges (brain covering). A scan of the spine can help clarify if back pain with neurological symptoms such as leg weakness is caused by bone metastases (in which case a tumor has grown out of the bone and is pressing on the spinal cord) or by a metastasis to the spinal cord itself, a more serious condition. Often a spinal tap or lumbar puncture must be performed to sample the spinal fluid and detect meningeal metastases.

General Evaluation of Metastases: Often doctors will want to look for disease in the entire body at once. One way that they can do so is by ordering a PET scan. PET scans usually look at how fast cells use up sugar; cells that are growing rapidly (like cancer cells) will show up as bright on a scan. PET scans cannot tell if bright areas are cancer or not, only that cells there are more active. A biopsy is still required to make a final diagnosis.

resources

CT AND PET SCANS

- Imaginis, CT Scan: Provides detailed information on this scan.
    http://imaginis.com/ct-scan

- Radiology Info, PET Imaging: Provides detailed information on this scan.
    http://www.radiologyinfo.org/en/info.cfm?pg=pet&bhcp=1

Prognosis for Distant Metastasis

Not everyone with distant metastasis wants to know her prognosis — that is, an estimate of how much longer she is expected to live. Nonetheless, having some idea about survival time may help you make wise decisions in living your life and in planning for death, whether death is months or many years away. Studies show that cancer patients are often unaware of their prognosis, particularly if they have advanced cancer, and that those with late-stage cancer make inaccurate estimates of their survival time. Since doctors often take their cue from patients and wait to be asked about prognosis, it takes a proactive patient to find out this kind of information (40).

An individual's prognosis for metastatic breast cancer can be difficult for physicians to determine since the disease's progression is highly variable. When someone is first diagnosed with spread to distant organs, her prognosis may not be clear. While physicians try to be forthright, estimating how long someone has to live is complicated and is based on a number of factors, including where the metastases are located, how well the person can tolerate therapy, and what other medical conditions may be present. It is also influenced by a person's response to chemotherapy or hormonal therapies, and it usually takes an interval of time to assess if treatments are effectively arresting the disease.

As a group, patients diagnosed with metastatic disease are living longer today than even ten years ago, with an approximately 30 percent improvement in survival since the addition of Herceptin and aromatase inhibitors to treatment (41). As shown in figure 2, a prognosis is more favorable the longer the time between an initial diagnosis of breast cancer and the discovery of a distant recurrence. In most cases the sooner a breast cancer recurs, particularly if it recurs within two years of initial diagnosis, the more aggressive the tumor is. This aggression may be due to many factors specific to the cells of the tumor. When death due to any cause is tracked, it appears that women who have greater than ten years between initial diagnosis and recurrence may be dying not from breast cancer but from other diseases associated with age.

Additionally, the site of metastasis correlates with length of survival, with the longest survival time seen in people who have metastases to the bone only and the shortest survival time seen in those with metastases to the brain. This is shown graphically in figure 3. Everyone, of course, is alive at the zero point when the metastasis was diagnosed. The line with xs

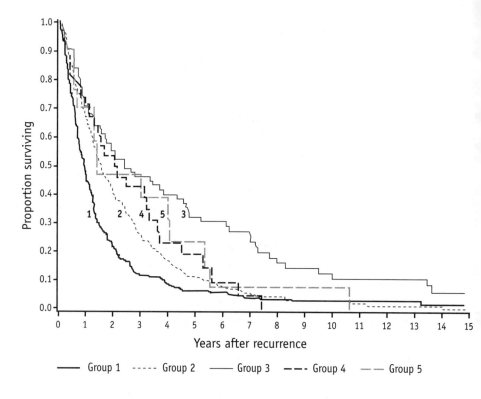

2. Survival times following recurrences in 529 patients, separated by time of recurrence. Group 1: less than or equal to two years from time of diagnosis to recurrence; group 2: 2–5 years to recurrence; group 3: 5–10 years to recurrence; group 4: 10–15 years to recurrence; group 5: greater than fifteen years to recurrence. From T. G. Karrison et al., "Dormancy of Mammary Carcinoma after Mastectomy," *Journal of the National Cancer Institute* 91, no. 1 (1999): figure 2.

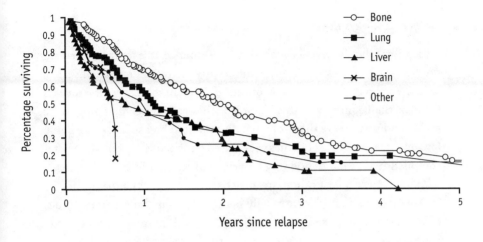

3. Survival following relapse by distant site of recurrence in a cohort of women followed from 1989 to 2002. From E. Elder, C. Kennedy, L. Gluch, et al., "Patterns of Breast Cancer Relapse," *European Journal of Surgical Oncology* 32, no. 9 (2006): 922–27, figure 5.

represents those in this study with brain metastasis. In following that line from the zero point you can see that no one was alive one year after diagnosis, whereas more than 2 percent of the people with bone metastasis, represented by the line with circles, were alive five years after diagnosis. It is important to remember that these data were accumulated prior to the widespread use of new hormonal therapy, immunotherapy and chemotherapy agents, and modern radiotherapy techniques; average survivals now are likely to be longer.

BREAST CANCER PROGNOSIS

- Nexcura NexProfiler Treatment Option Tool for Breast Cancer: Provides a tailored tool that produces a prognostic profile with links to the scholarly articles used to produce the results. You need to have your pathology report handy to answer a questionnaire.

    https://www.cancerprofiler.nexcura.com/Secure/InterfaceSecure
        .asp?CB=174

    http://www.nexcura.com/AboutTools_PharmaandMed.asp

resources

There Is Always Hope

A prognosis should never be looked at as a sentence. It is far from a certain prediction. People can react quite differently to treatments, and much is unknown about the progression of cancer. Keep in mind, too, the caveats listed at the beginning of this chapter with regard to reading prognostic tables. Indications are that women with advanced breast cancer are living longer now than in past decades (42). Based on the most recent SEER data, compiled from 1988 to 2003, 13.6 percent of women initially diagnosed with metastatic breast cancer are alive ten years after their diagnosis.

New treatments are continually being tested in clinical trials to determine which ones can prevent recurrence and improve survival time. You may want to familiarize yourself with clinical trials in chapter 2 and discuss with your oncologist whether or not you would be a good candidate for enrolling in one. Thanks to funding from organizations such as the National Cancer Institute, Susan G. Komen for the Cure, National Breast Cancer Coalition, National Association of Breast Cancer Organizations (NABCO), and the Breast Network of Strength, scientists across the country have been awarded grants to conduct biomedical research that someday may turn metastatic breast cancer into a chronic rather than fatal disease.

Further Reading

After Breast Cancer: Answers to the Questions You're Afraid to Ask, by Musa Mayer. Patient Center Guides, 2003.

After Breast Cancer: A Common-Sense Guide to Life after Treatment, by Hester Hill Schnipper. Bantam Books, 2003.

The Johns Hopkins Breast Cancer Handbook for Health Care Professionals, by Lillie D. Shockney and Theodore N. Tsangaris. Jones and Bartlett Publishers, 2007.

Living beyond Breast Cancer: A Survivor's Guide for When Treatment Ends and the Rest of Your Life Begins, by Marisa Weiss and Ellen Weiss. Three Rivers Press, 2010.

CHAPTER 2

Immediate Concerns and Best Care

Since the house is on fire, let us warm ourselves.

—Italian proverb

Nobody has ever measured, even poets, how
much a heart can hold.

—Zelda Fitzgerald

If you have just learned you have metastatic cancer, your world may be crashing down around you. Your plans and priorities for the next day, month, year—indeed for the rest of your life—are called into question. You come face to face with the reality that we do not have control over many aspects of our lives.

The news can be incapacitating. Unresolved issues with loved ones can immediately surface and intensify. If the metastasis is a recurrence, you may feel as devastated, or more so, as when you were first told you had breast cancer, and family and friends, not realizing the seriousness of a distant recurrence, may not acknowledge your difficulty as they may have when they learned you had an earlier-stage cancer.

You are faced with important choices about your physical and emotional well-being that you need to make with as clear a head as possible, yet you are in the midst of crisis. This chapter can help you make smart decisions at this difficult time. It begins with advice about absorbing the shock of the diagnosis, followed by how to tell others, and it concludes with guidance for securing the best medical care, including ways to research medical providers, facilities, treatments, and clinical trials.

At this difficult time it may be heartening to know that much help is available to you. Know too that many women with metastases live quality lives for a number of years (1). Survival times can vary widely, and one never knows what the future might bring. The next treatment breakthrough may make a significant difference in the course of your disease, or, though rare, you may experience an unexplained remission. Though the diagnosis of late-stage cancer is initially shattering, people often come to have profound understandings about themselves and life as the result of facing metastasized breast cancer. Some even experience newfound serenity and vibrancy in living.

Emotional Self-Care

Undoubtedly you are under considerable stress if you have been told that cancer has spread in your body, so taking care of yourself is paramount. You can handle this stress by consciously eating in a healthful manner, resting, garnering support, and acting on the many aspects of your life that are in your control. It is important as well for you to tend to an aspect of living not fully in your control: your emotions. To access your deepest emotions, give yourself moments of solitude and quiet. Take time to get out into nature; go for a long walk. Anger, sadness, pity, or envy may arise. Be open to all of your feelings without judgment. Do not try to feel any certain way. If you cannot get in touch with your emotions, let that be fine as well.

People benefit from talking with others about their emotions. As best as possible select people who can listen to your feelings without judging them or attempting to change what you are experiencing. If those closest to you are not available or able to do this, seek someone who can—perhaps someone in the clergy or a professional cancer counselor. Cancer centers usually can advise you how to contact both. Many women find solace and hope in talking with others who have been diagnosed with late-stage cancer. No one knows better what the experience of advanced cancer is like than those who have walked down that road. People with metastatic cancer are as close as a phone call or mouse click away. In the next resource box you will find a breast cancer hotline, online chat groups, and links that will enable you to learn if a support group meets in your community. Whether you talk with loved ones or strangers, connect with people who can nurture you; excuse yourself from, or avoid, those whose lack of support is troublesome. Put yourself first at this time.

Be especially gentle with yourself, avoiding self-criticism. Maintain your routines as well as you can, but allow yourself additional time to relax. Make a point to feed your soul with whatever you find uplifting: prayer, meditation, poetry, inspirational literature, music, dance, gardening, work, exercise, or helping others. Remember that all human beings

endure suffering, and countless people have led the way before you in confronting crises. In person or through readings, seek those who have faced
life-threatening predicaments in a manner that you admire. You are not
alone or unloved. If you feel isolated, know that many people, even ones
who do not know you, are able to offer help and unconditional love. Seek
their kindness.

EMOTIONAL SUPPORT

- Network of Strength: Offers twenty-four-hour phone support.
  800-221-2141 (English), 800-986-9505 (Español)
  http://www.networkofstrength.org

- CLUB-METS-BC: An online support group
  http://www.acor.org/club-mets-bc.html

- Breast Cancer Support: Look for the virtual meeting place for those with
  recurrence.
  http://bcsupport.org

- breastcancer.org: Indexed and ongoing discussion forums.
  http://community.breastcancer.org

- Inflammatory Breast Cancer Mailing List
  http://www.ibcsupport.org

- Sisters Network, a National African-American Breast Cancer Survivorship
  Organization: Offers support and information specific to African-American
  women, including links to affiliate chapters.
  http://www.sistersnetworkinc.org

resources

Telling Others

Among the first decisions that arise after learning you have late-stage
cancer is whom to tell and how, and when to tell them. If you receive the
news of the spread, or possible spread, of your cancer in the absence of
a loved one, do not delay in confiding your situation with at least one
or two others who care deeply for you and in whom you trust. Perhaps
someone will be able to help by being present as you move through any
additional testing and as you learn about treatment possibilities. When

telling those closest to you, consider asking them to keep the news confi-
dential so that you can better control when a wider circle of people, such
as your employer and coworkers, learn about your illness. To save others
and yourself unnecessary worry, have a confirmed diagnosis, such as a definitive pathology report, before divulging the news of metastatic cancer
to a great many others.

It may be particularly hard to tell those who will be most affected by your
diagnosis, such as a spouse, partner, children, parents, and dear friends.
If you find yourself considerably anxious about telling specific loved ones,
ask yourself whether you are wisely protecting yourself, or whether you
might be avoiding intimacy by "protecting" them from this difficult news.
The Golden Rule may be helpful. If the situation were reversed, would you
like to know if they were diagnosed with your condition? If so, you likely
will rest easier if you gather your courage and either tell them yourself, or
ask someone who knows you all to break this news. Keep in mind, though,
that if telling someone will likely make your life more difficult, delaying
the news until you have developed the support you need to deal with that
person's reaction may be beneficial.

You can help soften the emotional blow for those closest to you by informing them of your situation before they learn the news through a third
party. Intimate family and friends will likely be hurt if they learn that
acquaintances knew about your illness before they did. If they suspect
something is wrong, it is easier for them to adjust to knowing that you
have late-stage cancer than to be held in uneasy suspense. Those who love
you may find your news devastating; at the same time, at some level they
will likely be appreciative of your desire to be close to them by sharing a
life event of such magnitude. In doing so, you give them the opportunity
to offer their love, thus enriching each other's lives.

How to Tell Others

If you have the presence of mind to do so, you can help those closest to you
hear your news while easing their distress in a number of ways. If possible,
pick a time to tell them when they can best absorb what you have to say,
such as early in the day, when they have some free time, and when others
are available to support them. You may want to tell two or three loved
ones together. Tell those closest to you in person, and when that is not
possible, on the phone. If you cannot reach someone right away, it is best
not to leave an upsetting message on someone's voice mail, answering

machine, or e-mail. A message like "Please give me a call sometime today when you are free" would be appropriate. If you find contacting others too difficult and/or if other issues preoccupy you, you may want to ask certain loved ones to inform others about your illness.

When telling a loved one, take control of the conversation from the start and lead into what you have to say. You could begin with something like, "At my last checkup the doctor found something suspicious," and follow with a sentence or two saying what tests you had before reporting the results. Do not take more than a minute or so to get to the point. Share your feelings as well, unless you feel the person with whom you are talking cannot listen without interfering. Do not be embarrassed to cry, wail, swear, or do whatever you need to do. Do not misrepresent the news by minimizing or overdramatizing your condition as this will break down trust between you and those who care for you. If you want to open your-self up to more intimacy and you are ready for a heartfelt response, you can welcome your loved ones to express their feelings in return. They may be overcome with sadness, fear, or anger. They may be stunned. Sharing moments of devastation together can ease loneliness. Before ending the conversation, your loved ones will probably feel better if you tell them what the next step is. You also can refer them to help, such as the organizations listed in the resource box "Support for Caregivers" in chapter 8.

When telling a child, keep your explanation simple and short. You may be inclined to hide the truth from a child, but never more so than now, children need to know that you will be honest and up front. Children will likely be reassured if you let them know that you will keep them informed of what the doctor tells you. Furthermore, let them know that even though you are facing a serious illness from which people die, you will be there with them for as long as you can be, and it could be a very long time. Tell them and show them you love them. Ask them how they feel. Listen. Let them have whatever reaction they have, from crying to anger to no reaction. It is common for children to have little reaction since they come to understand the meaning of such news gradually.

Sometimes all does not go smoothly. Loved ones can overreact in ways that are more hurtful than helpful. Some may offer unsolicited advice or attempt to take control of your decisions. Those closest to you may feel guilty and helpless and infantilize you. Without meaning to, they can compromise your independence by taking over tasks that you are quite capable of doing. Some, not having dealt with their own fears of illness and death, may attempt to minimize your condition or withdraw from you. As such situations arise, put yourself first. Though you cannot control others' actions, you can take action yourself by telling people what you do and do not want from them.

As time goes by, you may become exhausted from repeatedly sharing updates about your condition and attempting to stay in touch with everyone who wants to hear from you. Some have found it helpful to invite people to become part of an online e-mail list that you, or someone who is willing to help you, use to send messages about how you are doing. No doubt family and friends who express a willingness to be on such a list will appreciate receiving periodic updates on your condition. Another possibility is to set up an invitation-only Web site where you can let people know how you are doing.

resources

SETTING UP AN INVITATION-ONLY WEB SITE

- CarePages
    http://www.carepages.com

- LiveJournal
    http://www.livejournal.com

Getting the Best Care

Quality medical care consists of many factors, including finding an experienced, respected oncologist and a state-of-the-art facility, interrelating well with your doctor, learning about your disease, and understanding your options. In most cases, there is no need to panic and rush into treatment when breast cancer has spread to organs in the body. Unlike with a local recurrence, immediate medical attention is not as critical for treating a metastatic recurrence unless you have major symptoms of malfunctioning organs, since the cancer has already clearly spread beyond the breast. For this reason, the course of your disease is not likely to be altered if you take a number of days to investigate and consider where you would like to receive treatment. Depending upon the amount of disease present and where it is located in your body, you may be able to wait several weeks before starting treatment. Investigate whether or not you would like to be enrolled in a clinical trial; if you wish to, you need to select an oncologist or center where the trial is offered. The resources in the remainder of this chapter can help you in considering your options.

Choosing Doctors and Facilities

When you are diagnosed with a recurrence, take time to consider whether or not it is desirable for you to move forward under the care of a different oncologist. It is critically important that your oncologist has extensive experience treating your type of metastatic breast cancer or that she or he is in close consultation with experts who have that expertise. Do not simply rely on referrals from your primary care doctor, your health plan, or acquaintances since research indicates that people who carefully select their oncologist usually find better care (2). For any oncologist you are considering, ask her or his office how many patients with your diagnosis the doctor has treated in the last year. A reasonable figure would vary, but think about looking further if your doctor has seen fewer than twenty such people (3, 4). Changing doctors may not be easy. You may feel a sense of camaraderie, even loyalty, to your physician; however, good physicians have as their top priority their patients' health, even if that means losing a patient so that someone with more expertise can treat her.

In selecting a doctor, be aware that simply because someone has a license to practice does not mean that she or he is up to date and respected by patients and colleagues. One measure of expertise is for a doctor to be board certified. Medical specialty boards award board certification, which ensures that a doctor has met national standards, including passing the tests set by the board and having a designated amount of experience in that specialty. To maintain certification, a doctor must periodically attend medical education programs and pass demanding recertification exams. You may also want to know where a doctor obtained her or his medical degree and completed medical training, how long that doctor has been practicing in your area, and where the doctor practiced before. Sometimes doctors move to avoid sanctions in a particular state. Look into whether the doctor you are considering has been reprimanded by a state or professional medical board, whether others have filed complaints about her or him, and whether the doctor has been successfully sued. You can sometimes get this information by calling the doctor's office and asking questions, though it may be more reliable to use the links in the resource box at the end of this section.

Learn with which hospital(s) a doctor is affiliated, not only to gauge whether the hospital's location is convenient for you (since you will likely use its services), but also to gauge the doctor's standing. Affiliation with a good hospital indicates that the doctor is well qualified. You can use the Web sites in the next resource box to gather information about hospitals such as an overall quality score for their treatment of particular diseases like cancer. These Web sites, or the hospital itself, can also often provide further information, such as the number of times a particular procedure or surgery is performed annually, the overall hospital infection rate, and the patient-to-nurse ratio, all of which are indicators of the hospital's level of care. Patients who go to hospitals that have repeatedly administered the treatment or performed the surgery or procedure that they will undergo fare better than patients who go to hospitals with less experience (5–9).

It is advantageous to have an oncologist who practices in a breast clinic where multidisciplinary teams of surgeons, radiation oncologists, and medical oncologists work collaboratively. In such settings doctors often confer with each other about patients and keep one another current on research findings. Having these specialists together in one facility can also save you time and energy in terms of transportation and record keeping, and it may speed up the process of getting test results.

If you are fortunate enough to live near a comprehensive cancer center, you would be wise to take advantage of the considerable expertise at your disposal. You can see where these are located using the last link in the next resource box. Cancer patients who are treated at comprehensive centers have slightly better survival rates than those who are not (2). These centers are teaching institutions. The oncologists at comprehensive cancer centers usually devote their clinical practice and research to a particular type of cancer, so they are familiar with the most cutting-edge treatments and research findings. Also, these facilities often have the most modern equipment. Sometimes it is easier to enroll in clinical trials through these centers since the very doctor you are seeing may be the head investigator for a trial. Nonetheless, you can receive excellent care from the many dedicated and highly competent oncologists who are not affiliated with such centers. It may be more to your liking and more convenient to be treated by a nearby oncologist who can refer you to a large cancer center if necessary.

Last but important, other factors such as availability and interpersonal style can matter significantly when choosing a physician. You may want to ask the doctor's office how large his or her patient load is, how patients are cared for when the doctor is unavailable, and to what extent the doctor is involved in a patient's end-of-life care.

Knowing that you and your doctor will be dealing with life and death matters, consider how important it is to you to have an empathic oncologist. You need to feel comfortable enough to share relevant personal information. Having a physician with a good bedside manner is highly desirable, but take into account that many of your emotional needs can be addressed by other health-care professionals and loved ones. It is not essential to like your doctor, but it is essential to trust in her or his expertise and ability to listen to your concerns.

Before you finalize any decision to change doctors or facilities, check to be sure that your public or private insurance will continue to help cover your medical expenses. If you determine it is best for you to seek new medical care, it is courteous to inform and thank your current doctor. You will need to contact your current doctor's office to have your records transferred to the new doctor's office in advance of your first medical appointment, and you may need to repeat some tests. Take into account that your new oncologist will need time to come to know you and your medical history. Be ready during exams and consultations to provide your new physician with pertinent information about your illness. It is to your benefit to build a strong relationship with your health-care providers and not to change doctors with frequency without cause. It stands to reason that the more hospitals, physicians, and nurses that become involved in your care, the more likely people will not be knowledgeable about your medical history, and the more likely medical error can occur.

RESEARCHING DOCTORS AND HOSPITALS

- American Board of Medical Specialties (ABMS) Certified Doctor Verification Service: Lists doctors' board certifications, free with registration.
  http://www.abms.org

- Federation of State Medical Boards: Lists the state medical boards under the "State Medical Board Info" link; depending on your state's laws and policies, you may be able to learn without cost whether a doctor has malpractice suits and complaints filed against her or him.
  http://www.fsmb.org

resources

resources

(Resources, continued)

- Federation of State Medical Boards DocInfo: For a small fee this site allows direct access to information about physicians' backgrounds and disciplinary infractions.
  http://www.docinfo.org/docinfo_faq.html#q12

- American Medical Association, Physician Select: Lists doctors who are and are not members of this association.
  http://webapps.ama-assn.org/doctorfinder/home.html

- Dr. Score: Allows you to rate doctors and view others' ratings; the results are an informal and unscientific means to attempt to assess patient satisfaction.
  http://www.drscore.com

- HealthGrades.com: Offers reports on hospitals and doctors for a small fee, including information such as a hospital's accreditations, services, and safety ratings and a physician's education, training, board certification, and possible professional misconduct.
  http://www.healthgrades.com

- Centers for Medicare and Medicaid Services: Allows you to make hospital comparisons for free. Veterans facilities are not included.
  http://www.hospitalcompare.hhs.gov

- Commonwealth Fund: Performance data on hospitals at no charge.
  http://www.whynotthebest.org

- U.S. News and World Report: Lists "America's Best Hospitals" and ranks hospitals by type of illness.
  http://www.usnews.com

- National Comprehensive Cancer Network (an alliance of nineteen state-of-the-art cancer centers in the United States): Lists member institutions.
  http://www.nccn.org/members/network.asp

Working in Collaboration with Health-Care Providers

Your doctors' and other health-care professionals' responsibility is to provide you with the best medical care possible, as humanely as possible.

For your physical and emotional well-being build a relationship of mutual trust and respect. Doctors and patients can have different expectations and styles of relating. Some patients want their doctor to be a friendly partner; others want a distant, unemotional decision maker. You may need to examine what you want and tell your doctor, who has no doubt seen patients who are happy with different approaches. Perhaps your doctor can accommodate the type of relationship with which you are most comfortable.

Your manner is likewise important in relating to your physician. As with any relationship, honesty and kindness are helpful. You must be up front. If you suspect that you will not follow a treatment regimen, say so. If you have a financial worry or sexual concern, say so. Speaking up is your best assurance of getting your needs addressed. People who are clear with their health-care providers more likely will receive the tests and treatments they need and avoid unnecessary ones. Acknowledge the wealth of information and experience physicians, physician assistants, and nurses bring to your care. Nonetheless, in the final analysis, this is about your body and your life; you are ultimately responsible for the decisions and choices that you make in regard to your health. Helpful guidelines for doctor and patient interaction, which were first drafted by six oncologists, are outlined in "The Wellness Community Physician/Patient Statement" below.

The Wellness Community Physician/Patient Statement

The text of the statement is as follows:

As your physician, I will make every effort to:

Provide you with the best medical care that is most likely to be beneficial to you.

Inform and educate you about your situation and the various treatment options available to you. I will provide a detailed explanation for any question you may have, but you need to let me know about how much or how little you wish to know.

Encourage you to ask questions about your illness and its treatment and answer your questions as clearly as possible. I will also attempt to answer questions asked by your family. However, my primary responsibility is to you, and I will discuss your medical situation only with those people authorized by you.

Help you remain aware that you will make all major decisions about the course of your care. However, I will accept the responsibility for making certain decisions if you want me to.

Assist you in obtaining other professional medical opinions if you desire or if I believe it to be in your best interest.

Relate to you as one competent adult to another, always attempting to consider your emotional, social, and psychological concerns as well as your physical needs.

Spend a reasonable amount of time with you on each visit unless required by something urgent to do otherwise. I will give you my undivided attention during your visit.

Honor all appointment times unless required by something urgent to do otherwise.

Return phone calls as promptly as possible, especially those you indicate are urgent.

Make test results promptly available and indicate, at the time the test is given, when you can expect the results and whom you should call to get them.

Provide you with any information you request concerning my professional training, experience, philosophy of care, and fees.

Respect your desire to try treatment that might not be conventionally accepted. However, I will give you my honest opinion about such unconventional treatments.

Provide active support and focused medical attention throughout the course of the illness.

Maintain accurate records of your medical information and provide proper billing information to your insurer.

The Physician-Patient Relationship

As your physician, I hope that you, the patient, will make every effort to:

Adhere to our agreed-upon treatment plan.

Be as candid as possible about what you need and expect from me.

Let me know if you desire another professional opinion.

Inform me of all forms of therapy you are involved with, even those that are complementary, alternative, or unconventional.

Honor all appointment times unless required by something urgent to do otherwise.

Be as considerate as possible of my need to follow a schedule to see other patients.

Attempt to make all phone calls to me during working hours. Call on nights and weekends only when absolutely necessary.

Attempt to coordinate the requests of your family and confidantes, so that I do not have to answer the same questions about you to several different persons.

Provide my office with accurate information about your insurance and other pertinent information.

As mentioned in the statement, patients are responsible for keeping their health-care professionals informed of their ongoing physical state. You can reduce medical error by reminding your physician about your medical conditions and past treatment and keeping your doctor current about how you are responding to treatment. An aid in doing this is to maintain a body diary similar to the one suggested in chapter 6 under "Describing and Evaluating Pain." A symptom that might seem insignificant to you might be revealing to a professional. When your symptoms confuse or frighten you, do not hesitate to call the doctor's office. If you are worried about being seen as a hypochondriac, you most likely are not. Bottom line: err on the side of caution and call. It can be helpful to have a nurse contact at your physician's office who can advise you whether or not you need to be seen by the doctor. Neither exaggerate nor underplay your symptoms or feelings. You need not apologize for your illness or for taking up a professional's time. If you repeatedly have false alarms, ask your health-care practitioner to help you in judging when to call or seek counsel to alleviate your anxiety.

Keep communication with your physician honest. Sometimes patients' concerns go unvoiced. For example, cancer treatments can lead to sexual dysfunctions that may be difficult to bring up during an appointment. If you feel uncomfortable speaking directly to your doctor about a problem, talk with your doctor's assistant or nurse. Be forthcoming and straightforward with your emotions as well. If you are feeling particularly fragile, hurt, or angry, let your health professional know that at the beginning of an appointment. Ask for what you need. For example, it might help you to hold someone's hand during a painful procedure, or you may want to request a moment to compose yourself. Last, it is vitally important to inform your doctor if you are involved in complementary or alternative treatments, even if you sense that your doctor does not want you to partake in them. A number of treatments and supplements, including some vitamins and minerals, are known to interact adversely with medicines and radiation, canceling out beneficial effects and sometimes creating dangerous side effects.

Use the questions in chapter 3 under "Questions to Consider When Deciding Treatment" to discuss medical decisions with your oncologist. Ask your physician what reasoning led her or him to suggest a particular treatment protocol. If you have other health conditions and previous treatments, ask if there might be other choices. For example, if you have osteoporosis, you may need to carefully weigh the risks and benefits of aromatase inhibitors in comparison with other medications. Doctors sometimes need your prompting to consider your case from other angles (10). As you weigh the pros and cons of a treatment, it will be helpful to understand the difference between relative and absolute benefit, which is explained in appendix A. When possible, ask your oncologist to give you the chance of benefit in absolute terms rather than relative terms.

Preparing for Appointments

Prepare for your appointments. To avoid emergencies that could increase your wait time, schedule them early in the day. Review your body diary and bring it with you, or, a few days in advance, e-mail or fax a concise, brief written statement that offers pertinent information about your health. Even if the doctor does not have time to read it in advance of your appointment, she can refer to it when you are being seen. Include dates, clear descriptions of occurrences and symptoms, and conclude with questions you may have. Be selective in your questions, typically limiting yourself to five to seven at most, putting the most important ones first. Handling your appointments in this professional manner will earn you the respect and gratitude of your health-care providers, along with securing you quality care.

When you are facing potentially distressing news or difficult decisions, try to arrange for someone to accompany you to your appointment. It is hard to think clearly under stressful circumstances and hard to remember accurately what the doctor says. An additional person can take notes and ask questions that might not occur to you. Before your appointment is over, find out what the next step is. When your care involves tests and scans, ask when you can expect to hear the results, from whom, and in what manner—for instance, by e-mail, phone, standard mail, or in person. If you do not hear from your doctor or the office when expected, it is important to take the initiative to contact the office. Do not be reluctant to call since this will ensure you receive attention while reducing the chance of medical error.

Keeping Records and Making Requests

In July 2004, the United States government began a process that encourages physicians to keep electronic medical records (EMRs). The hope is that by 2024, scans and records will no longer be physically transferred among hospitals and clinics; instead, medical providers will have instant access to a patient's medical record over the Internet. This same Internet storage will allow you to view and keep track of your records as well. Until that time, you can create your own physical file or computer file that includes notes from your appointments and the results of tests and scans. Currently some medical facilities and health insurance companies, along with some private companies including Google Health, offer space on the Internet for you to store and organize your medical information. Some facilities are offering USB computer storage "keys" that contain electronic medical records and that can be put into a USB port on any computer. No system as yet is, or maybe ever will be, completely safe from all possible breaches of privacy or loss of data, though this is true of paper records as well.

Be aware that in the United States, by law, clinics cannot show or send your records to outside parties without your approval. Clinics do have the right to keep your original records, but they must provide you with copies at your request. If the provider does not comply with a verbal request, send a written one. Each state has laws determining how much a health care provider can charge for duplicating your records. Learn about your state's laws governing costs and your rights to medical records in chapter 7 in the resource box titled "Legal Assistance Regarding Medical Rights."

Being Proactive and Protecting Yourself

In the early 2000s, the Institute of Medicine reported that in the United States more people die annually because of medical errors than because of automobile accidents (11). In 2002, the Joint Commission of Accreditation of Healthcare Organizations and Centers of Medicare and Medicaid took action and devised ways for patients to participate in their care to reduce the number of mistakes. As part of this effort it created a pamphlet titled "Speak Up," which you can obtain through accessing the first link in the next resource box. The commission urges patients to be proactive and voice their concerns when they think something might be amiss in their medical care. Medications are a particular concern. To prevent mistakes, ask questions; for example, when given an intravenous treatment in a bag, ask how long it should take for the bag to clear and be aware of its progress. When going to appointments, bring a written list of the medications you are taking, the medical conditions you have, and what you are allergic to. If you are not sure why you are being given a drug, or why a procedure has been ordered, ask about it. When a test has been ordered that you had a short time ago, inquire whether it is possible to use the previous results. In addition to thwarting mistakes, by asking questions you can reduce unnecessary and duplicate tests and procedures.

Having an operation or other invasive procedure puts you in a vulnerable position. Before having surgery, ask for an explanatory handout telling you how to prepare for your procedure and what to expect afterward. Find out if you will need someone to drive you to and from the hospital. Ask what precautions you need to take, if any, when you return home and under what circumstances you should call the doctor's office. If the surgery involves removing a tumor, ask whether this tumor should be frozen. Sometimes frozen tissue samples are saved so that later they can be tested to determine whether new chemotherapy, biological, and genetic treatments may be effective for your particular cancer. While you are under anesthesia or are groggy, try to arrange for a family member or friend to ask about you, someone who can be sure that you are not forgotten, who can check on your medications, and who can keep track of your needs. Also, this person could take notes about what the doctor says immediately following your surgery.

Being human, health-care professionals will not handle every situation flawlessly. If a professional has done something that troubles you, assume that person and others in that workplace want to give you the best care and would like to know about your concern. You can tell them simply by filling in the blanks of the following statement either verbally or in a note: "When X happened, I was concerned about Y, or felt Y, and would be pleased if Z happened instead." You may be offered an explanation that pleases you, and perhaps you will see a change in the problematic conditions or behavior that will benefit you and others. If it becomes clear that the unprofessional conduct is not being addressed after you have discussed the problem with your health-care provider, contact the administrators of the clinic or hospital. If you still receive no consideration, you can use the Web sites in the previous and next resource boxes to file a complaint with medical boards, and you can consider going elsewhere for your care. Though it may be stressful to make a change, it might be more stressful not to. You may need some time to talk with trusted confidants to weigh this decision.

The health-care system can be daunting for anyone. To better assure that you get the best care and are less overwhelmed by the bureaucracy, consider having an advocate help you with medical and practical concerns. Some medical centers will provide you with one at your request. You also may want to seek the services of someone connected with a national advocacy organization that you can contact using the links in the following resource box.

HEALTH SAFETY AND HEALTH ADVOCACY

HEALTH SAFETY

- Joint Commission of Accreditation of Healthcare Organizations: Offers links for the general public, including tips on finding the best health care and registering a complaint about a health-care organization; also included is a downloadable pamphlet titled "Speak Up." Alternatively, call 877-223-6866 to request a copy.

  http://www.jointcommission.org

- U.S. Food and Drug Administration: Allows you to report and learn about dangerous drug interactions and troublesome side effects.

  http://www.fda.gov/medwatch

- National Coalition for Cancer Survivorship: Provides a free copy of "Teamwork: The Cancer Patient's Guide to Talking with Your Doctor."

  http://www.canceradvocacy.org
  http://www.canceradvocacy.org/resources/publications/teamwork.pdf

HEALTH ADVOCACY

- Center for Patient Partnerships: Provides an application process to obtain an advocate to help you with medical, legal, and financial matters. Komen advocates are available to aid breast cancer patients.

  http://patientpartnerships.krambs.com

resources

(Resources, continued)

- Patient Advocate Foundation: Aids patients in getting access to good care, maintaining employment, and preserving financial stability.
  http://www.patientadvocate.org

- National Patient Advocate Foundation: Provides information and supports access to health care.
  http://www.npaf.org/about-npaf/index.html

Researching Your Disease and Treatment

Educating yourself about your disease not only reduces the possibility that you will be a victim of medical error, but it also helps you find the most up-to-date treatment for your cancer, helps you better weigh the trade-offs of various treatments, and helps you speak with confidence when talking to health-care professionals. Studies have shown that the more informed patients are, the better their care and higher their satisfaction (12). In being knowledgeable about your disease and treatments you are better able to engage in shared decision making with your doctor. You can make a more informed choice about a treatment's effect on your quality of life with increased knowledge of the treatment's benefits and risks. Since doctors have limited time to consult with each patient, you will be able to ask more specific questions and spend less time going over basic information.

Researching your own disease, however, can be daunting. This book can help. Chapter 3 covers the standard treatments for metastatic breast cancer as of this writing. Chapter 4 explains the development of cancer and how emerging therapies attempt to intervene in the process. Throughout those chapters and at the end of this section are Web links that lead to the most current information, as well as sites that discuss ways to research cancer. You can go into great depth when investigating cancer, such as reading medical journals, or you can read quick, simple explanations on sites designed for the general public. You do not have to become an expert; in fact, that would take a considerable commitment over many years. Fortunately, oncologists have already done so. Fortunately, too, many Web sites for breast cancer patients offer easy access to basic treatment information. If researching your disease becomes burdensome and is keeping you from enjoying life, you might solicit help from others to look up information, seek a second opinion on your case, or simply decide to entrust more of the decision making to your doctor and look up additional information when you most feel the need.

When exploring the research that has been conducted on breast cancer, you will quickly discover that the good and bad news is that you have access to a mountain of information. When you type the key words "breast cancer" into a Google search box, over 50 million sites will appear in twenty-two hundredths of a second. To be a savvy, selective researcher you need to keep two guiding principles in mind. First, make sure you gather information from a credible source; second, note how current the research is.

Though the Internet is a route to the most up-to-date information, it is also the quickest route to misinformation. Do not solely base your treatment decisions on personal testimonies or advice shared in breast cancer listservs and chat rooms. Other cancer patients' experiences can be idiosyncratic; their genetics and previous medical history can be different from yours in important ways, and their knowledge of medicine and biology could be very limited. Keep in mind that few, if any, Internet sites check users' backgrounds to see if they are even who they purport to be. Be critical of nonmainstream Web sites. Anyone with a bit of know-how and a few resources can create a Web site, and some people have means for getting their sites to be among the first you see when doing a search.

On a credible Web site you should be able easily to identify the person or organization that authored the site. Sites ending with ".com" have commercial interests, and ".org" and ".edu" sites can sometimes have biases. One way you can find out what those biases are is to read the mission statement of the organization. You can also look at who heads the organization, or who is on the board. Make sure the site includes a working e-mail address or phone number to contact the organization. Be suspicious of any site that does not provide all the above information. Finally, do not forget to check when the site was last updated since treatment information rapidly changes. You can also check the credibility of some sites using the Health on the Net Foundation link in the next resource box. The most authoritative sites for research purposes are search databases that index medical journals; an example is PubMed (listed in the next resource box). These sites bring you to articles in peer-reviewed journals where research findings are first reported. Medical journal articles, however, are written for other experts and can be hard to understand. The Health and Human Services Department of the U.S. government has Web sites that put the most noteworthy information into language more suitable for the general public. Some credible Web sites and subscription breast cancer news agencies do likewise and are listed in the last resource box in this chapter, "Keeping Up to Date with Breast Cancer Developments." If you have trouble finding the information you would most like, or would like to see this information in print form, go to your public library and request help from a reference librarian. Reference librarians are trained to assist the public, and their assistance is usually without charge.

When you are looking at the results of a study, know the gold standard in medical research studies: they involve large enrollments—that is, seven hundred or more people—and they are double-blind, meaning that participants are randomly assigned to a particular treatment, and they and their doctors do not know which treatment they are receiving. However, experimental clinical research begins with fewer subjects, and fewer people are enrolled as well when a rarer condition is researched. When reading about different studies for the same condition or treatment, do not be surprised to discover contradictory results. One way to sort out what is happening in such situations is to look for an academic article that is a comprehensive analysis of many studies, sometimes called a meta-analysis, or an article that summarizes much of the key material, such as a review article. Keep in mind that studies quickly become outdated and that oncologists devoted to your specific disease can offer you recent information. Furthermore, oncologists can critically assess the results of medical studies to uncover flaws or limitations in the findings. Doing your own research is empowering, but this is an aid to, rather than a substitute for, a candid discussion with your doctor.

The results of research studies occasionally make big news in the popular press. Frequently the breaking news stories present a rosier picture of cancer advancements than is the reality. In some cases, cancer breakthroughs reported in the media can be a decade or more from finding their way into the clinical setting; in other words, doctors may not be able to use the breakthrough medicines with patients for many years. Only a small percentage of substances that look promising in lab and animal studies ultimately is found to be safe and effective in humans. Those writing for the media are generally reporters, not cancer experts, so important details may be overlooked in their stories, and the brevity of the medium requires simplification. Discoveries often end up revealing how complex cancer is instead of being the "cure for cancer" that everyone hopes for. That said, we live in a time of exciting developments and extraordinary advances, including the mapping of the human genome. Some of what was standard care even a few years ago is not now. It is not far-fetched to believe that experimental treatments may someday enable those with metastatic cancer to live a normal lifespan.

AUTHORITATIVE SOURCES FOR BREAST CANCER RESEARCH

- U.S. National Library of Medicine and National Institutes of Health: Offers a link for the public that searches lay periodicals and a link, "Health Care Professionals," that searches medical journals.
    http://www.nlm.nih.gov

- PubMed, U.S. National Library of Medicine and National Institutes of Health: Offers a search engine for a database consisting of medical journals. Look for articles under the "Review" tab.
    http://www.ncbi.nlm.nih.gov/entrez/query.fcgi?DB=pubmed

- LiveHelp: Answers general cancer questions or assistance in navigating the NCI's Web sites; available Monday–Friday 9:00 a.m.–11:00 p.m. Eastern Time.
    https://cissecure.nci.nih.gov/livehelp/welcome.asp

- PDQ® (Physician Data Query), NCI's Comprehensive Cancer Database for Recurrent and Metastatic Breast Cancer: Provides peer-reviewed summaries on a host of cancer topics, such as cancer treatment and screening.
    http://www.nci.nih.gov/cancertopics/pdq/cancerdatabase

- NCI's Breast Cancer Page: Offers a host of links leading to information about treatment, screening, statistics, and more.
    http://www.cancer.gov/cancertopics/types/breast

- CancerGuide, Researching Your Options: Offers extensive guidance and links for finding information about cancer.
    http://cancerguide.org/research_home.html

resources

resources

(Resources, continued)

- Health on the Net Foundation: Enables you to type in a Web address to see if the site is certified by this organization. Sites authorized to display their emblem must meet a code of conduct and are monitored for adherence to the code.
  http://www.hon.ch

Exploring Treatment Options

You do not want to delay in getting treatment, but before you begin, you should consider whether or not you should get a second opinion. You should also look into whether or not you are eligible for a clinical trial designed for your condition and, if so, carefully weigh the advantages and disadvantages of enrolling in it.

Second Opinions

As mentioned in chapter 1, treatment protocols for metastatic cancer are more varied than treatment protocols for earlier stages of the disease. Pathologists do not always come to the same conclusions when interpreting slides and scans, and oncologists do not always agree on what is best for a particular patient. Many people wisely seek the advice of a second expert for a pathology report and/or treatment protocol. If you have insurance, check to see what your insurer will cover with regard to second opinions. Also, contact the second doctor's office to learn what a second opinion will cost. Some doctors' fees for second opinions are lower than the cost for a standard appointment. In some cases you may not have to be seen in person.

Certain situations make getting a second opinion crucial. If your oncologist's practice is not limited to breast cancer, if your pathologist does not specialize in breast cancer, or if either of your physicians is inexperienced, a second opinion is imperative. Rare kinds of breast cancer or other health conditions that could interfere with treatment also call for another opinion. Get a second opinion as well if your doctor wants you to enroll in a clinical trial in which she or he is an investigator. A second opinion is less imperative if your doctor is part of a team of physicians who specialize in breast cancer.

Seeking a second opinion is simply taking good care of yourself; it is not being unkind to your doctor. As your doctor knows, second opinions are part of the medical world, and she or he likely seeks and gives them as well. To be considerate, let your doctor know that you will be getting a second opinion. If after obtaining and discussing the additional opinion with your current doctor you believe a new doctor can give you better care, you owe it to yourself and your loved ones to change doctors. It is also possible that after discussing the second opinion with your current doctor, you and your doctor may modify the original treatment protocol. A second opinion can also confirm that your original treatment plan is the best one, giving you the peace of mind that you have done all that is possible to obtain the highest quality of care.

If you receive conflicting treatment opinions that cannot be resolved, consider which doctor is more current in her or his knowledge, and possibly seek a third opinion. Be careful, though, not to waste time and money by conferring with numerous specialists. Getting more than three opinions could be a denial of your condition or an avoidance of treatment.

As a last assurance that you are getting top-of-the-line treatment, use the resources in chapter 3 in the resource box titled "Treatment Strategies." Included are links to the NCCN, which offers treatment guidelines along with decision trees. You can also look over the NCI's PDQ for metastatic breast cancer; it offers guidance to physicians about treatment options.

Unconventional Paths

Oncologists use evidence-based therapies, tested in clinical trials, known to produce results. A minority of people shun this traditional medical model. They may decide to do nothing about their cancer, though the complications and pain of end-stage cancer can be hard to tolerate without outside care. Others may decide to partake solely in alternative care. Be aware that the distress of having late-stage cancer can lead to desperate health-care decisions that can be physically, emotionally, and financially harmful. Before you make a choice that excludes standard medical care, we suggest you read over the material in chapters 3–5, which cover both standard and complementary/alternative care.

The kind of treatment you seek can depend on how you conceptualize your illness. Illness is a physical manifestation, and allopathic (standard Western) medicine can alleviate symptoms and, at times, prolong life. But, in many people's eyes illness involves more than the physical. Some believe, whether consciously or unconsciously, that their illness may be caused by other factors. For example, those who think their illness is the result of psychological problems may meet with psychiatrists or counselors to work through unresolved issues or to help them deal with stress. Those who think their illness is punishment may seek a means of absolution through good deeds or prayer. Those who believe their illness is a metaphysical disruption may attempt to return to better health through psychic and spiritual healing techniques such as visualizations or Reiki. As of now, there is no clear evidence what nonphysical factors, if any, may cause or promote breast cancer. Still, illness is complex. It may be important to you to work on your disease in all dimensions: physical, emotional, and spiritual. Or, you may not give any meaning to your illness but want to cover your bases by choosing a variety of means to improve your health.

A few rare people forgo all treatment for personal, religious, or philosophical reasons and allow their illness to proceed naturally without outside intervention, as an undomesticated animal would in nature. Most likely, though, you will be considering treatment options and weighing the chances that a treatment will improve or prolong your life against the treatment's unpleasant or dangerous side effects. In doing so, you can always ask yourself and your doctor what would happen if you did not take the treatment.

Last, a small number of people who have diligently researched their disease sometimes want to try a medical protocol that has not been approved, or possibly even considered, by health authorities. Most oncologists will not venture outside of approved protocols, regardless of your willingness to sign countless waivers. Even if a doctor were willing to create a one-person trial, the institutional review board (IRB) of a hospital or clinic would likely not approve it as there would be no usable research data obtained from such a trial and the risk-benefit would be difficult to assess for a single person. In addition, hospitals are aware that some people have sued medical establishments and won, even though the patient and the patient's family had signed waivers, and may override any trial that the IRB approved. Still, a very few oncologists with their own clinics may be willing to assist you in an unorthodox approach. This is a risky path, only for the very adventurous and for those who can cover costs without the help of insurance.

Whatever you decide, it may help to remember that all the important decisions in life, including your treatment decisions, are made in the midst of some uncertainty. We can only make a best guess about which paths to follow. Since no one knows *the* way, the most you can do after gathering information, weighing the odds and trade-offs, and considering what is important to you, is to move forward with what you believe is likely to produce the outcome you desire, and rest assured, you have done what you could do.

KEEPING UP TO DATE WITH BREAST CANCER DEVELOPMENTS

- Medscape's Resource Center for Breast Cancer: Offers updates and access to scholarly articles, with free registration.

    http://www.medscape.com/pages/editorial/resourcecenters/public/breastcancer/rc-breastcancer.ov

- Medline Plus: Offers highly informative categorized links such as Latest News, Diagnosis, and Treatment.

    http://www.nlm.nih.gov/medlineplus/breastcancer.html

- breastcancer.org: Offers research news and free e-mail updates.

    http://www.breastcancer.org

- UpToDate: A noncommercial site for physicians that provides current medical information; a subscription is expensive ($100 or more), but the site is highly user-friendly and offers quick access to medical information.

    http://www.uptodate.com

- San Antonio Breast Cancer Symposium: Provides streaming webcasts and abstracts from the annual conference.

    http://www.sabcs.org

- BreastCancer.net: Offers weekly research abstracts over e-mail for a small subscription fee.

    http://www.breastcancer.net

- Breast Cancer Online Cambridge University Press: Offers an online journal and e-mail abstracts.

    http://journals.cambridge.org/action/displayJournal?jid=BCO

resources

(Resources, continued)

- Living Beyond Breast Cancer: Provides current breast cancer news.
  http://www.lbbc.org

- Mamm Magazine: Offers updates and magazine highlights and subscription information.
  http://www.mamm.com

Clinical Trials

In 1962, the U.S. Food and Drug Administration (FDA) was charged with establishing a systematic approach to evaluating new drugs in patients; the directive resulted in the testing of drugs in progressive stages, or phases, through clinical trials. Clinical trials exist for nearly every disease, though the majority of trials investigate cancer treatments. Few breast cancer patients are aware of the many possible clinical trials in which they may be eligible to participate, and many patients have little understanding of how clinical trials operate. For example, clinical trials are available for people who are at risk for developing cancer, for people who have early-stage cancer and hope to ward off a recurrence, for people who have advanced cancer, and for people for whom all standard treatments have failed. Some trials examine cancer and its connection with lifestyle factors, such as diet and exercise; others study complementary treatments, such as herbs, but most investigate untried but promising drugs or therapies, or new drug combinations or delivery systems. Once a treatment shows promise in stalling or curbing cancer in animals, clinical trials with humans commence. A new therapy is researched on humans most often in three phases.

Phases of Clinical Trials

Phase I: Phase I trials are the most cutting-edge, the most experimental. In these trials a therapy is tried on people for the first time, and the consequences are not known. These trials generally involve increasing the amount of medication to determine the maximum tolerated dose while monitoring the side effects. Phase I trials usually consist of small numbers of people and are often conducted at the National Institutes of Health in Bethesda, Maryland, or at NCI-designated cancer centers around the country. Phase I trials are often reserved for patients who are not re-sponding to conventional therapies and who want to take a long shot on a brand new possibility. Safety, not effectiveness, is the priority in these initial trials. Some unforeseen side effects can be debilitating, and, rarely, they can be fatal. Compared to the past, today's experimental treatments for breast cancer are often less toxic. While not the goal of a Phase I study, the remote but real possibility exists that the treatment may slow or stop the course of your cancer.

Phase II: Once a treatment has shown promise in fighting cancer and has shown itself not to cause more harm than the disease, it can graduate to a Phase II trial. Phase II trials aim to establish what dosage and what sched-ule of dosages are effective in reducing or stabilizing tumor size. The num-ber of participants is expanded to include more people than in Phase I. Once a recommended method for giving the medicine and the appropriate dose are arrived upon, the treatment can move into Phase III trials.

Phase III: Phase III trials are comparison studies. A new treatment is com-pared to a standard treatment to see whether the former exceeds the latter's effectiveness. Participants are often randomly assigned by a com-puter to receive either the new or standard treatment. The random as-signment controls for factors that might create a biased treatment group if people were assigned to treatment groups (called arms) in some other manner. If you enroll in a Phase III clinical trial, you may get the new treat-ment, or you may get the current standard treatment; neither you nor your doctor will know until the trial is complete. If you are chosen for the new treatment, you may be among the first women who possibly benefit from the new treatment. If you are not chosen, you still will be given the best standard treatment possible, the treatment you would receive if you did not enroll in the trial. If the newer treatment is clearly superior, the study may be halted so that all participants can have access to the better treatment. Though beneficial for the participants, halting a trial can keep researchers from learning if the results of the treatment are better in the long term and what the long-term side effects might be.

Phase IV: When a new treatment begins being used more widely in clinical settings, Phase IV trials are sometimes initiated to monitor its long-term benefits and side effects. This phase is often referred to as post-marketing surveillance.

In the United States the FDA approves all trials, including those initiated through businesses or private foundations. Most often clinical trials are proposed by oncologists, scientists at hospitals, clinical research organizations, and pharmaceutical companies. Each hospital or research facility has an institutional review board (IRB) that oversees trials and reports to the FDA. Once approved, the sponsor of the trial enrolls participants in a variety of ways, mostly through doctors informing their patients or through patients' requests. Trials taking place at only one facility—"local" trials—are typically small, with one hundred or fewer people. These trials usually require periodic travel to the site. Others, called cooperative or multi-center trials, involve hundreds of people and have sites all the over the country.

Each trial has eligibility criteria. Often the criteria are based on a participant's having a specific stage and type of breast cancer, along with having had, or not having had, certain kinds of previous treatment. If you want to be in a trial, you do not have to have your current doctor's approval. You can contact the doctor associated with the clinical trial yourself, but be sure your current doctor knows what you plan to do so that you do not jeopardize your care with conflicting treatments or drug interactions. The trial company or lab will not administer the treatment; rather your doctor, or a participating doctor who is not an employee of the company or lab, will administer the treatment.

It can take from a week to a few months to find and enroll in a trial, and you may want to regularly check even after enrolling in one to see if another one becomes available that is more suitable for you. Once you have spotted a suitable trial, the process of determining eligibility and joining is often quicker if a facility near you is enrolling people and if you have not had a great deal of prior treatment. Prior treatment can make you ineligible; it also involves the transfer of more records and often more evaluation, such as your going to interviews and possibly having additional testing.

Considerations

Only about 5 percent of cancer patients in the United States participate in clinical trials, though the percentage of participation is probably higher among those with late-stage cancer. This scant figure, much lower than the percentage of Europeans who enroll in trials, may be a result of doctors not informing patients about protocols. Given the great number of patients and the great number of trials, it is not possible for oncologists to be aware of all the trials in which a particular patient could enroll. Therefore, you need to inform yourself about them and approach your doctor. Participating in a clinical trial requires thoughtful consideration. Few therapies are shown to be effective in fighting cancer in Phase I trials; about one experimental drug in five goes on to be used in a clinical setting, and usually the gains in treatment are modest (13).

Make your decision to participate in a trial with open eyes by weighing the likelihood that you will personally benefit from the treatment. Carefully consider the informed consent form so that you know to what extent you may be sacrificing the quality of your remaining life in an attempt to prolong it. Keep in mind that you can drop out of a trial at any time. Before agreeing to participate, talk with your doctor, and ask the doctor conducting the trial the questions below, adapted from *The Alpha Book on Cancer and Living*, by Brent G. Ryder (14). Also consider asking for a trained advocate or nurse to help you weigh the benefits and risks.

> What is the purpose of the study?
> What testing and treatment are involved?
> What is likely to happen to me with this treatment? Without it?
> Are there other treatments? What are the advantages and disadvantages of those treatments?
> How long will the study last?
> How will the treatment affect my daily life?
> What side effects might I have?
> If I am harmed by the study, what treatment will I receive?
> Does the study cost me money, or does it provide free care?
> Does the study include long-term care? What kind?
> Will I have free access to the drug or check-ups once I am off the study?

You may also want to know whether or not the trial is already underway and, if so, what the results thus far have shown and whether or not ongoing results will be accessible to you and made public. Many of these questions will be answered by a document called a "consent form." The sponsor of the trial, whether the NIH, another funding agency, or a pharmaceutical company, is required to be clearly listed in the first two or three paragraphs of this form.

Participating in a trial may cost you money. If you have health insurance, check to see if it will cover all or some of the costs of the trial in which you wish to participate. Usually your insurers will be billed as if you were receiving standard care for your type of cancer. Still, because no evidence exists that the trial therapy is effective, some insurers will not pay, even though it costs them no more than the standard care. However, since many trials are funded by taxpayer money, in some states, by law, Medicaid or Medicare will help cover costs. The pharmaceutical companies that fund trials may also subsidize the expense. If you live far from the trial site, check into free travel resources such as those mentioned at the end of the following resource box.

The hoped-for benefit of a trial is that a new therapy will prolong your life or add to its quality. Even if it does not, enrollment in a clinical trial pretty well assures that you will be closely observed and conscientiously monitored. Additionally, some who enroll in trials, particularly those who enroll in Phase I trials, have the great satisfaction of knowing that their participation will benefit others in the future, even though it probably will not benefit them.

It is likely that you are a beneficiary of the patients who enrolled in clinical trials over the years. They made it possible for many women to have lumpectomies as opposed to radical mastectomies, for others to benefit from Taxol, for oncologists to know the best ways to administer chemotherapy drugs; in fact, all that is standard treatment currently has been established through clinical trials, then reported in medical journals. As of this date, no one site lists all trials; the sites below cover a wide range of both public and private trials.

CLINICAL TRIAL INFORMATION

- National Cancer Institute: Offers a search engine leading to cancer clinical trials sponsored by the government and private industry.

  http://www.cancer.gov/clinicaltrials

- National Institutes of Health: Offers a search engine leading to clinical trials sponsored by the government and private industry for all diseases; this is the same database as in the above link.

  http://www.clinicaltrials.gov

- Center Watch Clinical Trials Listing Service: Tracks both government and industry trials worldwide.

  http://www.centerwatch.com

(Resources, continued)

- Current Controlled Trials: A site directed to health-care professionals that provides access about ongoing clinical trials worldwide.
  http://www.controlled-trials.com

- BreastCancerTrials.org: Allows you to register for a free service that matches your health record with breast cancer clinical trials.
  http://www.BreastCancerTrials.org

- National Comprehensive Cancer Network: Links to cancer centers so that you can learn what trials may be occurring at a site near you.
  http://www.nccn.org/clinical_trials/patients.asp

- National Association of Hospital Hospitality Houses: Helps with housing for those needing treatment away from home.
  800-542-9730
  http://www.nahhh.org

- National Patient Travel Center: Helps patients cover costs for airline travel for treatment.
  800-296-1217
  http://www.patienttravel.org

Further Reading

Breast Cancer Sourcebook: Health Reference Series, 3rd ed., edited by Karen Bellenir. Omnigraphics, 2009.

A Cancer Survivor's Almanac: Charting Your Journey, by Barbara Hoffman, JD. Chronimed Publishing, 1995.

Dear God, They Say It's Cancer, by Janet Thompson. Howard Books, 2006.

Healing Lessons, by Sidney J. Winawer with Nick Taylor. Routledge, 1999.

It's Not about the Hair: And Other Certainties of Life and Cancer, by Debra Jarvis. Sasquatch Books, 2007.

The Lonely Patient: How We Experience Illness, by Michael Stein. Harper Perennial, 2008.

The Measure of Our Days: A Spiritual Exploration of Illness, by Jerome E. Groopman, MD. Viking Press, 1997.

Talking with Doctors, by David Newman. Analytic Press, 2005.

Waiting for Wings: A Woman's Metamorphosis through Cancer, by Heidi J. Marble. James Stevenson Publisher, 2006.

When Words Heal: Writing through Cancer, by Sharon A. Bray. Frog, 2006.

YOU: The Smart Patient; An Insider's Handbook for Getting the Best Treatment, by Michael F. Roizen and Mehmet C. Oz, MD. Free Press/Simon and Schuster, 2006.

CHAPTER 3

Medical Treatments

The cost of a thing is the amount of what I call life
which is required to be exchanged for it.
—Henry David Thoreau

Even the confrontation with disease should be
approached with the realization that many of the
sicknesses of our species are simply conveyances
for the inexorable journey by which each of us
is returned to the same state of physical, and
perhaps spiritual, nonexistence from which we
emerged at conception. Every triumph over some
major pathology, no matter how ringing the
victory, is only a reprieve from the inevitable end.
—Sherwin Nuland, *How We Die: Reflections on Life's
Final Chapter*

Devoted medical researchers are working to turn metastatic breast cancer
into a less deadly, more manageable disease, and little by little they are
making progress. Though a cure has been elusive, current treatments can
improve the quality of life and sometimes prolong it. Current remedies
shrink and eradicate tumors. Even if the treatment you receive does not
considerably extend your life, it can relieve much of the pain and some of
the limitations that cancer may cause. For example, rather than the loss
of mobility because a bone tumor has destroyed a hipbone, it is possible
to reduce the size of the tumor through drugs and radiation, enabling a
patient to function more normally. And, there is always hope that a newly
discovered treatment will offer significantly more time for people to live.
You can investigate clinical trials (see chapter 2) and possibly be among
the first patients who benefit from an experimental drug or procedure
that helps turn breast cancer into a chronic rather than a life-threatening
disease.

This chapter will familiarize you with a number of therapies used to treat metastatic breast cancer. This background, along with the most current information you can obtain by using the resources in this chapter, will better enable you to collaborate with your oncologist in making treatment decisions.

Physical and Emotional Considerations in Determining Treatment

Treatment for metastatic breast cancer is highly individualized. Oncologists take into account a number of physical factors in considering what therapies may help a patient. First, the type of cancer dictates treatment possibilities. Breast cancer is most accurately thought of as a collection of cancers originating in the breast. Samples from your tumor reveal sensitivities that indicate which medicine will likely be effective. For example, if the tumor is sensitive to hormones, a number of hormonal therapies may shrink the tumor, or if your tumor overexpresses (produces too much) HER2/neu, the cancer is likely to respond to antibody or other targeted therapy.

Depending on your symptoms at the time your metastasis is discovered, you will be examined for spread to other parts of your body (see chapter 1, "Detecting and Confirming Distant Metastases"). If your metastasis appeared two or more years after an initial diagnosis of breast cancer, you will need to have the new tumor's characteristics reassessed by biopsy and testing of ER, PR, and HER2 at a minimum, as estrogen receptor positivity can be lost and HER2 overexpression gained. In one study, 36 percent of patients whose initial cancer showed positive estrogen receptors had lost positive receptor status at the time of recurrence (1). Another study showed that a significant percentage of metastatic tumors — 12 percent — were HER2 overexpressing, while the primary tumors were not (2).

In addition to the type of breast cancer, other physical factors are taken into account in determining what treatment should be prescribed for an individual, such as the number of metastases, their location, and a person's general physical condition. If you have a few areas of metastasis, surgery or radiation may be helpful. Surgery and radiation are less helpful if the metastases are spread throughout an organ, as is the way breast cancer often appears in the lungs, liver, and bone. The affected organ(s) also indicate which treatments will provide the most relief; for instance, bisphosphonate therapy is used in particular for bone metastases. Your overall health, other medical conditions, and any previous treatment affect your suitability for various therapies. Many of the newest treatments are offered first-line only, meaning that if you have had other treatment for metastatic disease, you would not be eligible to have them. Sometimes too much of a treatment can cause more harm than good. For instance, there is a limit to the amount of Adriamycin that an individual can tolerate before this drug causes heart damage, so the current state of a person's heart and previous use of the drug must be taken into account. However, a different formulation of the drug, Doxil or Myocet, may be given even after someone has received the maximum total dose of Adriamycin.

Currently few treatment regimens individually are known to prolong survival more than a few months, although when one regimen fails, it is possible to move to a new regimen that may extend your life again by a number of months. It is difficult to determine how long a patient might live given multiple treatments. Which treatment will work and the side effects of a particular treatment vary widely from person to person. Determining an effective regimen requires close monitoring and includes some trial and error. Most oncologists prescribe therapy to which your particular cancer will likely respond while balancing how much that therapy will compromise your quality of life. Once an effective treatment is found, it is continued until your cancer no longer responds, or you develop unmanageable side effects. At that time, your oncologist will likely suggest changing to another drug to which the tumor has a high chance of responding. Generally this process is continued until all options are exhausted, you become too ill to take further treatment, or you wish to stop. Breast cancer patients are fortunate in comparison to those with most other cancers; when one treatment fails, many options usually remain available to them.

In addition to physical considerations, your feelings about how aggressively you want to be treated should be taken into account. This is especially important with late-stage cancer. Compared with earlier stages of breast cancer, treatment for metastatic cancer is less standardized and therefore more dependent on your and your oncologist's background and priorities. At one end of the continuum are health-care professionals and patients who focus on maintaining a good quality of life, striving foremost to reduce symptoms of cancer and side effects of treatment. At the other end of the spectrum are oncologists and patients attempting to extend life at any cost, administering the most aggressive treatment that a patient can withstand while hoping to capitalize on the odds that the treatment may significantly prolong life. Somewhere between the two ends of the spectrum are doctors and patients attempting to lengthen life while minimizing troublesome symptoms and treatment side effects.

Your doctor's approach may be different from your own. Ask your on-cologist what her or his priority is—to attempt a cure? To prolong your life with minimal side effects? Find out how aggressively your oncolo-gist plans to treat your metastasis and why. Consider how aggressively you would like it to be treated. What are your priorities? To be pain-free? To remain alive until a particular event? To be mentally alert? To be as physically autonomous as possible? How important to you are such things as maintaining your manual dexterity or continuing to appreciate food and smells? Different treatments may compromise different aspects of your life. Clarify what matters to you. Write down your wishes, and give a copy of your wishes to your doctor so that together you can make choices that will help you live, as much as possible, as you would like. Of course, you and your doctor want to prolong your life, but you need to weigh the chances of living somewhat longer against the unpleasant side effects of a therapy. You need to feel comfortable with your oncologist, her/his team, and their approach. If you do not, consider finding another oncologist with whom your priorities are more closely aligned.

Asking your doctor the following questions and talking with others can help you decide whether or not you are willing to take a specific drug or undergo a particular surgery. Nurses in your treatment facility are also an excellent resource. In addition, you could contact other patients through online support groups, or through your treatment facility, who have ex-perienced a particular treatment (see chapter 8, "Reaching Out to Others for Emotional Support"). Remember, though, that people's reactions and tolerance can vary greatly; therefore, consider soliciting the thoughts and experiences of several individuals.

Questions to Consider When Deciding Treatment

1. What are the side effects of a particular treatment? How might these side effects affect the quality of my life?
2. How long will the side effects last?

3. How much time, particularly quality time, might this treatment give me?
4. To what degree will the treatment be effective in reducing symptoms?
5. What are the worst- and best-case scenarios of the treatment, and what research or experience is the basis for these scenarios?
6. What are the chances of tumor shrinkage?
7. How will I be monitored?
8. What are the other options?

In arriving upon a treatment plan, do not discount your feelings. Examine whether you are agreeing to a treatment because you want to, or because others want or expect you to. If you need help sorting out your feelings or asserting your wishes, you can ask to speak with a counselor. Most cancer centers offer this type of support service, and if you request it, they will arrange an appointment for you to speak with counselors experienced in working with cancer patients, sometimes without charge. Whatever you decide, remember that you can change your mind. Perhaps after you experience a therapy you will decide that it detracts too much from the quality of your life. Be aware, though, that the side effects for some drugs may lessen, or worsen, after the initial doses. You have the right to refuse, stop, or, if it is appropriate, start any approved treatment. The decision-making process is just that, a process, meaning that it is continually in flux. Keep your communication open with your doctors and family members.

If you personally research various treatments for metastatic breast cancer, you may be disheartened to read that most approved treatments extend life by only a few weeks or months, but this can be misleading. Individual drugs get approved for use based on results from clinical trials that evaluate their benefit when given alone, but cancer drugs (also called agents) are generally given one after another and sometimes in combinations, which may mean that people's lives are prolonged for longer than research studies may suggest. For example, a drug that increases survival by four months when given alone to patients with late-stage metastatic breast cancer might increase survival by a year or more when given together with other agents. The NCCN Practice Guidelines are based on results of clinical trials of agents that have shown either improved overall or progression-free survival. Remember that cancer is different from many other health conditions since rarely is only one kind of drug used in treatment.

What follows are widely accepted approaches to managing late-stage breast cancer. The information is necessarily general since management of metastatic breast cancer is tailored to each patient. Furthermore, treatment regimens are continually being modified or replaced in light of ongoing research results. For the most up-to-date treatment strategies we encourage you to work with an oncologist whose practice largely consists of breast cancer patients or to obtain a copy of the NCI's state-of-the-art patient and doctor treatment statements and to investigate the links below.

TREATMENT STRATEGIES

* National Comprehensive Cancer Network: Includes information about testing, along with treatment guidelines with decision trees. Click on NCCN Clinical Practice Guidelines in Oncology.
  http://www.nccn.org

* American Cancer Society's link into Nexprofiler: Offers a treatment tool that uses information from your pathology report to suggest possible treatments. You will need to sign into this site, but there is no fee.
  http://www.cancer.org/docroot/ETO/eto_1_1a.asp

* UpToDate: Offers general principles for the treatment of metastatic breast cancer.
  http://patients.uptodate.com/topic.asp?file=cancer/5162

* PDQ, NCI's Comprehensive Cancer Database for Recurrent and Metastatic Breast Cancer: Offers guidance to health professionals on treatment options.
  http://nci.nih.gov/cancertopics/pdq/treatment/breast/
  HealthProfessional/page8

* National Cancer Institute: Offers links for specific kinds of treatment.
  http://nci.nih.gov/cancertopics/treatment/breast

resources

Local Treatment Aimed at Specific Tumor Sites

If your metastasis is confined to one or two areas, you may have local treatment, meaning surgery or radiation aimed directly at tumors, followed by systemic treatment, meaning whole body therapy, usually consisting of drugs. If your metastases are widespread, you will probably begin with systemic treatment—either hormonal therapy, chemotherapy, or biological therapy—followed by local treatment of any area that may be causing particular problems.

Surgery, which is a local treatment, is more often used to remove an initial tumor in the breast rather than breast cancer tumors that appear in other organs. Unless a metastasis is confined to one spot and it is not likely to spread to other spots, surgery is not a viable treatment option. One study found that when breast cancer recurred, it appeared in multiple sites 44 percent of the time for estrogen receptor negative patients and 31 percent of the time for estrogen receptor positive patients (3). However, good data support prolonged survival with the surgical removal of single brain metastases, single or few liver metastases, and single lung metastases (4–7). In the case where multiple tumors are present, no evidence suggests that cutting out each tumor provides benefit, and it may in fact cause harm due to surgical complications. Surgery does not address the fundamental problem of the cancer cells moving throughout the bloodstream and spreading to other organs. Surgery can be helpful, though, in supporting or stabilizing a weight-bearing bone that has been weakened by disease, alleviating pain and maintaining mobility. Again, both the specifics of your disease and the whole picture of where the cancer is in your body will determine how extensively surgery might be combined with other approaches.

Other local treatments, such as radiation and heat therapies, may be used to shrink or eliminate tumors. A radiation beam is often used to reduce the size of a tumor in bone or the brain. For example, external beam radiation is a procedure in which high-energy x-rays are aimed at tumors. The actual radiation treatment is painless, just like having an x-ray. Immediate side effects are typically not seen, but over time variable side effects may be seen, depending on the site, area, and dose of radiation. The exposures to other organs in the field of the tumor being treated will determine what side effects someone experiences. For example, treatment of lymph nodes in the chest may cause some burning of the esophagus and difficulty swallowing. Radiation that encompasses a large amount of bone marrow may result in low red blood cell counts, causing anemia. Your radiation oncologist will discuss with you the potential side effects prior to each treatment.

Treatment by Tumor Site

Treatment for tumors varies by what organ the tumor is inhabiting and may involve various kinds of surgery and radiation.

Bone Metastases

External beam radiation may be used to treat individual tumors if the tumors are causing pain or impinging on the spinal cord. Injections of bone-targeting radioisotopes, such as strontium-89 chloride (Metastron) and samarium-153 lexidronam (Quadramet), may be helpful in the reduction of pain. If x-rays reveal a tumor is weakening a bone, particularly one of the long bones of the arm or leg (humerus or femur), surgery may be recommended to stabilize the bone and keep it from fracturing. Surgery is typically followed by external beam radiation to the site.

Liver Metastases

Radiofrequency ablation (destruction) or MRI-guided Laser-Induced Interstitial Thermotherapy (LITT) can be used to eliminate or shrink tumors when they are primarily confined to the liver. These treatments can sometimes lengthen survival by years (8). Additionally, resection (surgical removal) of isolated liver tumors in the setting of otherwise stable disease can provide long-term survival benefits (9).

Brain/Spinal Metastases

Tumors can grow in either the interior of the brain, called the parenchyma, or the lining of the brain, called the meninges. Treatment of tumors in these two areas is different. For treatment of tumors that have grown inside the brain, surgery may be used if only one tumor is present, and it is followed usually by whole-brain external beam radiation. If multiple tumors or large tumors (greater than 3 cm) are present, or if a single tumor is in a place that cannot be reached by surgery, then either whole-brain radiation can be performed or stereotactic radiosurgery, also called Gamma Knife radiation, may be used. Tumors that have recurred may be treated with radiosurgery, a very specific targeting of an area in the brain with a high-dose beam of radiation that minimizes side effects to the surrounding brain. Usually whole-brain radiation cannot be repeated due to possible toxic side effects such as dementia. Some chemotherapies (those given intravenously or as pills) may cross to a small extent from the blood into the brain (crossing the "blood-brain barrier") and may be used to treat recurrent tumors. Many clinical trials are ongoing in the treatment of breast cancer brain metastases.

Tumors that have grown on the surface of the brain or spinal cord—called leptomeningeal disease, leptomeningeal carcinomatosis, or carcinomatous meningitis—are usually treated with local chemotherapy in conjunction with radiation to sites of tumors that can be seen on scans. Often a small catheter, called an Ommaya or Rickham reservoir, is placed beneath the scalp, allowing injection of chemotherapy directly into the fluid surrounding the brain, the cerebrospinal fluid. This is called intrathecal administration of chemotherapy. If the cerebrospinal fluid (CSF) flows without obstructions, sometimes the chemotherapy will be administered via lumbar puncture, an injection into the CSF between the lower bones in the spine. Some radiation oncologists advocate craniospinal irradiation, or radiation to the brain and entire spinal cord, which has also been shown to be successful. Some small studies have shown the benefit of systemic (intravenous or oral) chemotherapy that can cross into the cerebrospinal fluid. Studies are ongoing with newer drugs given intrathecally (into the CSF) and systemically (through pills or intravenously).

Lung Metastases

As in the brain, tumors can grow in either the interior of the lung, called the parenchyma, or the lining of the lung, called the pleura. Solitary metastases, or single tumors, inside the lung may be surgically removed if cancerous tumors have not appeared in other organs. Large areas of disease in the lung that are blocking breathing tubes (bronchi) may be reopened with surgery and a tube called a stent or the breathing tubes may be treated with external radiation.

When fluid accumulates outside the lung, it is called a pleural effusion. Effusions may be caused by a cancerous tumor (a malignant effusion) or by other causes such as heart failure or side effects of chemotherapy (a benign effusion). To determine the cause of the effusion, your oncologist will likely perform a thoracentesis—a procedure in which a thin needle is inserted into the pleural space (the space between the lung and the rib cage) to withdraw fluid. If you are short of breath, a large amount of fluid can be removed this way, usually reducing your symptoms. This fluid can be analyzed to determine whether cancer or some other problem is causing the fluid buildup. Thoracentesis can be done in the office with a local anesthetic.

If the fluid keeps recurring in the pleural space and causing breathing difficulties, placement of a chest tube into the space may be necessary. Once the fluid is mostly drained, a chemical (usually talc) is administered through the tube to scar the pleural cavity; the scarring causes the lining of the lung to stick to the chest wall, removing the space for fluid to accumulate. Pain medication is necessary when recovering from this procedure. For a more rapid result, or if the fluid is not free-flowing, a thoracic surgeon may use a thoracoscope (VATS) to view and drain the pleural space and scar the lining. This procedure can result in significant long-term relief from pleural effusions.

Abdominal Metastases/Ascites

Ascites is a buildup of fluid in the abdomen that may result from either liver metastases or from metastases to the lining of the abdomen. This fluid can cause abdominal discomfort, difficulty eating, and difficulty breathing. The fluid may be removed with a small needle, called a paracentesis, up to two liters at a time. If the fluid continues to build up, a permanent catheter can be placed into the abdomen to drain the fluid off. These catheters can drain either to the outside of the body (with either a Tenkhoff or Pleurx catheter) or to the inside of the body into one of the large veins (with a Denver shunt). The external catheter placement can usually be done on an outpatient basis under local anesthesia, while the Denver shunt may be placed either with local or general anesthesia, depending on your specific situation.

resources

LOCALIZED TREATMENTS

- American Cancer Society for Radiation: Offers an overview of radiation treatment, including how radiation works, types of radiation, and side effects.

    http://www.cancer.org/docroot/ETO/eto_1_3_Radiation_
    Therapy.asp

(Resources, continued)

* World Health Organization: Provides information on pain reduction for metastases.
  > http://www.whocancerpain.wisc.edu/eng/15_4/research.html

* City of Hope, External Beam Irradiation: Provides information on stereotactic brain irradiation for brain metastases.
  > http://www.cityofhope.org/patient_care/treatments/
  > radiation-oncology/Pages/specialty-treatment-programs.aspx

* Musella Foundation for Brain Tumor Research: Provides an explanation of stereotactic radiosurgery.
  > http://virtualtrials.com/jhrs.cfm

* National Institutes of Health: Provides information on radiofrequency ablation for liver metastases.
  > http://www.cc.nih.gov/drd/rfa

* Radiological Society of North America (RSNA): Provides information on radiofrequency ablation of liver for liver metastases.
  > http://www.radiologyinfo.org/content/eh/info.cfm?pg=rfa

* MedlinePlus Medical Encyclopedia: Thoracentesis: Provides information on thoracentesis for pleural effusions.
  > http://www.nlm.nih.gov/medlineplus/ency/article/003420.htm

Treatment Aimed at Cancer Cells throughout the Body: Systemic Treatment

There are three basic types of systemic treatment: *hormonal/endocrine therapies*, *chemotherapy*, and *targeted/biological therapies*. Hormonal therapies most often reduce and block hormones that are associated with tumor growth to keep cancer cells from dividing. The side effects are generally mild. Chemotherapy interferes with the cell division of all rapidly dividing cells in the body. Along with killing cancer cells, chemotherapy affects other rapidly dividing cells in bone marrow, the lining of the mouth, stomach, and intestines and can thus cause more problematic side effects than hormonal therapies. Targeted therapies directly target receptors or proteins that bind to these receptors (often called ligands) found in and on cancer cells. These therapies include angiogenesis inhibitors, which target the growth of new blood vessels that are vital to support tumor growth. The side effects of targeted therapies are usually mild, but more severe side effects have been noted, including cardiac problems, interstitial lung disease, bleeding, or intestinal perforation.

Hormonal/Endocrine Therapies

Hormonal treatments are increasingly being used instead of chemotherapy as first-line treatment for advanced breast cancers. If you are postmenopausal, if your breast cancer is confined to a few spots, and if your tumor tested positive for estrogen and/or progesterone receptors, you are likely to begin treatment with anti-hormonal therapy. The more estrogen and progesterone receptors that are on your cancer cells, the more likely your cancer will respond to hormonal drugs — in other words, the more likely the tumors will shrink. In addition, your cancer is more likely to respond to hormonal treatments if you have had a long disease-free interval before having a recurrence, if you are older, and if your metastasis is to the bone. This is an important distinction in the case of breast cancer as bone disease tends to progress more slowly and respond better to hormonal therapy.

If your tumor is sensitive to estrogen and progesterone and you are still menstruating, your ovaries are still producing estrogen, so you may be put into a temporary chemically induced menopause by injection of Lupron or Zoladex, which shuts down pituitary gland signals to the ovaries. (Menopause reduces the levels of circulating estrogen in your blood, providing an environment less hospitable to ER-/PR-positive cancer cells.) The effects of the injection are reversible, and thus they must be given every one to three months to be effective. Premenopausal women may also undergo chemotherapy before hormonal therapy. In addition to reducing the number of cancer cells, chemotherapy often induces menopause in menstruating women. Whether or not this happens depends on a number of factors, including your age and the length and kind of chemotherapy you receive. However, the younger you are, the more likely your period will return (10). Learning that you are faced with an early menopause can be startling. In addition to adjusting to the news of late-stage cancer, you will be adjusting to this life change. However, know that reducing estrogen will fight your disease, offering you more quality time.

The aim of hormonal therapy is to keep the body from producing estrogen or to block the cancer cells' hormone receptors. Either works to sabotage cell division and, therefore, growth of the tumor cells. After about ten to eighteen months of therapy the cancer cells often adapt to the drug, though the time it takes for a hormonal therapy to become ineffective can vary greatly. If the cells adapt to one drug, it helps to change the hormonal environment in your body by stopping one medicine and switching to another. Sometimes when beginning a hormonal treatment, you can experience a "tumor flare"—that is, for up to a month your symptoms get worse instead of better. Though a worsening of symptoms can be frightening, a flare-up is actually a good sign that your cancer is responding to the medicine and that you may eventually feel relief.

Hormonal therapies, as research results show, are quite successful at reducing tumors and prolonging survival, and they are less toxic than chemotherapies. A number of oncologists think all women with estrogen receptor positive metastatic disease should begin with this gentler treatment as opposed to chemotherapy. You may need to discuss this type of treatment with your doctor. Some oncologists have more knowledge and experience with chemotherapies than with hormonal therapies. Hormonal therapies may not act as quickly on tumors as chemotherapy, so if you have a large amount of cancer that may threaten your organ function, your oncologist will likely want to shrink tumors down with chemotherapy prior to starting hormonal therapy. Seek a second opinion if you believe you are a candidate for hormonal therapy and your oncologist does not want to discuss this option with you.

What follows are descriptions of the most frequently prescribed hormonal therapies. They fall into three main categories: *aromatase inhibitors, estrogen blockers or selective estrogen-receptor modulators (SERMs),* and *luteinizing hormone-releasing hormone (LHRH) analogs.* Most are taken daily in pill form, and while you are taking them, you and your doctor will monitor your response in monthly check-ups. Combining hormonal drugs has not been shown to enhance their effectiveness.

The side effects of hormonal drugs are not usually troublesome and go away in a few weeks after your body adjusts to the medicine. However, in a minority of women the hormonal therapy is not well tolerated, so be certain to mention any troublesome symptoms to your doctor since you likely can be switched to a different medicine. Once the considerable number of hormonal drugs has been exhausted, your oncologist may recommend chemotherapy or another type of therapy.

Aromatase Inhibitors

These drugs reduce the amount of estrogen circulating in your body by inhibiting aromatase, a naturally occurring enzyme. Aromatase converts androstenedione and testosterone to estrogen in multiple tissues in post-menopausal women. Many breast tumors also produce their own aromatase. These drugs are only for women who are postmenopausal since they do not affect estrogen produced by the ovaries.

Approved Drugs

> **Anastrozole (Arimidex; AstraZeneca):** 1-mg pill taken daily, with or without food; approved by FDA for use in metastatic breast cancer December 1995 and for adjuvant treatment of breast cancer in September 2002.

> **Exemestane (Aromasin; Pfizer):** 25-mg pill taken daily after a meal; approved by FDA for use in advanced breast cancer in October 1999 and for adjuvant treatment of breast cancer in October 2005.

> **Letrozole (Femara; Novartis):** 2.5-mg tablet taken daily, with or without food; approved by FDA for use in advanced breast cancer in July 1997 and for adjuvant treatment of breast cancer in December 2005.

resources

UNDERSTANDING AROMATASE INHIBITORS

- National Cancer Institute: Information on aromatase inhibitors
    http://www.cancer.gov/clinicaltrials/developments/
    aromatase-inhibitors-digest

Estrogen Blockers or SERMs

These drugs work by attaching to a cell's loading docks (receptors) for estrogen before your own estrogen can. Your own estrogen moves from these receptors into the center of the cell and activates cell division. These blockers occupy those spots, keeping the cell from dividing. SERMs act as anti-estrogens in some tissues, such as breast cancer cells, and as estrogens in others, such as the endometrium (the uterine lining). Estrogen-receptor antagonists, or pure anti-estrogens, act only as anti-estrogens in tissues.

Approved Drugs

> **Tamoxifen (Nolvadex; AstraZeneca):** A SERM and the oldest approved standard therapy, available in a generic form. Taken in 20-mg doses by mouth daily. Not recommended as first-line therapy for metastatic disease unless a woman is premenopausal.
>
> **Toremifene (Fareston):** A SERM, taken in 60-mg doses by mouth daily.
>
> **Faslodex (Fulvestrant; AstraZeneca):** A pure anti-estrogen given intramuscularly by injection once a month. Blocks estrogen's effect on cancer cells by inactivating estrogen receptors and may overcome tamoxifen resistance.

UNDERSTANDING ESTROGEN RECEPTORS AND SERMS

• National Cancer Institute: Information on estrogen receptors and SERMs
http://nci.nih.gov/cancertopics/understandingcancer/
estrogenreceptors

resources

LHRH (GnRH) Agonists or Analogs

These drugs alter the hormonal climate of the body by stopping the signal from the brain to the ovaries that causes the ovaries to produce estrogen. They may be used instead of surgical oophorectomy (ovary removal) in premenopausal women. Initially these drugs raise the level of estrogen for about a month until the ovaries shut down.

Approved Drugs

> **Leuprolide acetate (Lupron; TAP Pharmaceuticals):** May be given monthly or every three months (doses of 7.5 or 22.5 mg respectively) as an intramuscular injection; FDA approved for the treatment of endometriosis and fibroids in women.
>
> **Goserelin acetate (Zoladex; AstraZeneca):** May be given monthly or every three months (doses of 3.6 or 10.8 mg respectively) as subcutaneous injection; FDA approved for the palliative treatment of advanced breast cancer in pre- and perimenopausal women.

Chemotherapy

Chemotherapy, also know as cytotoxic therapy, generally works by interrupting cell division. By definition cancer is uncontrolled cell division. You can think of cytotoxic drugs as acting like crop dusters flying in to kill the infestation of rapidly dividing cells. Each treatment reduces the percentage of rapidly dividing cells, but it is nearly impossible to destroy every cell. The hidden ones continue to multiply. The remaining cells can eventually grow again. Still, affected organs function more normally than they could otherwise, improving the quality of life, particularly once the side effects of chemotherapy diminish.

The first chemotherapy, called nitrogen mustard, came into use in the 1940s and gave rise to modern drugs like cyclophosphamide (Cytoxan). Since those early days many new substances have been discovered that work as chemotherapy agents. More than ten cytotoxic drugs are known to be effective against breast cancer—a large number in comparison to other cancers. The number of effective agents is advantageous since oncologists can prescribe different combinations and different drugs when tumors no longer respond to the therapy a person is currently on, or (in the case of some cytotoxic drugs) when someone has reached the toxicity limit for a particular drug.

Chemotherapies are administered orally or intravenously, individually or in combination, at periodic intervals. Often cytotoxic drugs are given once every week, or every few weeks, over a period of months. A particular chemotherapy drug and dose are usually given in the order of what will most likely create the most complete shrinkage of tumors for the longest time. What is prescribed depends also on other variables, such as what previous chemotherapy someone has had, how long ago it was administered, and a person's current physical condition. Unlike hormonal therapy, these drugs sometimes work better in combination, though combining them can exacerbate side effects such as nausea. Some clinical trials are underway to explore the efficacy of combining hormonal, molecular, and chemotherapies.

The majority of breast cancer patients—50–70 percent—respond to one or more cytotoxic drugs, meaning that their tumors shrink or disappear for more than three months. In general, chemotherapy works better in estrogen receptor negative patients. Genetic factors that may help oncologists tailor chemotherapy to suit an individual's type of cancer are now under study, and hopefully gene signatures will become widely available to predict which chemotherapy would be best suited for a patient's treatment. Currently it is possible to take a woman's cancer cells, culture them in a Petri dish, then determine which chemotherapy agents kill the cells. Unfortunately this technique, known as an *in vitro* drug assay, does not clearly reveal to which drugs the cells will respond in your body, and none of the advertised tests currently appear promising. If the chemotherapy regimen that shrank someone else's tumor is not shrinking yours, remember that there is much variability in the way people respond to medicine. Two women given the same dose of a drug would likely have different levels of the drug circulating in their bodies. Though it is undoubtedly discouraging to find that your cancer is resistant to a drug, it is quite possible other drugs given in different combinations will work for you.

On the day of your chemotherapy treatment your vital signs and weight will be checked, and you will have your blood drawn to determine the levels of your white cells, red cells, and platelets, as well as blood chemistries. If one or more of these levels is abnormal, it signals that the chemotherapy is having some effect on your body. If the cell counts become too low—in other words, if the chemotherapy is making you highly anemic or too susceptible to infections—you may be given supportive medicines and/or your treatment for that day may be postponed.

It usually takes about two months to know if your tumors are responding to a chemotherapy protocol. If a treatment is effective for you, you will likely remain on the same medicine until your tumor begins to grow. The cancer cells can become resistant to a drug, just as bacteria become resistant to antibiotics, and at this point a new drug may be tried. In general, most breast cancer specialists advocate single-drug (agent) regimens, except in the case where large areas of disease need to be reduced quickly. So far studies have shown that high doses of cytotoxic drugs, as are given in regimens requiring bone marrow or stem cell support, do not enhance their ability to combat breast cancer. Other variables that are being manipulated to increase effectiveness include how a drug is administered—in pill form, intravenously, or through a patch—and the frequency of administration—daily, weekly, or monthly. You can learn more about how chemotherapy works to stop cell division in chapter 4 and by using the Internet links in this section.

Standard Chemotherapy Agents Used
for Metastatic Breast Cancer

All of the following are intravenous agents unless otherwise stated.

Alkylating agents: Cyclophosphamide (Cytoxan)—both intravenous and oral

Anthracyclines: Doxorubicin (Adriamycin); Epirubicin; Liposomal doxorubicin (Doxil, Myocet)

Anti-metabolites: Methotrexate; Gemcitabine (Gemzar)

Fluoropyrimidines: Capecitabine (Xeloda)—oral only; 5-FU/Fluoro-uracil

Platinum compounds: Carboplatin; Cisplatin

Taxanes: Docetaxel (Taxotere); Paclitaxel (Taxol); albumin-bound nanoparticle paclitaxel (Abraxane)

Vinca alkaloid: Vinorelbine (Navelbine)

Camptothecin: Irinotecan (Camptosar)

Epothilone analog: Ixabepilone (Ixempra)

Preferred Single Agents (from NCCN clinical guidelines)

Doxorubicin	Docetaxel
Epirubicin	Capecitabine
Pegylated liposomal doxorubicin	Vinorelbine
	Gemcitabine
Paclitaxel	Albumin-bound paclitaxel

Other Agents That Are Effective in Breast Cancer

Cisplatin	Fluorouracil continuous infusion
Carboplatin	Ixabepilone
Etoposide (oral)	Ixabepilone plus capecitabine
Vinblastine	

Common Combinations

Docetaxel and doxorubicin
Doxorubicin and paclitaxel
Docetaxel and capecitabine
Gemcitabine and vinorelbine
Docetaxel or paclitaxel and carboplatin

Preferred Combinations (from NCCN clinical guidelines)

CAF/FAC (cyclophosphamide/doxorubicin/fluorouracil)
FEC (fluorouracil/epirubicin/cyclophosphamide)
AC (doxorubicin/cyclophosphamide)
EC (epirubicin/cyclophosphamide)
AT (doxorubicin/docetaxel; doxorubicin/paclitaxel)
CMF (cyclophosphamide/methotrexate/fluorouracil)
Docetaxel/capecitabine
GT (gemcitabine/paclitaxel)

**Preferred Combinations with Trastuzumab
(Herceptin) (HER2-Positive Disease)**

Paclitaxel with or without carboplatin
Docetaxel
Vinorelbine

Preferred Combination with Lapatinib (Tykerb) (HER2-Positive Disease)

Capecitabine

Preferred Combination with Bevacizumab (Avastin; Genentech)

Paclitaxel

Chemotherapy Ports/Catheters

As noted in the preceding material, many cytotoxic drugs are given intra-venously. Some people prefer to be given these drugs through a port that is inserted into the body, rather than through a needle inserted into a vein. A port is advantageous if you have small or weak veins, or if you may be on chemotherapy over an extended period. Insertion of a Porta-cath or Infusaport requires same-day surgery under light anesthesia. The port is often inserted into the subclavian vein (near the collarbone), and Infusaports are often placed in the arm. On treatment days a needle is placed through the skin overlying the port into the reservoir beneath. The port is flushed with saline (sterile salt water), and then chemotherapy is infused, all of which is a relatively painless procedure. The development of a blood clot or infection is possible with ports, but the risk is small in most people.

PORTS AND CATHETERS TO ADMINISTER CHEMOTHERAPY

- breastcancer.org: Offers an explanation about ports.
  http://www.breastcancer.org/tre_sys_chemo_ports.html

- American Pediatric Surgical Association: A medical overview of catheters.
  http://www.eapsa.org/parents/resources/catheter.cfm

- Cancer Links: Offers patients' views of ports.
  http://www.cancerlynx.com/comments_ports.html

Chemotherapy Side Effects

Many side effects of cytotoxic drugs are cumulative. If the drug you are prescribed causes hair loss, you may not lose any hair after the first dose, but as you continue treatments, you will increasingly lose hair. Likewise, though you may not be fatigued at first, over the course of many treatments you may experience significant fatigue. Nausea usually is most intense shortly after a treatment; then the feeling slowly subsides until the next treatment. Your level of discomfort during and following a treatment can vary each time. When treatment stops, the side effects generally subside as time goes by.

Common side effects of chemotherapy are listed below, but the side effects of particular chemotherapy agents differ. You can learn about them specifically and how to manage them by using the Internet links in this chapter for chemotherapy and for individual drugs. Keep in mind that chemotherapy side effects may differ not only by what drug you are taking, but also by the strength of the dose, the other medicines you are taking, and your body's unique reaction to the drug.

Bone Marrow Side Effects: Chemotherapy can lower your red blood cell count, possibly causing anemia, fatigue, and shortness of breath. It can also lower your white cell count, suppressing your immune system and making you more susceptible to infections and illness. Last, it can lower your platelet count, causing you to bruise or bleed more freely.

Gastrointestinal Side Effects: After a chemotherapy treatment you can become nauseated and vomit, but newer medications make this a less frequent side effect. You may find tastes and smells unpleasant, somewhat metallic, or chemical-like. Chemotherapy can also cause mouth and throat dryness, mouth sores, thrush, and diarrhea or constipation.

Nails, Skin, and Hair Side Effects: Chemotherapy may cause hair loss; skin dryness; and lined, brittle nails. Some chemotherapies may cause nail loss or changes in the palms and soles. Doxil and Xeloda commonly cause a reddening and pain in the palms and soles that is called hand-foot syndrome. This resolves once the medication is stopped and/or the dose reduced.

Neurologic Side Effects: Some chemotherapies such as taxanes, vinca alkaloids, and platinums can cause numbness and/or tingling in your hands and feet, called peripheral neuropathy. This side effect can be worse if you are diabetic. In most cases, this resolves; however, the more severe or long-standing the neuropathy, the less likely it is to completely resolve after stopping the chemotherapy. Be sure to tell your treatment team if you begin to have numbness/tingling in your fingers or toes.

While undergoing chemotherapy, drink plenty of fluids, particularly near the time you receive your treatment. Avoid large crowds of people and those with contagious illnesses if you are taking a treatment that your doctor or nurse says may lower your white blood cell count. To the extent you are able, engage in moderate exercise daily, which will help combat fatigue, and continue to eat a balanced diet. Some chemotherapies may cause people to either gain or lose weight. Ask your treatment team what to expect from your particular regimen.

CHEMOTHERAPY

- American Cancer Society: Offers helpful general information.
    http://www.cancer.org/docroot/ETO/content/ETO_1_2X_
        Chemotherapy_What_It_Is_How_It_Helps.asp

- National Cancer Institute: Offers self-help for managing chemotherapy side effects.
    http://nci.nih.gov/cancertopics/chemotherapy-and-you/page4

- breastcancer.org: Suggests ways to manage the side effects of chemotherapy.
    http://www.breastcancer.org/treatment/chemotherapy/
        side_effects.jsp

resources

Targeted Molecular Approaches

Targeted therapies, which are designed to bind to or block a specific mole-cule important to cell division, are not new. The earliest targeted therapies were chemotherapies, including nitrogen mustard agents and methotrex-ate, that mimic cellular building blocks or block their production. Hor-monal therapies are also a targeted therapy since they target estrogen receptors or the enzyme aromatase. With newer discoveries in cancer mo-lecular biology, more targets are being discovered that lend themselves to "rational" drug design—that is, the design of drugs that bind so specifi-cally to their targets that healthy tissue is less likely to be affected by the treatment. New targeted therapies are not without side effects, but the side effects are of a different variety than with standard chemotherapy.

Monoclonal Antibodies—An Effective Targeted Therapy

Advances in immunology coupled with advances in understanding the mechanisms of cancer progression have led to the development of thera-pies that target specific proteins, such as growth-factor receptors in or on a cancer cell. These therapies can be in the form of either small molecules, which can be taken by mouth, or monoclonal antibodies, which must be given in the vein. A monoclonal antibody is an immune protein that can attach to a specific area of a cell that may be causing uncontrolled cell growth. These antibodies are created to identify a specific protein(s) on a cancer cell—for example, a signaling receptor—and then the antibodies bind to that protein. The binding of the monoclonal antibody stops the normal function of the protein and, in the case of receptor-associated tar-gets, stops the messages from the receptor that cause the cell to divide. The process also "programs" your immune system to look for and destroy the antibody. In the case of breast cancer, two monoclonal antibodies are currently approved by the FDA for use in patients—trastuzumab (more commonly referred to by its trade name, Herceptin) and bevacizumab (known as Avastin).

Drugs Targeting Cell Growth

Herceptin was the first monoclonal antibody to receive FDA approval as a treatment for metastatic breast cancer, and it marked the beginning of this new category of anti-cancer drugs. Because this kind of therapy is intended to target just the cancer cell, it does not create many of the difficult side effects of chemotherapy. Monoclonal antibodies, unlike earlier chemotherapy, do not attack all rapidly growing cells in the body, whether cancerous or not, causing hair loss and destroying bone marrow. However, Herceptin can cause heart failure, particularly in combination with drugs such as Adriamycin.

Herceptin can be effective in the 20–30 percent of breast cancer patients whose tumors overexpress the HER2 protein. Tumor cells in this type of breast cancer have an abnormal number of HER2 receptors on the cells' surface, causing the cells to divide uncontrollably. It has been a challenging type of breast cancer to care for in the past. Herceptin is not effective for tumors that lack an increased amount of HER2 protein.

Herceptin given alone or in combination with chemotherapy has been shown to improve overall survival. A study published in 2001 that enrolled 469 women with metastatic breast cancer found that those taking Herceptin plus either Adriamycin and Cytoxan, or with Taxol, lived on average about five months longer than those randomized to chemotherapy alone (11). A high rate of cardiac dysfunction (27 percent) was found in women taking Herceptin and Adriamycin; studies are now underway to see whether this problem will occur with other formulations of anthracyclines such as liposomal doxorubicin or other related anthracyclines such as epirubicin. Herceptin is usually combined with chemotherapy, such as Taxotere, Taxol, or Navelbine, unless chemotherapy has already been administered and was not effective. Even if your tumor overexpresses HER2 and you do not respond to Herceptin, treatments such as chemotherapy and other targeted therapies may be helpful.

Recently small molecules have been developed that also bind to HER2 and a related receptor, EGFR. These small molecules have some advantages over monoclonal antibodies: they are given orally, and they may overcome resistance to antibody therapy. In general, the small molecules target the part of the receptor that is inside the cell, and the antibodies target the part of the receptor that is outside the cell. A small molecule, lapatinib (Tykerb; GlaxoSmithKline) has shown impressive results combined with capecitabine in the treatment of breast cancer, with an approximately 50 percent improvement in progression-free survival and time to progression compared to capecitabine alone (12). Lapatinib is a dual tyrosine kinase inhibitor of EGFR and HER2. It appears to be effective as a single agent in women whose disease has progressed on Herceptin (13).

HERCEPTIN AND TYKERB

• National Cancer Institute: Information on trastuzumab (Herceptin).
  http://nci.nih.gov/cancertopics/understandingcancer/
  moleculardiagnostics/Slide23

• National Cancer Institute: Information on lapatinib ditosylate (Tykerb).
  http://nci.nih.gov/cancertopics/druginfo/lapatinibditosylate

Angiogenesis Inhibitors: Drugs Targeting Blood Vessel Growth

Angiogenesis inhibitors, another type of targeted therapy, disrupt the formation of blood vessels that feed a tumor, a process known as angiogenesis. In 2004, the first breast cancer clinical trial that tested an angiogenesis inhibitor produced promising results. This trial, involving 722 women, showed that women who took bevacizumab (Avastin), an antibody against a protein needed to create blood vessels (the protein is called vascular endothelial growth factor, VEGF), in combination with paclitaxel, a chemotherapy, had an advantage of a six-month longer disease-free survival, in comparison to women taking paclitaxel alone. Whether this extends survival or just arrests the disease for some time period has not yet been demonstrated (14). Side effects of Avastin can include holes in the lower intestinal tract, high blood pressure, impaired healing of cuts and bruises, and bleeding or clotting problems.

Approved Monoclonal Antibodies

Trastuzumab (Herceptin; Genentech): Intravenous doses, once a week to every three weeks. Herceptin targets and binds with the extracellular domain of HER2, a tyrosine kinase receptor. FDA approved for breast cancer.

Bevacizumab (Avastin; Genentech): Intravenous doses, target VEGF. FDA approved for use in colorectal cancer and non-small-cell lung cancer. FDA approved for use in breast cancer in combination with Taxol.

Approved Small Molecules

Lapatinib (Tykerb; GlaxoSmithKline): Oral, small-molecule inhibitor of EGFR and HER2. Effective in women whose disease has progressed on Herceptin. FDA approved for use in breast cancer with capecitabine.

ANGIOGENESIS INHIBITORS

- National Cancer Institute
    http://www.cancer.gov/cancertopics/understandingcancer/
        angiogenesis

- National Cancer Institute: Summary of bevacizumab trial results.
    http://nci.nih.gov/newscenter/pressreleases/AvastinBreast

- Food and Drug Administration: Questions and answers about bevacizumab (Avastin).
    http://www.fda.gov/cder/drug/infopage/avastin/avastinQ&A.htm

- National Cancer Institute: Clinical trials with angiogenesis inhibitors.
    http://www.cancer.gov/clinicaltrials/developments/anti-angio-table

Additional Treatment and Supportive Drugs for Metastatic Breast Cancer

For Bone Metastases: Bisphosphonates

This is a class of drugs used for bone metastases to reduce fracture and pain, as well as reduce the need for radiation. They are given intravenously generally every four to twelve weeks. They may cause kidney impairment, and kidney function needs to be checked prior to each dose. If you are taking these drugs, consult with both your oncologist and dentist before having dental work. Patients on bisphosphonates can develop a rare but serious condition known as osteonecrosis of the jaw, a loss or breakdown of the jawbone. A thorough dental exam should be performed prior to therapy. Be aware of abnormalities of your gum and teeth such as (but not limited to) infection, bleeding, pain, or a heavy feeling in your jaw, and report these immediately.

Approved Bisphosphonates

Zoldedronic acid (Zometa)
Pamidronate (Aredia)

resources

BONE METASTASES

• American Cancer Society's Guide for Bone Metastases: Explains causes, detection, and treatment.
  http://www.cancer.org/docroot/CRI/content/CRI_2_4_1X_What_ Is_bone_metastasis_66.asp

For Reduction of Inflammation

Non-Steroidal Anti-Inflammatory Drugs (NSAIDs): Include non-prescription pain relievers such as aspirin, ibuprofen, and naproxen.

Steroids: Dexamethasone (Decadron) or prednisone. These steroids are also used to reduce swelling of the brain from brain metastasis or of the area surrounding the spinal cord in cases of cord compression by tumor.

For Chemotherapy Side Effects

To Fight Infection

  Antibiotics: To treat or prevent bacterial infection
  Antifungals: To treat fungal infections such as thrush
  Antivirals: To treat viral infections, such as shingles

To Boost White Cells

  Filgrastim (Neupogen)
  Peg-filgrastim (Neulasta)
  Sargramostim (Leukine)

To Boost Red Cells (Fight Anemia)

  Epoetin alfa (Procrit)
  Darbepoetin alfa (Aranesp)

To Fight Nausea

  Ondansetron (Zofran)
  Granisetron (Kytril)
  Dolasetron (Anzemet)
  Palonosetron HCI (ALOXI)
  Dexamethasone (Decadron)
  Aprepitant (Emend)

  Prochlorperazine (Compazine)
  Promethazine (Phenergan)
  Lorazepam (Ativan)
  Dronabinol (Marinol)
  Metoclopramide (Reglan)

To Improve Appetite

> Megestrol acetate (Megace)
> Cyproheptadine hydrochloride
> Dronabinol (Marinol)

LOOKING UP DRUG INFORMATION AND SUPPORTIVE DRUGS

DRUG INFORMATION

- MedlinePlus Drug Database: A service of the U.S. Library of Medicine and the National Institutes of Health.
  http://www.nlm.nih.gov/medlineplus/druginformation.html

- Cancerlinks: Organizes information about drugs using the U.S. Library of Congress classifications, allowing the reader to critically assess information on Web pages.
  http://www.cancerlinks.org/drug.html

- CancerQuest: Offers detailed but user-friendly information on cancer treatment, as well as scientific animated visuals.
  http://www.cancerquest.org/index.cfm?page=521

- WebMDHealth: Offers simple, concise information on drugs.
  http://www.webmd.com/drugs/index-drugs.aspx

- WebMDHealth: Offers explanations of drugs used specifically for late-stage breast cancer.
  http://my.webmd.com/drugs/search.aspx?stype=CONDITION&query=
  breast+cancer&go.x=12&go.y=15

SUPPORTIVE DRUGS

- Cancer Supportive Care Programs, Supportive Chemotherapy Drugs: Explains what drugs are used to combat specific side effects, including nausea, mouth sores, anemia, and cardiac toxicity (among others). The dose, side effects, and cost are listed in a user-friendly table.
  http://www.cancersupportivecare.com/chemotherapy.html

resources

Monitoring Treatment

While under treatment, you will be examined regularly to see how you are feeling and to see how well you are tolerating therapy. Various methods will be used to assess whether your tumors are responding to the medicine, to check whether your symptoms warrant a change in medication, and to consider whether cancer may have spread to another organ. Though your known metastases will be closely monitored, often it is not sensible in terms of enhancing comfort and survival to discover other metastases early if they are not causing you trouble. Additional tests may be ordered only when it is suspected that uncovering a new metastatic site could lead to treatment that may enhance your quality of life.

In monitoring you, your doctor will be looking for how much your cancer shrinks in response to treatment. You and your doctor will be hoping for one of the following responses, which are classified into four levels:

> **Complete response:** The tumor(s) is no longer detectable.
> **Partial response:** The tumor(s) has shrunk to at least half its size.
> **Minor response:** The tumor(s) has decreased less than 50 percent.
> **Stable disease:** Though there was no reduction in the size of the tumor(s), the disease is not progressing.

In all instances, the change, or lack of change, must last three months to be considered a response. Some treatments are slower to act than others, but a slow treatment can be as effective as a fast one.

Scans are used to detect the shrinkage of tumors on the average of every two months. These are the same scans discussed in chapter 1, "Detecting a Local or Regional Recurrence." Sometimes blood tumor markers—such as CA 15-3, CA 27.29 (tests that detect elevations in MUC-1 protein products), or occasionally CEA—are followed if your tumor markers were elevated at the time you were diagnosed with metastatic disease. More recently, the CellSearch (Veridex) test has been approved; it counts the number of tumor cells circulating in the blood and can give an idea of disease response as well as survival time. The results from these tests, along with your accounts of your health, are what your oncologist will use to monitor the effectiveness of the medicine you are taking. Your self-reports about levels of fatigue, pain, and breathing are also used to judge the effect of treatments.

If you are experiencing unpleasant side effects from a drug, call your doctor's office so that the dosage can be altered. It is best to do this early since if the side effects become severe, you may need to go off the drug, a change that is less desirable than adjusting the dose. Do not be fearful about taking a needed break from chemotherapy since it may not affect your long-term prognosis.

MEASURES OF TREATMENT EFFECTIVENESS

• Veridex: Provides an overview of information on the CellSearch system.
  http://www.veridex.com/Systems/Systems.aspx?id=1

Supportive/Palliative Treatment

When medicines are no longer effective or are compromising the quality of your life, you will likely arrive at a time when you wish to consider a different course of treatment. Often doctors frame decisions of this type as a choice between "curative" and "palliative" treatment. Curative treatment refers to medicine that attacks the cancer, such as chemotherapy and targeted therapies, though such treatment very rarely provides a cure in the case of metastatic breast cancer. Palliative (supportive, comfort) treatment refers to medicine that relieves pain and reduces problematic symptoms. The line between curative and palliative treatments is not distinct since the same treatments aimed at keeping cancer at bay also reduce pain and other symptoms. However, at the point at which curative cancer-fighting medication is no longer producing results or has too many side effects, palliative medication can become the primary focus of treatment.

Changing one's treatment focus to only supportive medication is understandably difficult for most people. Though there is always hope, stopping chemotherapy or other active therapies can signal the reality that one's time is limited, a situation that many people are reluctant to face. Research has shown that patients in the later stages of cancer tend to overestimate how much longer they have to live. According to results reported by researchers affiliated with the Dana-Farber Cancer Institute, 82 percent of cancer patients who statistically have six months to live think they have longer (15). These patients are twice as likely to request or agree to aggressive treatment rather than comfort care. According to this study, doctors are 70 percent accurate in estimating patients' survival time, but they may be uncomfortable relaying the prognosis, may relay prognostic information in a manner that is not clear, or may feel that a patient would be too overwhelmed to hear such unwelcome news.

As the above research indicates, your doctor may be reluctant to recommend that you focus on palliative treatment and to advise you that the therapies that directly fight your cancer may not be beneficial. You may need to be the one to broach the topic about when to move to treatment that reduces unpleasant symptoms, rather than trying another therapy aimed at fighting the cancer. The NCCN recommends considering stopping active treatment if a patient is resistant to two chemotherapies. However, most medical oncologists feel that is too few if someone's quality of life is still good. Some doctors never want to stop active treatment. They may hope to win the war with the disease or to learn more in the battle. Other doctors may stop treatment when you want to try something more. It is important to maintain clear communications with your oncology team about your needs and desires. In your deliberations and discussions, keep in mind that a remission is not the same as a cure and that any prognosis is a best guess.

It will be helpful to you, your loved ones, and your doctor if you take time to consider what you want. You can make your decisions more easily if you explore your priorities, values, and feelings about the possible manner and timing of your death. You can learn more about the choices at the end of life by reading chapter 6, which includes a discussion of pain relief and hospice, and you can learn how others have met the psychological challenge of facing death in chapter 8. When you are ready, pose the following questions to yourself: How would you like to spend your final time in this existence? Do you want to pursue experimental treatment to contribute to more understanding about cancer treatment, hoping a new drug may extend your life but increasing the chance you may die under treatment in a hospital and may suffer unpleasant drug side effects? Would you prefer possibly dying sooner with a clearer mind and a more peaceful end? Do you want time away from the medical world, only to return to it as needed?

Making the choice to focus solely on palliative care will depend on a host of factors, including possibly your age and life circumstances. If you have small children, trying to add one month of life may matter more to you than it may for an elderly person. Once you clarify what you want, you are in a better position to take into consideration what the doctor and your loved ones want. In considering options, be aware of your relationship to those closest to you. How candid and open are you with one another? Whatever others suggest or assume you should do, be certain you do not lose track of what you want.

Whatever you decide, your choice is part of a process. Your feelings about the risks and benefits of various treatments may change. You are always free to negotiate what you think is in your best interests. Telling your doctor what your preferences are is a part of the process. Armed with your oncologist's best estimate of your remaining time and with the information about a treatment's side effects and potential to extend your life, you can best decide what to do.

Further Reading

Handbook of Metastatic Breast Cancer, by Stephen Johnston and Charles Swanton. Informa HealthCare, 2006.

Molecular Oncology of Breast Cancer, edited by Jeffrey S. Ross and Gabriel N. Hortobagyi. Jones and Bartlett Publishers, 2004.

100 Questions and Answers about Advanced and Metastatic Breast Cancer, by Lillie D. Shockney, Gary R. Shapiro. Jones and Bartlett Publishers, 2008.

CHAPTER 4

Understanding Cancer Development, Treatment, and Emerging Therapies

We are within striking distance of writing the detailed life histories of many human tumors from start to life-threatening finish. These biographies will be written in the language of genes and molecules. Within a decade, we will know with extraordinary precision the succession of events that constitute the complex evolution of normal cells into highly malignant, invasive derivatives.

—Robert Weinberg, professor of biology and noted cancer researcher, MIT Whitehead Institute, 1996

The human body is a little universe
Its chill tears, so much wind-blown sleet
Beneath our skins, mountains bulge, brooks flow
Within our chests lurk lost cities, hidden tribes
Wisdom quarters itself in our tiny hearts
Liver and gall peer out, scrutinize a thousand miles
Follow a path back to its source, else be
A house vacant save for swallows in the eaves.

—Shih-shu (ca. seventeenth century–early eighteenth century)

Armed with new understandings about the human genome, the processes of cell duplication, and cellular environments, researchers are investigating a multitude of new cancer therapies. Before the 1980s, scientists exposed cancer cells to treatments and observed whether the treatments stopped or slowed the rate of cell division. Now that more is known about cell division, components of the immune system, and how malignant cells develop a blood supply, research is focused on pinpointing molecular

mechanisms that give rise to cancer and on discovering means to intervene in these processes.

As cancer's complexity reveals itself, it appears unlikely that a magic
bullet will be discovered that cures all cancers. Instead, oncologists and
their patients increasingly have at their disposal a more varied and targeted arsenal of possibilities that could turn fatal cancers into chronic
diseases. Oncologists and patients have known for some time that what
works well for one person with cancer may not work as well for another,
and the reasons for such differences are now starting to become clear.
Ideally, this new knowledge will lead to more targeted treatments. Cancer
therapies are increasingly being tailored to each patient, depending upon
what cellular process has malfunctioned and led to uncontrolled growth.
What gave rise to one person's uncontrolled breast cancer cell growth can
be different from another person's. Many of the new molecular treatments
are being tested in clinical trials, and in the next decades some will become
conventional practice. New treatments will make current procedures such
as radiation and chemotherapy more potent and less toxic. To understand
how the new therapies work is in large part to understand how cancer develops.

Understanding Cancer Development

Any tissue in the human body can develop into cancer; therefore, there are
as many different types of cancer as there are types of cells in the body.
Each individual cancer arises from a particular set of gene mutations and
possesses unique characteristics. The universal term "cancer" is more accurately thought of as a collection of diseases with two common features—
uncontrolled cell growth and invasive cell growth. Normally cells operate
under a very strict set of checks and balances that keep too many cells
from growing in one area. When cells become cancerous, they lose this set
of checks and balances, resulting in unrestrained growth and, often, loss
of the ability to undergo normal cell death. If we use the analogy of cancer
as an automobile, we can say that the disease can result from too much
weight on the accelerator, too little pressure on the brake pedal, or a combination of both. In the case of cancers that form solid growths, decades
may pass before the process results in the formation of a palpable tumor
(a mass that can be felt). In order to be called a cancer, these tumor cells

must also become invasive. Normal cells are kept in their highly structured areas of growth by barriers called basement membranes, which act like fences among organs, blood vessels, and lymphatic channels. Cancer cells develop ways to eat through these fences, entering the blood and lymph streams and invading organs.

Cancer always has genetic origins, meaning that changes in genes cause it, but cancer is not always hereditary, meaning that the gene changes are not always passed on from parents. In fact, the majority of human cancers are not hereditary; rather, they arise from aging and environmental exposures that cause the genetic instructions — DNA — to change and operate in a defective manner. There are a number of ways in which gene function can change and cause cancer. Extra copies of a gene may be made, causing an excess of protein that can increase cell growth, division, or metastasis. Genes may be silenced or stopped from being read appropriately. Parts of a gene may be deleted, giving rise to a nonfunctional protein or one that is produced to overly high levels. Gene mutations can also give rise to substitutions in the resulting protein, causing a gene to function abnormally or without its normal regulatory switches.

Cancer is not one event but a complicated process. Many theories have been posed in an attempt to understand how cancers develop in a healthy individual. The most accepted theory is that cancer arises after cells have accumulated a number of malfunctions, both genetically and biochemically, usually over the course of many years. Currently, it is widely believed that cancer starts with a single mutated cell. Of the trillions of cells in the body, one of the many cells that contain a genetic mutation escapes the proofreading checkpoints in the cell, and this cell and its descendants further escape the detection of the immune system. If unchecked, these descendants can continue to mutate and exponentially reproduce, resulting in life-threatening tumors in essential organs. When pathologists examine tumor cells, they are looking for certain molecular cell features to determine how advanced and aggressive the cancer is. This molecular development theory is divided into stages, each heralded by a genetic change, and it is described below and illustrated in figure 4.

First Stage

Somewhere in the body a change occurs in the DNA of a cell, and that small change interferes with the cell's life cycle, causing the cell to dupli-

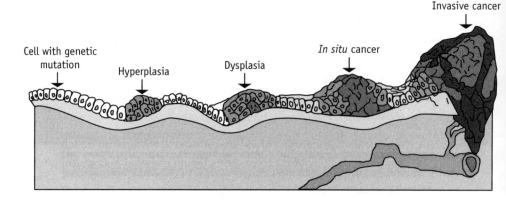

Cell with genetic mutation **Hyperplasia** **Dysplasia** **In situ cancer** **Invasive cancer**

4. The stages of tumor development. A malignant tumor develops across time and appears to be the result of four types of mutations: (a) The tumor begins to develop when a cell experiences a first mutation that makes the cell more likely to divide than it normally would. (b) The altered cell and its descendants grow and divide too often, a condition called hyperplasia. At some point, one of these cells experiences a second mutation that further increases its tendency to divide. (c) This cell's descendants divide excessively and look abnormal, a condition called dysplasia. As time passes, one of the cells experiences a third mutation. (d) This cell and its descendants are very abnormal in both growth and appearance. If the tumor that has formed from these cells is still contained within its tissue of origin, it is called *in situ* cancer. *In situ* cancer may remain contained indefinitely. (e) If some cells experience fourth and further mutations that allow the tumor to invade neighboring tissues and shed cells into the blood or lymph, the tumor is said to be malignant. The escaped cells may establish new tumors (metastases) at other locations in the body. From National Institutes of Health and the National Cancer Institute, http://science.education.nih.gov/supplements/nih1/cancer/guide/understanding1.htm (accessed December 31, 2005).

cate itself more than the body needs. Not all DNA changes are harmful to the body, but ones that interfere with the cell's life cycle can lead to uncontrolled cell growth. A change might be the result of a mistake in replication of the DNA brought about by a cell that has aged and replicated many times, or it can be brought about by an inherited anomaly, or an environmental irritation, or possibly an interaction of these. Some chemicals (such as formaldehyde and asbestos), radiation (such as that from the sun or from X-rays), and viruses (such as the human papilloma virus) are environmental toxins or irritations that can give rise to DNA mutations (changes) or changes in enzyme function, leading ultimately to cancer.

Inappropriate DNA changes occur regularly in our bodies and occur more frequently as our cells age. Usually our immune system recognizes the resulting wayward cells and destroys them, or the cell itself self-destructs (undergoes apoptosis). Even when the immune system does not eliminate these wayward cells, usually the excess cell proliferation leads to benign growths, such as cysts, warts, or fatty tumors. Such growths can be found in every part of the body and rarely change further into invasive cancer.

Second Stage: Hyperplasia

The descendants of the first altered cell look quite like their normal counterparts. If they continue to overduplicate, however, after years it is possible that one of these cells (one in a million) will have a second genetic change, making this cell less normal and even more prone to duplicate rapidly.

Third Stage: Dysplasia

If viewed under a microscope, it can be seen that the cells that are offspring from the second stage are abnormal in shape compared with typical cells of that tissue. Over time, a third series of changes may occur, and these offspring will become increasingly abnormal and rapidly dividing.

Fourth Stage: *In Situ* Cancer

The cells springing from the third stage eventually comprise a tumor. If these cells remain contained within a barrier called the basement membrane, the tumor will remain contained (*in situ*), and it could possibly remain contained indefinitely. However, sometimes a fourth change occurs that enables a cell and its descendants to penetrate nearby tissue (the process of invasion) and connect with the blood and/or lymph systems.

Invasive Carcinoma

The descendants of the invasive cells can now make their way to the blood and lymph vessels, which serve as mediums for them to travel to other organs in the body. These highly abnormal cells then can acquire further genetic changes that promote metastasis, or travel to other organs in the body. This process can be debilitating and eventually lethal. The cancer cells become parasitic, competing with healthy cells for body nutrients, glucose, and oxygen. The tumors eventually crowd out the normal cells of the organ in which they reside, causing it to malfunction.

A Closer Look at the Genetic Changes in Cancer

Understanding how treatments intervene in the cancer process requires understanding how the first change in a cell may occur. This calls for a closer look at the cell and its life cycle. Figure 5 shows the inner workings of a normal cell. Every cell in the body has a nucleus, and within the nucleus are chromosomes. The chromosomes are comprised of strands of DNA molecules. A gene is a section of the DNA strand that directs the synthesis of proteins. Genes also exert control over the proteins, including special proteins (called enzymes) that trigger chemical reactions in the cell. A protein is a sequence of chemical bases known as amino acids. There are twenty amino acids; two well-known examples are lysine and tyrosine. In summary, a gene is a portion of a DNA molecule that instructs amino acids to combine, causing the cell to create a particular protein. When a gene is triggered to do its work, the cell produces that protein. When a genetic change occurs, the gene's instructions are altered, causing the process of protein creation to go awry. The result is that no protein is produced when it is called for, or the subsequent protein is different from, or more plentiful (overexpressed) than, what a normal cell would produce. These changes can interfere with the normal process of cell division and duplication.

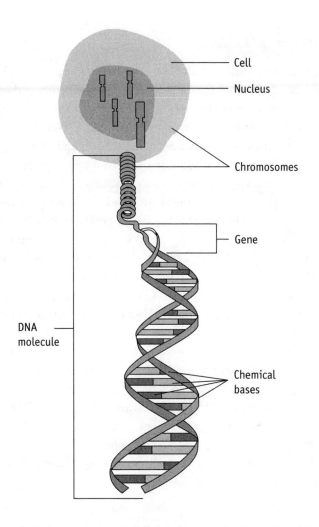

Cell

Nucleus

Chromosomes

Gene

DNA molecule

Chemical bases

5. Nucleus of a Cell. From Access Excellence Resource Center, National Health Museum, http://www.accessexcellence.org/AE/AEPC/NIH/gene02.html (accessed October 8, 2006).

Cell Division and Duplication

The duplication of a cell is an elaborate event. Cellular proteins play a part in either starting or stopping duplication at various points in the process. Cell division is usually prompted when a cell secretes a growth-stimulating protein. These growth-stimulating proteins bind to receptors (antenna-like molecules) sticking out of a nearby cell. Once bound, the receptor then sends a message into the cytoplasm of the cell that initiates a chain of protein-driven messages. The messages eventually reach the cell's nucleus, telling the nucleus to duplicate its DNA and divide itself in two. These events are divided into four stages that are described below, outlined in table 3, and simply illustrated in figure 6. To see an animation of a normal cell passing through the stages and creating a duplicate cell, go to the Cancerquest site in the next resource box and click on "The Cell Cycle."

Conventional chemotherapies and radiation interrupt the cell cycle in a variety of ways, as discussed under "How Current Treatments Fight Cancer" in this chapter. Recent findings about how proteins stimulate and halt cell duplication have produced opportunities to develop treatments that target specific malfunctions. While understanding the science can be challenging, it is highly rewarding and illuminating to have a basic knowledge of the workings of cancer cells in order to understand how new and emerging therapies work. Knowledge of cancer development also enables you to realize what has happened and is happening in your body. The sites in the next resource box offer a more complete explanation of the biology of cancer.

Table 3. Stages of cancer

Stage	Approximate Length of Stage
G1: The cell enlarges and prepares to copy DNA	6–12 hours
G0: The cell rests	Indefinite time
S (synthesis): DNA copying takes place	6–9 hours
G2: The cell checks DNA for mistakes and prepares for division	3–4 hours
M (mitosis): The cell divides in two	1–2 hours

Note: The times indicated are examples that reflect the durations observed for cancer cells growing in culture (that is, outside of the body). Cancer cells grow much more slowly inside the body, spending the majority of time in the G0 resting phase.

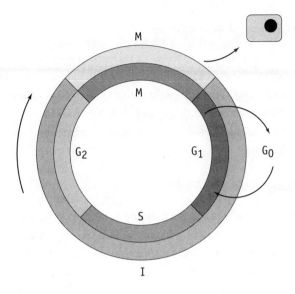

6. The Cell Cycle. By Richard Wheeler (Zephyris), 2006. http://en.wikipedia
.org/wiki/Image:Cell_Cycle_2.png.

CANCER BIOLOGY

- Cancerquest: A layered site that teaches the biology of cancer, including
  visual presentations (video clips) on cell division, tumor biology, and
  more.
    http://www.cancerquest.org/index.cfm?page=51

- Mayo Clinic: How Cancer Spreads video.
    http://www.mayoclinic.com/health/cancer/MM00638

- National Cancer Institute, Understanding Cancer: Offers graphically rich
  tutorials.
    http://nci.nih.gov/cancertopics/understandingcancer
    http://nci.nih.gov/cancertopics/understandingcancer/
      cancergenomics/Slide49

- National Institutes of Health and National Cancer Institute: Offer a variety
  of ways to learn about cell biology and its relationship to cancer.
    http://science.education.nih.gov/supplements/nih1/cancer/
      default.htm

resources

The Development of Breast Cancer

Cancer, as is clear from the preceding sections, always has a genetic origin. A gene malfunction can be of many types, caused by a number of factors, such as a cell's aging, environmental toxins, and (less often) a hereditary genetic disposition. Once this genetic malfunction occurs, over time in the breast a tumor is formed. What follows is a brief look at this development in the breast.

Hereditary Breast Cancer

The first gene associated with hereditary breast cancer, BRCA1, was mapped to the long arm of chromosome 17 in 1990 and cloned in 1994 (1, 2). A second breast cancer gene, BRCA2, was identified in 1994 on the long arm of chromosome 13 (3). Together, mutations in these genes account for about 10 percent of all breast cancers and 50 percent of all hereditary cases of breast cancer. They are found much more commonly in women with strong family histories of breast and/or ovarian cancer, in women with bilateral breast cancer, and in women who develop breast cancer at a young age (under age fifty). Mutations in BRCA2 are considered the major genetic risk factor for male breast cancer, with some increased risk of male breast cancer with BRCA1 mutations. Certain ethnic groups, such as Ashkenazi Jews, are more likely to inherit a mutated copy of either BRCA1 or BRCA2. The abnormal gene may be inherited from either parent, and it appears that a second mutation is needed in the normal copy of the gene for cancers to arise. Both genes appear to be tumor-suppressor genes—that is, when the gene functions normally it stops the process of cell division and replication.

In hereditary breast cancer families that do not carry mutations in either BRCA1 or BRCA2, there is an increased presence (5–13 percent) of a specific mutation in CHEK2, a gene encoding a protein involved in cell-cycle checkpoints and repair (4). This mutation increases the risk of female breast cancer twofold and male breast cancer tenfold. Other genes give rise to hereditary breast cancer as well. Mutations of the tumor-suppressor gene TP53 in normal cells cause a hereditary cancer syndrome called Li-Fraumeni syndrome. People with one inherited copy of an abnormal TP53 gene can develop numerous types of cancers at a young age, including breast cancer, brain cancer, soft tissue sarcoma, osteosarcoma, and adrenocortical carcinoma. Similarly, mutations in another tumor-suppressor gene, PTEN, give rise to Cowden syndrome, a rare disorder that causes multiple noncancerous growths. Women with one abnormal inherited copy of PTEN are at increased risk for development of breast cancer, thyroid cancer, and endometrial cancer.

Non-Hereditary (Sporadic) Breast Cancer

Most breast cancers (around 90 percent) do not have an inherited basis; rather, they result from multiple genetic changes that have accumulated over time in breast tissues. In general, it is impossible to tell what caused these multiple genetic changes in each individual person or, for that matter, in each individual cancer. Observational studies — studies that follow a group of people over a long period of time to look for disease occurrence — have shown that risk of breast cancer changes with various dietary and environmental exposures throughout life. Many of these exposures affect risk only during certain developmental periods, such as pre-puberty. Some of these influences are listed in table 4, and you can learn more about environmental factors in the following resource box. We assume that these exposures lead to genetic changes that eventually cause (or prevent) cancer, but again, we cannot with certainty say that exposure, for example, to DDT at an early age caused a genetic change that then caused a breast cancer. Perhaps future research will enable us to track the genetic footprints of environmental damage, but for now we can only guess at causes of most breast cancers.

ENVIRONMENTAL FACTORS AND BREAST CANCER

resources

- Sprecher Institute, Breast Cancer and Environmental Risk Factors: Offers many learning resources, statistics, and links to information on environmental factors and breast cancer.
  http://envirocancer.cornell.edu

- Breast Cancer Fund, State of Evidence: Offers yearly reports titled "The Connection Between Breast Cancer and the Environment."
  http://www.breastcancerfund.org/site/pp.asp?c=kwKXLdPaE&b=206137

- Silent Spring: Offers a way to potentially gauge breast cancer risk based on exposure to carcinogens.
  http://sciencereview.silentspring.org/index.cfm

Table 4. Increased and decreased breast cancer risk factors.

Increased Risk	Decreased Risk
Chemicals	*Chemicals*
Estrogen + progesterone	NSAIDs, including aspirin
Tobacco smoke	Vitamin D
DDT	*Diet*
Dioxin	Alpha- and beta-carotene
Heptachlor (insecticide)	(not supplements)
Benzene	Dietary fruit and cereal fiber
BPA (bisphenol A)	*Lifestyle*
Diethylstilbestrol (DES)	Breast feeding
Phthalates	Daily exercise
Parabens	
Diet	
Alcohol consumption	
Grilled meat and fish consumption	
Lifestyle	
Overweight and obesity	
Overnight shift work	
Radiation	
Ionizing radiation	

Many different tissues in the breast can give rise to breast cancers, including ducts, lobules (dilated sections of duct to hold milk), nipples, fat, the pectoralis major muscle, and the chest wall/rib cage. The two most common breast cancers are invasive ductal carcinoma (80 percent) and invasive lobular carcinomas (15 percent) (5). With the exception of rare cancers, such as inflammatory breast cancer, scientists estimate that it takes years for cancer to develop to a size that is palpable (able to be felt). The average doubling time for breast cancer is sixty days, increasing with increasing age of the tumor (6). A tumor of 1 cm would be comprised of approximately one hundred billion cells. Given this, it would take many years before a cancer grew to the size of about half a centimeter and could be detected by a mammogram and another year before it doubled to a size of 1 cm, barely palpable. The average doubling time, however, is a very rough estimate, with many cancers growing slower or faster and possibly in spurts.

Invasive Ductal Carcinoma

Invasive ductal carcinomas are breast cancers that look like the cells lining the ducts (see figure 1, chapter 1). While a great deal of research is underway to determine why normal breast cells develop into invasive breast cancers, the appearance of cells as they make this transition has been fairly well described.

First, cells in the duct undergo hyperplasia, meaning that there are many more cells than usual, but they all appear normal. Hyperplasia can be caused by inflammation or infection. This can be commonly seen in combination with fibrocystic disease. Florid ductal hyperplasia carries with it a slight increased risk of subsequent invasive cancer.

Next, the hyperplastic cells become atypical. This means that the cells start to look more abnormal and less like normal breast cells. Sometimes it is difficult to assess an area of hyperplastic cells in the breast with a needle biopsy or fine needle aspiration, in which case a larger biopsy is called for. Atypical ductal hyperplasia confers an increased risk of breast cancer, four to five times that of the general population.

Next, the atypical cells develop into cancer cells that are confined to the duct. This is called ductal carcinoma *in situ* (DCIS). Though cancer cells are present in DCIS, they have not penetrated the wall of the duct (basement membrane) into the surrounding tissue. This is considered a Stage 0, or a pre-invasive, lesion/tumor. In some women these cancerous cells will never leave the confines of the duct. For others, the lesion/tumor will develop into an invasive cancer. Because oncologists cannot predict who is going to have the more aggressive form, they operate on the safe side and assume the cancer may spread. DCIS is therefore treated with removal of the abnormal area, and radiation therapy and hormonal therapy are considered.

When the cancer cells spread outside of the duct, they are considered an invasive ductal carcinoma. This does not mean that the cancer is metastatic (present in other areas of the body). Rather, this means that the cancer managed to get out of the duct and spread to local tissue. This is what is typically considered breast cancer. At this point, the cancer is "staged" using Roman numerals I to IV as a means to characterize how much the disease has spread. Currently breast cancer staging is largely determined by the size of the tumor and the extent to which the cancer cells have spread to neighboring lymph nodes and other places in the body (see chapter 1, "Predictors of Recurrence"). Therapy for invasive cancer can include a combination of surgery, radiation therapy, chemotherapy, and hormonal therapy.

Finally, if the breast cancer cells have spread past the breast and nearby lymph nodes, the cancer is considered metastatic. This means that the cancer has spread to other organs of the body, which can include the bones, lungs, liver, and brain. When breast cancer has spread to these areas, it is currently considered impossible to cure. Rather, oncologists change the goal of therapy from curing to controlling the cancer for as long as possible while working to maintain a good quality of life for the patient. Many therapies are available for metastatic breast cancer patients, and if they respond to these therapies, patients can live for years.

Invasive Lobular Carcinoma

Invasive lobular carcinomas are breast cancers that resemble cells found in the lobules of the breast, where milk is produced. Sometimes these cancers are more difficult to see on a mammogram. The lobules tend to be much larger and more elastic than ducts (see figure 1, chapter 1). When cancer cells are confined inside the lobule, this is considered lobular carcinoma *in situ* (LCIS). LCIS is being detected more frequently now that more biopsies of abnormal areas on mammograms are being performed. Like DCIS, LCIS is a Stage 0 breast cancer. It is considered more a marker of increased breast cancer risk in either breast. Since LCIS is not considered a direct precursor to invasive breast cancer, as DCIS is, it is not routinely excised. Women diagnosed with LCIS are observed closely and may be advised to consider further chemoprevention strategies, such as tamoxifen.

Invasive lobular carcinoma develops when cancer has spread outside of the lobule to the surrounding tissues. It is staged based on the size of the tumor and whether any neighboring lymph nodes are involved. It is treated with a combination of surgery, chemotherapy, radiation, and possible hormonal therapy.

When invasive lobular carcinoma escapes the breast into other areas of the body—typically the bone, lungs, lining of the abdomen, liver, and brain—it is considered metastatic. As with invasive ductal carcinoma, the goal of therapy switches from cure to control of the disease. Invasive lobular carcinoma is as sensitive to chemotherapy and radiation as invasive ductal carcinoma, and if it is sensitive to other therapies, it can be treated for years.

How Current Treatments Fight Cancer

At the time of this writing, the removal of tumors, when possible, remains the most potent treatment for cancer. Adjuvant (treatment following surgery) hormonal therapy and chemotherapy have been shown to account for about half of the reduction in deaths due to breast cancer in 2000 (an absolute benefit of about 15 percent) (7).

The well-established therapies of surgery, radiation, and cytotoxic chemotherapy have been in use together for several decades. Though the effectiveness of chemotherapy and radiation has been enhanced and their side effects reduced, they have the drawback of attacking rapidly dividing healthy cells along with rapidly dividing cancer cells. Molecularly targeted therapies have been designed to preferentially attack cancer cells. Treatment is rapidly moving from a focus on indiscriminate destruction to a focus on targeting and controlling; however, some of the most effective cancer therapeutics remain those identified in the drug screening of natural products that have multiple mechanisms of action. What follows are brief explanations of how the traditional but still effective cancer treatments work to stop the multiplication of cancer cells.

Radiation

Cancer cells are more susceptible than healthy cells to the effects of radiation (x-rays, gamma rays, electron beam). Following exposure to ionizing radiation, cells can die by the activation of programmed cell death pathways, such as apoptosis or autotrophy, or by necrosis or mitotic catastrophe. A number of chemotherapies and targeted therapies can work with radiation to "radio-sensitize" cancer cells, making radiation more effective.

Radiation therapy has made a number of advances in recent years, allowing for more directed radiation with less surrounding organ damage. Some of these advances include the use of 3-D planning, better patient immobilization procedures, and new machines that offer computer-controlled dosing.

Intensity Modulated Radiation Therapy (IMRT)

IMRT is a precise method of external beam radiation therapy that delivers high doses of radiation directly to the tumor while sparing surrounding healthy tissue. IMRT allows doctors to customize the radiation dose by modulating, or varying, the amount of radiation given to different parts of the treatment area. This modulation is done in highly accurate, three-dimensional detail, according to the shape, size, and location of the tumor.

Stereotactic Radiosurgery

Stereotactic radiosurgery is not surgery; rather, it uses multiple beams of radiation to deliver large doses of radiation to focused areas of cancerous cells in the body or brain.

Hyperthermia

Hyperthermia is a treatment in which body tissue is exposed to high temperatures (up to 113° F). Hyperthermia is almost always used with other forms of cancer therapy, such as radiation therapy and chemotherapy.

RADIATION THERAPY

• National Cancer Institute: Offers a fact sheet on radiation therapy.
  http://www.cancer.gov/cancertopics/factsheet/Therapy/radiation

Chemotherapy

The chemotherapies used in standard practice for the treatment of breast cancer have an array of mechanisms by which to slow and kill rapidly dividing cells. Current chemotherapies cause cancer cells to destruct by altering the cells' DNA, thus triggering apoptosis (programmed cell death). Many of these mechanisms were discovered fortuitously in cancer screens (testing a substance in a Petri dish against cancer cells); however, a number were a result of early targeted therapy research.

What these chemotherapies have in common is that they can destroy rapidly dividing cells, including healthy ones, such as the red blood cells, white blood cells, and platelets produced in the bone marrow, the cells lining the digestive tract, and hair cells. Normal cells and cancer cells have almost the same genetic structure, so that what is aimed at one can damage the other. In addition to not being able to selectively target just the cancer cells, these conventional cytotoxic chemotherapies are not able to selectively intervene in a specific genetic malfunction that is causing a person's cancer. All of the drugs listed below are FDA-approved, meaning that they should be widely available anywhere in the United States. Federal legislation passed in December 2008 broadens the Medicare payment for "off-label" use of chemotherapy that is FDA-approved—that is, use of a chemotherapy in a situation in which it has not undergone Phase III testing, such as in fourth-line treatment of breast cancer. The following is a summary of how these agents do their work.

Anti-Tumor Alkylating Agents

Cyclophosphamide (Cytoxan): These agents bind with particular DNA building blocks, halting the replication of DNA and causing programmed cell death.

Anti-Metabolites

Methotrexate, 5-fluorouracil, capecitabine (Xeloda), gemcitabine (Gemzar): Methotrexate inhibits the production of folic acid, which is needed to produce thymidine, one of the building blocks of DNA. Without thymidine, no DNA can be made. 5-fluorouracil, capecitabine, and gemcitabine are all analogs of pyrimidines, other building blocks of DNA. They replace the normal building blocks in a new strand of DNA and prevent the addition of any further normal building blocks. In this way anti-metabolites keep the cell from creating DNA and cause apoptosis of the cell.

Topoisomerase I Inhibitors

Irinotecan (Camptosar)

Topoisomerase II Inhibitors

Doxorubicin (Adriamycin), epirubicin (Ellence)

Topoisomerases are enzymes that allow DNA to uncoil to allow transcription and replication, both essential for cell replication/division. Topoisomerase I does this by cutting and reattaching one strand of DNA, while topoisomerase II cuts and reattaches both strands. The topoisomerase inhibitors interrupt this process, triggering programmed cell death.

Microtubule Disruptors

Vinca alkaloids—vinblastine, vinorelbine: These substances interfere with the formation of microtubules that make microfilaments that pull chromosomes to the sides of a cell immediately prior to division. By keeping the chromosomes from moving to the sides, microtubule disruptors can keep the cell from dividing.

Microtubule Stabilizers

Taxanes—Paclitaxel (Taxol, Abraxane), docetaxel (Taxotere); epothilones—ixabepilone (Ixempra): These substances cause microtubules to stabilize, preventing a cell from dividing. This causes the cell to continually replicate DNA and eventually undergo apoptosis.

Intercalating Agents

Carboplatin, cisplatin: Intercalating agents wedge between bases along the DNA. The intercalated drug molecules affect the structure of the DNA, preventing polymerase and other DNA-binding proteins from functioning properly. The result is prevention of DNA synthesis, inhibition of transcription, and induction of mutations.

New Chemotherapies Derived from Natural Products in Clinical Trials

Note: The following list is not comprehensive and changes quickly. Please see a site such as clinicaltrials.gov for the latest Phase I and II clinical trials for metastatic breast cancer. Typically a person must be enrolled in a clinical trial to receive any of these chemotherapies as they are not yet FDA-approved for use in breast cancer.

Geldanamycin

Geldanamycin was isolated from Streptomyces bacteria in the 1970s and found to inhibit a protein called heat-shock protein 90 (HSP-90). There are two geldanamycin analogs currently undergoing testing in breast cancer:

> Tanespimycin (17-AAG) 17-N-Allylamino-17-
> Demethoxygeldanamycin

17-Dimethylaminoethylamino-17-Demethoxygeldanamycin
(17-DMAG)

Taxanes

Xyotax™ (CT-2103): Polyglutamate paclitaxel
RPR109881—a semi-synthetic taxane, effective in taxane-resistant
tumors, currently in Phase III testing

Epothilone

Sagopilone (ZK-EPO): A synthetic epothilone

Halichondrin

Halichondrin was isolated from the marine sponge *Halichondria okadai* in
1986.

Eribulin mesylate/E7389—a synthetic halichondrin analog that
works via inhibition of microtubule polymerization; it is currently undergoing Phase III testing.

Vinca Alkaloid

Vinflunine: A semi-synthetic vinca alkaloid.

Other Mechanisms of Action

BZL-101: An extract from *Scutellaria barbata*, currently undergoing
Phase II testing in breast cancer.

Flavopiridol (NSC 649890): An experimental semi-synthetic flavonoid
derived from the indigenous Indian plant *Dysoxylum binectari-
ferum* and the first cyclin-dependent kinase (CDK) inhibitor to
be tested in clinical trials. (Flavonoids are compounds found in
plants; they modulate various biological activities.)

AFP464/Aminoflavone (NSC 686288): A synthetic material that is related to flavonoids.

UCN-01: A staurosporine analog that acts as a cyclin-dependent
kinase inhibitor. It was originally isolated in 1977 from the bacterium *Streptomyces staurosporeus*.

How Targeted Therapies Fight Cancer

The discovery of multiple common genetic abnormalities in cancer cells has enabled scientists and clinicians to capitalize on the important differences between cancerous and healthy cells. Targeted therapies are aimed at specific proteins or cellular pathways known to be abnormal in cancer cells, so targeted therapies do less damage to normal cells than traditional chemotherapy. Significant obstacles must be overcome to develop these therapies. New technologies, such as combinatorial chemistry, allow for the screening of thousands of potential small molecules to find the best fit to a protein target. One of the great challenges in the development of targeted therapies is finding a way to transport a drug into a cell. This can involve finding vehicles, such as viruses, to deliver substances, or genetically altering material to adhere to the surface or penetrate the interior of cancer cells. It is necessary, too, to find ways to keep the immune system from considering the delivery vehicle foreign matter and destroying it. Still, in laboratory experiments and in human clinical trials, emerging targeted therapies are showing promise and continue to be refined. Though nearly all treatments have some undesirable side effects, targeted treatments are generally more tolerable for people since they less often damage healthy tissue.

Targeted therapies can be classified into three general, not always mutually exclusive, types: *immunotherapy/biological therapies*, *molecular approaches*, and *anti-angiogenic approaches*.

Immunotherapy/Biological Therapies: Approaches to Stimulate or Use the Immune System to Deliver Destructive Compounds

In the late 1800s physicians noticed that malignant tumors shrank in patients who had bacterial infections. The idea that an infection could stimulate the immune system led a few curious doctors to inoculate cancer patients with a vaccine containing dead bacteria cells. Some patients' tumors regressed, but the results were so unpredictable that most scientists abandoned these early attempts at fighting cancer through immunology. Now that more is known about the immune system, the interest in immunotherapy has been renewed. The attempt to rouse the body's own immune system to fight cancer can be divided into four categories: *nonspecific immunotherapy*, *passive immunotherapy*, *active immunotherapy*, and *adoptive therapy*.

Nonspecific Immunotherapy

This therapy stimulates the immune system overall to attack cancer cells but does not attempt to stimulate a particular aspect of the system. In the 1970s and '80s scientists realized that the body produced certain protein molecules to combat viral and bacterial invasions. These molecules, called cytokines, are proteins divided into families such as interferons, interleukins, and tumor necrosis factor (TNF). Injection of a patient with a bacterium or virus to trigger more, or specific, cytokines, or the direct injection of cytokines, failed to fight specific cancer cells. Trials are underway to see if cytokine immunotherapy may be effective in combination with other therapies, such as traditional chemotherapy.

Passive Immunotherapy (Antibody-Based Therapy)

Antigens are proteins that mark cells, or other substances, as foreign to the body, and they trigger the immune system to attack the foreign matter. Different antibodies (proteins the body makes in response to antigens) that circulate in the blood system recognize and bind to specific foreign antigens. This binding allows other components of the immune system, such as macrophages, to engulf the foreign cells and destroy them. Additionally, the binding of the specific antibody may be used to disrupt a receptor from signaling a cell to divide; such binding is one of the mechanisms through which Herceptin works. Scientists have continued to isolate antigens specific to cancer cells and to identify ways to help the immune system target those antigens. Scientists are also attempting to use antibodies as a vehicle for delivering a number of destructive compounds specifically to the cancer cells, including chemotherapeutic chemicals, radioactive compounds, plant or bacteria toxins, and genetic drugs.

Active Immunotherapy (Vaccine-Based Therapies)

With active immunotherapy a vaccine is administered to stimulate the body to produce the antibodies needed to target antigens on cancer cells. These vaccines may consist of a variety of substances, such as specific proteins from one's own cancer cells. It is hoped that these proteins will bind to antigens on live cancer cells and signal a type of white blood cell called T-cells, and other cells that provide immunity, to destroy those cells.

Adoptive Therapy

In this therapy one's own T-cells are isolated in blood samples and then cultivated in the laboratory by exposing them to tumor cells and antigens. When a large number of an individual's own T-cells have been "manufactured" in the laboratory, they are then injected back into the person.

Side effects from immunotherapies can include flu-like symptoms, low blood pressure, and skin irritations where a needle was inserted to inject a treatment. All of these immunotherapies have shown promise, but none so far has proven to be highly effective in thwarting cancers in large numbers of people. Some of the stumbling blocks in creating effective and practical immunotherapy include the great cost and time needed to isolate antibodies, as well as the uncanny ability of cancer cells to alter themselves so that they are no longer a target for the immune system. Still, the therapy shows promise, and a number of vaccines are being evaluated in clinical trials.

IMMUNOTHERAPY/BIOLOGICAL THERAPY

- National Cancer Institute: Provides answers to questions about biological therapy.

    http://nci.nih.gov/cancertopics/biologicaltherapy

Molecular Targeted Therapy: Approaches to Stopping the Abnormal Cell Cycle

As explained earlier in this chapter, scientists are beginning to understand what conditions signal a cell to duplicate and overduplicate. Many events do, and do not, have to take place for cells to grow in an uncontrolled manner to form a tumor and for certain tumor cells to break away from a tumor to form distant tumors. The number and intricacy of these genetic and protein interactions are astounding, and they are one reason cancer remains a complex challenge to all those studying the disease. Nonetheless, researchers at universities and pharmaceutical companies are trying various means to restore normal cellular function to cancer cells. Though

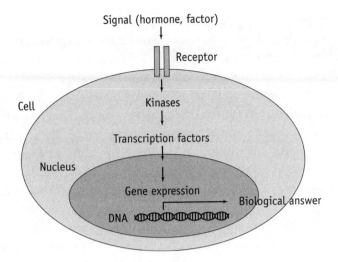

Signal (hormone, factor)

Receptor

Cell

Kinases

Transcription factors

Nucleus

Gene expression

Biological answer

DNA

7. Model of signaling within a cancer cell.

one genetic change may be the starting point for abnormal functioning, by the time a cancer is diagnosed, the cells are proliferating abnormally as a result of changes in several classes of genes. A major focus in current research is abnormal cell function associated with two classes of genes that are essential in coordinating the process of cell division: oncogenes and tumor-suppressor genes.

Oncogenes

"Oncogene" is the name for a mutant form of a gene that stimulates cell growth and division. An oncogene is only slightly different from its normal gene counterpart (a proto-oncogene), perhaps differing by only one amino acid, but this is enough to disrupt the cell's reproduction process.

Proto-oncogenes encode components of a cell's normal growth-control pathway. Some of these components are growth factors, receptors, signaling enzymes, and transcription factors. Growth factors bind to receptors on the cell surface; the receptors activate signaling enzymes inside the cell that, in turn, activate special proteins called transcription factors inside the cell's nucleus. The activated transcription factors "turn on" the genes required for cell growth and proliferation. This process is shown in figure 7.

Though many different genes can mutate and become oncogenes, scientists are focusing on the most commonly found oncogenes in human cancer as targets for potential drug therapy. Growth-factor receptors, which are frequently present in increased amounts (overexpressed) in cancer cells, have already been successfully inhibited in cancer treatment in the last decade. For example, the epidermal growth-factor receptor (EGFR) family has been successfully targeted in a number of cancers; it contains both EGFR and HER2 (EGFR2), both overexpressed in many with breast cancers. HER2 is the target of trastuzumab (Herceptin), discussed in more depth below. Another drug that has recently received FDA approval for the treatment of breast cancer is lapatinib (Tykerb), an oral dual tyrosine kinase inhibitor of EGFR and HER2, meaning that it blocks both EGFR and HER2 signals to the interior of a cell. Recent studies have shown that lapatinib is effective alone and in conjunction with chemotherapy in women with breast cancer that overexpresses either EGFR or HER2, although its greatest effect has been seen in tumors that overexpress HER2 (8). It is particularly effective in tumors that have grown despite treatment with Herceptin and may be effective in conjunction with Herceptin.

Another frequently mutated proto-oncogene is the Ras gene, found in approximately 20–30 percent of all cancers. The pathways that are controlled by activated Ras are designed to prolong cell survival and promote cell proliferation in response to an outside cell signal. A mutated Ras gene, or Ras oncogene, however, produces a protein that is always "on," sending this signal even in the absence of a trigger, continually telling the cell to reproduce. Less than 5 percent of breast cancers contain Ras mutations, but increased function of the Ras pathway is present in most breast cancers (9).

In studying the Ras gene, researchers have discovered that an enzyme called farnesyl transferase is required for the Ras protein to be "turned on" to send signals to the cell nucleus. Inhibitors of farnesyl transferase turn the Ras pathway off variably, but they may work best in tumors without Ras mutations. Farnesyl transferase inhibitors currently undergoing clinical trials in breast cancer include lonafarnib (SCH66336) and tipifarnib (Zarnestra). Dose-limiting toxicities include myelosuppression and neurotoxicity in tipifarnib and diarrhea in lonafarnib. The location of action of these agents is depicted in figure 8.

Tumor-Suppressor Genes

Tumor-suppressor genes produce proteins that signal a cell to stop dividing, and thus they normally prevent cancers. When these important

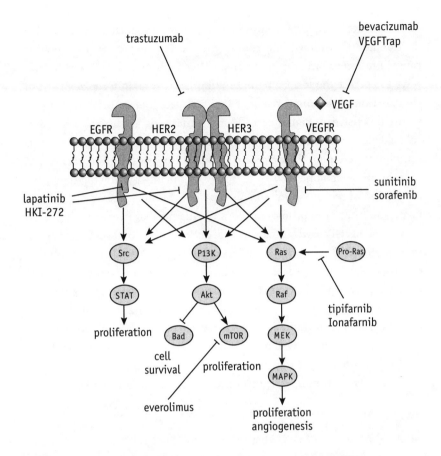

8. Simplified scheme of intracellular signal transduction pathways and targeted therapies. Ligand binds to the extracellular domain of membrane receptors, leading to activation of signaling proteins, which leads to cancer proliferation and angiogenesis. Each of these signaling proteins is a potential target for drug therapy: EGFR (epidermal growth-factor receptor); HER2 (human epidermal growth-factor receptor 2); HER3 (human epidermal growth-factor receptor 3); VEGF (vascular endothelial growth factor); VEGFR (VEGF receptor); Src (sarcoma protein); STAT (signal transducer and activator of transcription); PI3K (phosphoinositide-3-kinase); Akt (RAC-alpha serine/threonine-protein kinase or protein kinase B); mTOR (mammalian target of rapamycin); Bad (Bcl-2-associated death promoter); Ras (retrovirus associated sequences); Raf (receptor activation factor); MEK (mitogen-activated protein kinase); MAPK (MAP kinase).

genes mutate, their protein products no longer properly halt cell reproduction and they allow cancers to occur. Loss of control of the cell cycle
causes numerous later or "downstream" events in the cycle. There are two
ways to correct the loss of a tumor-suppressor function: replacement of
the function of the abnormal gene (as with gene therapy) or intervention
in the downstream signal cascade. Both methods are undergoing clinical trials in breast cancer. TP53 is a crucial tumor-suppressor gene that is
found mutated in up to 40 percent of breast cancers (10). The normal p53
protein prevents abnormal DNA from reproducing by slowing down the
replication of cells in order to allow repair; if this does not work, then cell
death (apoptosis) is promoted. Loss of this normal function allows for
uncontrolled cell growth. A recent trial of a cold virus (adenovirus) genetically engineered to contain a replacement normal TP53 (Adnexin; Intro-
gen Therapeutics) showed that when the virus was injected directly into
breast tumors and given at the same time as chemotherapy, it enabled
women with large breast cancers to undergo complete surgical resection,
meaning removal of the cancer (11). Further studies are planned with this
method of delivery, as well as with nanoparticle-delivered normal TP53.
At this point only local injection has been tested, making this treatment
suitable only for tumors that can be reached by an injection needle.

MOLECULAR DIAGNOSTICS AND TARGETED THERAPIES

- National Cancer Institute: Offers a detailed slide presentation about
  molecular diagnostics.
  > http://www.cancer.gov/cancertopics/understandingcancer/
  >   moleculardiagnostics

- National Cancer Institute: Offers a fact sheet on targeted therapies.
  > http://www.cancer.gov/cancertopics/factsheet/Therapy/targeted

Anti-Angiogenic Therapy: Approaches to Cut Off a Cancer's Blood Supply

Nearly every human cell is resting on, or near, a capillary, a vessel finer
than a strand of hair, thick enough for just one cell to pass through. The
blood circulating through the capillary brings nourishment to the cell and
takes away its waste. Because the endothelial cells, which line the inner

casing of the capillary, do not divide, capillaries do not enlarge or increase in number except when tissue must be repaired or in the uterus in preparation for menstruation. However, in the case of cancer, already mutant cells can undergo a further mutation. The resulting genes produce proteins that disrupt the cells' mechanisms for stimulating or halting capillary growth, allowing the vessels to break through tissue to reach and feed the mutated cancer cells. Cancers would remain small—less than a centimeter—and could remain harmless if they could not trigger capillaries to bring nourishment and if they could not use the capillaries to enter the lymph and blood system, enabling them to travel to other sites in the body.

It may take months or years for the cancer cells in an *in situ* carcinoma—cancer cells that have not broken through their surrounding basement membrane—to undergo the genetic changes that enable them to develop a blood supply and break out of their confined space. Once this proliferation of capillaries takes place, referred to as angiogenesis or neovascularization, the cancer can rapidly divide. In the process of angiogenesis, the normal endothelial cells lining the capillaries release cytokines or proteins that further spur mutant cancer cells' capacity to reproduce and travel.

Before angiogenesis, breast cancer tumors are hard to detect on a mammogram. Once a tumor undergoes angiogenesis, it can double in size rapidly. Some of the mutant cells that a tumor produces may be angiogenic, capable of inducing a blood supply, and others nonangiogenic. It is possible for a nonangiogenic tumor to form elsewhere in the body and lie dormant until something (as yet scientists are not sure what) triggers angiogenesis, at which point the cancer cells in the tumor become virulent and mobile.

Unlike the molecular approaches that fight cancer by intervening in the life cycle of a cell, anti-angiogenic substances interrupt a tumor's blood supply, shrinking the tumor and thwarting its capacity to metastasize. The first anti-angiogenic drug to be tested in human clinical trials was TNP-470 in 1992, with many more following. Many of these anti-angiogenic drugs work by stopping the proliferation of the endothelial cells that line the inside of the capillaries. Multiple targets for angiogenesis inhibition have been identified. One target for which multiple inhibitors have been developed is $\alpha v \beta_3$, an integrin found on the surface of fast-growing endothelial cells. Three classes of integrin inhibitors are currently in preclinical and clinical development: *monoclonal antibodies*, targeting the extracellular domain of the heterodimer (Vitaxin; MedImmune); *synthetic peptides containing an integrin specific binding sequence* (cilengitide; Merck); and *peptidomimetics* (S247; Pfizer), which are orally bioavailable nonpeptidic molecules mimicking the integrin specific binding sequence (12).

The vascular endothelial growth factor (VEGF) pathway has also been the target of multiple novel therapies. VEGF is critical in the formation of new blood vessels, binding to the VEGF receptor and causing intracellular signaling resulting in cell division and angiogenesis. The FDA recently approved bevacizumab (Avastin), a monoclonal antibody that binds to VEGF, for breast cancer treatment in combination with paclitaxel (Taxol). In combination with paclitaxel, bevacizumab doubled progression-free survival and response rates in women with metastatic breast cancer (E2100 trial) (13).

Sunitinib (SU11248) and sorafenib (BAY 43-9006) are both small molecule inhibitors of receptors involved in the VEGF pathway and are being used in combination with standard chemotherapies in multiple clinical trials for breast cancer. The location of action of these agents is depicted in figure 8.

Motesanib diphosphate (AMG 706) is a highly selective oral agent that is being evaluated for its ability to inhibit angiogenesis by targeting vascular endothelial growth-factor receptors 1, 2, and 3 (VEGFR1–3). It is also under investigation for its potential direct anti-tumor activity by targeting platelet-derived growth-factor receptor (PDGFR) and stem-cell-factor receptor (c-kit) signaling, which may also confer direct anti-tumor activity.

Drugs with such specificity generally have fewer side effects than current cytotoxic treatments; however, they appear to be most effective in combination with standard therapies such as chemotherapy. Because endothelial cells are less prone to mutation than already mutated cancer cells, the endothelial cells are less likely to develop immunity to treatment. Since one endothelial cell is needed to feed 10–100 tumor cells, killing endothelial cells can have pervasive effects on a tumor. As anti-angiogenic drugs enter mainstream treatment, they will likely be used in conjunction with conventional chemotherapies or hormonal therapies. In cancers that have metastasized, angiogenesis inhibitors may be used long term by patients, making cancer more a chronic than immediately life-threatening illness.

ANGIOGENESIS

- National Cancer Institute and National Institutes of Health
   http://nci.nih.gov/cancertopics/understandingcancer/angiogenesis

- Angiogenesis Foundation
   http://www.angio.org

New Targeted Therapies Currently in Clinical Trials

Note: The following list is not comprehensive and will change quickly. Please see a site such as clinicaltrials.gov for the latest Phase I and II clinical trials for metastatic breast cancer. As of this writing, typically a person must be enrolled in a clinical trial to receive any of these chemotherapies as they are not FDA-approved for use in breast cancer.

Temsirolimus (CCI-779): An intravenous mTOR inhibitor.

Everolimus (RAD001): An intravenous mTOR inhibitor.

GTI-2040: Antisense 20-mer phosphorothioate oligonucleotide, targeting the messenger ribonucleic acid for the R2 subunit of ribonucleotide reductase. Has orphan drug status under the FDA for renal cell carcinoma and AML.

Ispinesib: An oral small molecule inhibitor of kinesin spindle protein (KSP), a mitotic kinesin protein essential for proper cell division.

Vorinostat (Zolinza; Merck): An oral histone deacetylase inhibitor.

AG-013736: A VEGFR and PDGFR small molecule inhibitor.

Lenalidomide (Revlimid; Celgene): An oral thalidomide analog.

Combretastatin A-4: An intravenous angiogenesis inhibitor.

HKI-272: An oral EGFR small molecule inhibitor.

Imatinib (Gleevec): An oral small molecule inhibitor of bcr/abl and c-kit.

Denosumab: An intravenous monoclonal antibody that targets the receptor activator of nuclear factor kappa B ligand (RANKL) for bone metastases.

RAV12: An intravenous monoclonal antibody against RAAG12, a protein found frequently in adenocarcinomas.

PD-325901: A MEK inhibitor.

Bortezomib (PS-341, Velcade): An oral small molecule proteasome inhibitor.

MLN8054: An oral small molecule Aurora A kinase inhibitor.

Trastuzumab (Herceptin): An Example of a Successful Targeted Breast Cancer Therapy

The identification of the HER2/ErbB2 oncogene led to one of the first successful targeted therapies in breast cancer—trastuzumab, known by the trade name Herceptin. The normal HER2 gene produces the HER2 protein that forms a receptor on a cell's surface. Once a growth-factor protein simulates a bound HER2 receptor, a chain reaction commences, signaling the cell to divide. Normal cells have two copies of the HER2 gene, but some abnormal cells (in 20–30 percent of breast cancer tumors) contain more than two copies. The presence of extra copies is referred to as gene amplification or overexpression. As a result of the additional HER2 genes, more HER2 protein is produced, forming multiple HER2 receptors on the cell's surface. These multiple HER2 receptors trigger the cell to divide more rapidly than normal.

Trastuzumab appears to have three mechanisms of action. It binds to HER2 receptors to keep cells from reproducing, working as a targeted molecular approach. Trastuzumab is an antibody, thus it also likely triggers the body's immune system to attack the cell. Finally, it appears to work in synergy with classical cytotoxic chemotherapy. To uncover HER2 scientists had to painstakingly isolate a protein that occurs in high levels only in breast cancer cells, not normal breast cells, and that occurs in enough breast cancers that targeting this protein would be worthwhile.

Trastuzumab proved that targeted therapies could not only extend patients' disease-free survival time, but also overall survival time, particularly when used in combination with traditional chemotherapy. Targeted therapies may be more effective in combination with other therapies because chemotherapy and radiation can reduce the size of a tumor, thereby giving targeted approaches fewer cancer cells to fight. Additionally, the combination of targeted therapy with cytotoxic therapy provides two mechanisms of attacking DNA replication, increasing the likelihood of success.

The Future

The accumulated knowledge of cancer biology is increasing at a phenomenal rate. Humankind is uncovering the intricate molecular orchestration of bodily processes, and in doing so, we are learning how certain genetic mutations in these processes lead to cancer. This quest for knowledge is a colossal undertaking. The human genome consists of approximately twenty-five thousand genes, which produce over one hundred thousand proteins, all of which can interact with one another in exceedingly complex networks. Once protein mechanisms and interactions are better understood, we will be able to intervene more effectively and selectively in disease processes. Recent molecular knowledge has multifold beneficial effects for cancer patients. Advances are enabling researchers and clinicians to move toward a personalized approach to cancer diagnosis, prognosis, and treatment.

DNA Microarray

One technology aiding in the discovery of the orchestration of proteins that manage bodily functions is DNA microarrays. A DNA microarray, or gene chip, is a slide that can display what genes are active and inactive in a tumor at a given moment in time; in other words, it is a "snapshot" of the interactions of thousands of genes. The slide is a picture of "gene expression," the process required for DNA information to be converted into proteins. The study of the pattern of gene expression provides a gene expression profile that can be used to indicate not only whether a particular cancer is likely to metastasize, but also whether certain drugs can stop the cancer's growth. The profile is of a cancer; an individual can be tested to see whether her tumor matches the profile of particular cancers. For early-stage node-negative, estrogen-receptor-positive breast cancers, a twenty-one-gene-expression profile (OncotypeDX) is now commercially available, but the profile is not currently helpful to those with disease that has already spread.

MammaPrint® is a seventy-gene-expression profile that predicts distant metastases in young patients with node-negative disease less than 5 cm. Again, it does not yet have an application in metastatic disease.

Newer gene "signatures" that appear to predict responses to specific chemotherapies are being tested in adjuvant clinical trials. The results of these trials should determine whether the treatment of tumors based on chemotherapy signatures results in fewer recurrences and longer survival. If it does, then these same gene signatures could ostensibly be used to find appropriate drugs for treating metastatic cancer as well.

GENE EXPRESSION/SIGNATURE ANALYSIS

- OncotypeDX™
    http://www.oncotypedx.com

- MammaPrint®
    http://usa.agendia.com/index.php?option=com_content&task=
        view&id=27&Itemid=271

Nanotechnology

Nanotechnology also offers exciting ways to aid in screening and treatment. Nanotechnology is the creation of particles, sometimes consisting of organic matter and sometimes not, that are so small they are the size of molecules and atoms. This technology is currently being used in breast cancer diagnosis. Magnetic nanoparticles can be taken up by breast cancer cells; then imaging machines, such as an MRI, can illuminate whether or not the cancer cells have traveled into the lymph nodes, someday possibly eliminating the need for removing the lymph nodes surgically.

Nanotechnology is being used as well to deliver higher doses of chemotherapy with fewer toxic effects. For example, paclitaxel (Taxol) currently is combined with a derivative of castor oil in order for it to be dissolved into the bloodstream. Unfortunately, the castor oil has made paclitaxel more allergenic. Recently, however, it was found that paclitaxel could be combined with albumin, a natural substance in the body. The resulting new drug, Abraxane, makes it possible for patients to forgo taking significant premedications to tolerate paclitaxel; furthermore, Abraxane takes only thirty minutes to administer, as opposed to the three hours necessary for administering Taxol (14).

The encasing of chemotherapy in liposome coating is another example of nanotechnology aiding breast cancer patients. This protective coating allows patients to be given higher doses of chemotherapy. Some of these liposome coatings are heat-sensitive so that the coating remains on the chemotherapy until it comes in contact with heat. The coated chemotherapy circulates throughout the bloodstream, and when it reaches the heated area (usually the chest wall), the outer liposome dissolves, allowing the chemotherapy to move into leaky tumor vessels, directly applying a large dose of the drug where it is needed. This heat-sensitive technology is currently being evaluated in clinical trials.

NANOTECHNOLOGY

* National Cancer Institute
    http://nci.nih.gov/cancertopics/understandingcancer/nanodevices
    http://nano.cancer.gov/resource_center/tech_backgrounder.asp

* Molecular Diagnostics, Gene Expression, Microarrays, Proteomics,
    National Cancer Institute
    http://nci.nih.gov/cancertopics/understandingcancer/
        moleculardiagnostics

Future Means for Screening and Early Diagnosis

Other revolutionary avenues to aid cancer patients include the identification of simple markers that can detect cancer's presence early, before tumors have a chance to take shape. Such markers would also enable doctors to follow patients' response to treatments more quickly and with more precision than current methods that entail waiting for months and then looking for tumor shrinkage on scans. The use of bodily fluids such as urine, saliva, or blood to detect protein abnormalities that signal breast cancer has already shown promise. A recently approved method (CellSearch; Veridex) for detecting tumor cells in the blood (called circulating tumor cells) has been shown to predict length of survival in patients with metastatic disease (15). The relatively new science of proteomics—the study of the structure and function of proteins, including the way they work and interact with each other inside cells—along with the creation of proteomic profiles from blood samples will help predict cancer recurrences and perhaps predict cancer at much earlier stages.

New Methods, New Quandaries, Much Promise

Over decades the innovative methods we have discussed may slowly re-place the current scans, chemotherapy, and radiation, but for now and the near future, the new approaches often will be used in conjunction with old ones, enhancing effectiveness and sometimes reducing undesirable side effects. In addition to combining therapies, beneficial results have been shown from changing the timing, the dose, and the order of medicines so a fine tuning of known approaches will remain an important avenue of study in the efforts to control cancer.

Though the future of cancer treatment is a bright one for patients, it is not without clouds. The discovery, production, and administration of experimental medicines are enormously costly. It takes a great deal of time and advanced technology to investigate mutations and how mutated genes produce, or fail to produce, proteins that can be implicated in the development of cancer. The resulting therapies initially are available only through clinical trials. Afterward, pharmaceutical companies want to re-coup their expenditures for development costs, as well as generate profits for shareholders, so the expense of drugs can limit their accessibility to people depending on their country's health-care system, insurance plans, and national laws. Additionally, a drug that is the only one of its type on the market will be more expensive than one that is in competition with similar drugs. Furthermore, none of the new therapies is a "cure-all"— each new therapy becomes one more option, of many options, for sup-pressing the disease. Because of the many ways cancer cells overduplicate, protect themselves from the immune system, and mutate so that a treat-ment becomes impotent, switching treatments can keep cancer in check.

Cancer treatment is a race, with researchers and clinicians trying to stay a step ahead of the disease. Cancer patients are now being treated over the course of longer lifetimes. Such ongoing treatment will raise the cost of cancer care. The cost of long-term treatment, combined with the significant expenditures necessary for developing new treatments, creates inequitable access. Countries and people with the most resources usually have the most access to the best care. Governments and the public must wrestle with how to more fairly distribute therapies that can save lives. As an individual, you can raise the chances of getting good care by staying up to date with cutting-edge treatment and current clinical trials. (See the resource box in chapter 2 on "Keeping Up to Date with Breast Cancer De-velopments.") If you are without enough money to pay for treatment, you may be able to find financial assistance through various organizations. (See chapter 7, "Paying for and Managing Medical Expenses.")

In addition to unequal access, cutting-edge medicine generates other ethical and emotional dilemmas. Would you or a close relative want to know in advance that she may develop the type of cancer you have? How far in advance would you like to know if you are likely to develop a disease or have a recurrence? How certain of getting the disease might you want to be before taking preventive measures that may be undesirable? Deciding whether to undergo a newly approved treatment also raises questions. Though clinical trials demonstrate the immediate benefits of a drug in controlling cancer and assure the relative safety of that drug for the five or ten years participants took it in a clinical trial, long-term consequences are not known for many more years. Weighing the benefits of a drug against its known side effects and possible long-range adverse side effects is already a topic of much discussion among medical professionals and patients.

In addition to the dilemmas posed by treatments, the media and the public's notions of medical research can be problematic. Cancer patients should be skeptical about news reports touting "breakthroughs" and "cancer cures." News stories can exaggerate or misrepresent new findings and inspire unfounded hope. The true impact of a breakthrough is rarely apparent from a single study; rather it is proven over time with the accumulation of results from multiple studies. In 2005 Herceptin was heralded in the press as a "cure" for breast cancer. More accurately, Herceptin was found to help prevent cancer recurrence for the 20–30 percent of women who have HER2-positive or HER2-overexpressing breast cancer.

Those who follow research studies know that experiments that show promise on cancer cells in test tubes or in mice can end up as front page stories that give the impression a new therapy will be available in short order. However, most lab and animal studies do not end up being useful in clinical practice. The process of finding a helpful medicine is a long one, rife with roadblocks. It can begin with scientists identifying a target gene or protein, followed by development of an inhibitory drug, then identification of a delivery system. Early animal and human trials gauge safety and potency, and later ones determine effective treatment regimens for humans. During the trials clinicians report whether the treatment shrinks or dissolves tumors or extends progression-free survival and overall survival. On average, it takes more than twelve years for a treatment to be developed and approved by the FDA for clinical use.

Currently much cancer research is conducted in the United States, Europe, and Asia at universities and pharmaceutical companies, often in conjunction with one another. In 1993, Congress designated $210 million for breast cancer research administered, curiously enough, by the Department of Defense. Each year since then a similar amount has been designated for research, totaling almost $2.4 billion through the fiscal year 2009. The major contributors to breast cancer research include the U.S. government, pharmaceutical companies, and a number of business and nonprofit organizations, such as Avon and Susan G. Komen for the Cure. Thanks to the effective lobbying of groups like the Breast Cancer Coalition, funding in the United States has increased dramatically in the last few decades.

Another public force in breast cancer politics are skeptics who question the sincerity of the medical establishment in helping patients and who fear its influence. Some claim that pharmaceutical companies, physicians, hospitals—indeed anyone who makes a living in cancer research and care—have a vested interest in not finding a cancer cure. Some skeptics therefore advocate that patients turn solely to alternative care and refuse newly developed therapies. However, the vested interest accusation can be leveled against complementary and alternative specialists as well. The vast majority of researchers and clinicians are ethical, dedicated individuals. Speaking from our personal experience, we can say that most clinical oncologists would be pleased to be out of a job treating cancer and instead be working on preventing cancer.

It is, of course, important that the public, particularly those with cancer, look for signs that cancer caretakers are putting self-interest ahead of their patients' well-being. It is possible that some doctors or medical institutions could be slow in upgrading to new treatments because of the considerable trouble and expense such a change may require. It is also possible that in a competitive, career-driven environment, researchers may be reluctant to share information with one another in a timely way since it may harm their professional advancement or their company's profits. To reduce such problems, patients, caretakers, and scientists need to encourage an academic and industry ethos that rewards and is conducive to collaboration in an effort to help those suffering from diseases. Patients need to remain aware of and request the latest treatments from their healthcare providers. In addition to securing research funds, breast cancer activists can advocate for the timely and fair implementation of cutting-edge treatments.

Although the new developments in medical care prompt ethical and financial predicaments, much progress has been and is being made. New therapies have alleviated much physical and emotional pain for those with cancer and those who love them. They have improved the quality and length of lives. This time of explosive understanding is one of great hope.

Further Reading

The Biological Basis of Cancer, by Robert G. McKinnell, Ralph E. Parchment, Alan O. Perantoni, and G. Barry Pierce. Cambridge University Press, 1998.

The Biology of Cancer, by Robert A. Weinberg. Garland Science, 2006.

HER2: *The Making of Herceptin, a Revolutionary Treatment for Breast Cancer*, by Robert Bazell. Random House, 1998.

Life Script: How the Human Genome Will Transform Medicine and Enhance Your Health, by Nicholas Wade. Simon and Schuster, 2001.

Molecular Biology of Cancer: Mechanisms, Targets, and Therapeutics, by Lauren Pecorino. Oxford University Press, 2008.

One Renegade Cell, by Robert A. Weinberg. Basic Books, 1999.

CHAPTER 5

Complementary, Alternative, and Integrative Care

> Everything is under the influence of
> everything else.
> —Thich Nhat Hanh, *No Death No Fear*

> Medicine and sickness mutually
> correspond. The whole universe is our
> medicine. What is the self?
> —Yun-men

A great number of people with cancer seek "natural" ways to fight their disease and to enhance their quality of life. Such remedies and lifestyle choices are frequently referred to by the catchall term "complementary and alternative medicine," or CAM. Studies suggest that worldwide somewhere between 30 to 75 percent of cancer patients partake in CAM therapies (1). People engage in this type of care since CAM approaches often address a person's whole being: body, mind, and spirit (2), in contrast to conventional (allopathic or Western) medicine, which primarily targets the disease. CAM therapies are often, but not always, less toxic than conventional medicine and frequently call for active participation on the part of the patient. They may provide comfort, control, and empowerment. Those with cancer also sometimes turn to CAM therapies in desperation when standard Western medicine cannot offer them a cure or when they do not have access to conventional care. While multiple CAM therapies have been shown to improve quality of life in people living with advanced cancer, no CAM modality has been shown to prolong life or cure metastatic disease.

In exploring these modalities, you will quickly discover that the scope of CAM is vast. It includes an astounding array of supplements, medical systems, body therapies, energy therapies, and mind-body interventions. Strictly speaking, when these therapies are used in place of conventional modern medical treatment, they are termed "alternative." When these same therapies are used along with modern treatments, they are called "complementary." Therapies that have scientific proof of efficacy and are used in conjunction with standard Western medicine are often referred to as "integrative." For simplicity's sake, we use the commonly accepted abbreviation "CAM" throughout this chapter as an umbrella term that includes therapies that are also sometimes referred to as alternative and/or integrative. We refer to medicine based on clinical trial evidence accepted by most Western oncologists by a number of terms, including "conventional," "standard," "evidence-based," and "allopathic."

Because some CAM therapies and practices have been demonstrated to reduce symptoms or improve cancer patients' quality of life, they have been a great aid to countless people and are well worth investigating. However, we do not advocate the use of any CAM therapy to the exclusion of standard cancer therapy. Doctors who practice integrative medicine continue to advise patients wanting to combat cancer to use scientifically proven medical treatments and to use therapies that are not standard medical practice with caution, as a complement, not an alternative, to standard cancer care (3).

This chapter begins with a comparison of CAM and conventional medical care, followed by brief explanations of various CAM therapies often used by breast cancer patients; these are divided into categories suggested by the National Center for Complementary and Alternative Medicine (NCCAM), a branch of the National Institutes of Health. Because CAM is less regulated than conventional medicine, we also offer cautions and, as with conventional medicine, ways that you can investigate therapies and therapists. The link in the following resource box offers a good starting point for familiarizing yourself with complementary care. Our hope is for you to discover approaches that enhance the quality of your life and for you to make informed choices when doing so.

CAM CARE OVERVIEW

• American Cancer Society: Offers a general overview of complementary care with links.

> http://www.cancer.org/docroot/ETO/ETO_5.asp?sitearea=ETO

Comparison of CAM and Standard Western Medical Practices

As mentioned previously, CAM often differs from conventional medicine by addressing the overall well-being of an individual. In this vein, many CAM therapies are aimed at prevention rather than cure. Many practices focus on strengthening one's natural defenses and improving one's nutritional status. In contrast, allopathic medical practice is typically aimed at treating patients for what is an immediate threat to their health, often only intervening once an illness is diagnosed.

In general, CAM therapies also differ from conventional medicine by the rigor and quantity of scientific testing assessing their effectiveness and safety. Fundamentally, what separates CAM practices from conventional medical treatment for combating cancer are the levels of evidence proving a substance or practice is effective and safe. Some experts have gone so far as to say that there should be no "alternative" medicine; instead, "There is only medicine that has been adequately tested and medicine that has not, medicine that works and medicine that may or may not work" (4).

In conventional medicine, before a cancer treatment becomes the standard of care its value and safety have been proven through large clinical trials. Specifically, a treatment must result in at least one of the following outcomes without causing more harm than good: a reduction in the chance of a recurrence, a reduction of tumor size or number, an improvement in the quality of life or in prolonging survival. The effectiveness claims of CAM treatments frequently are not founded on the results of studies that test for the above outcomes. Their efficacy is typically based on personal testimonials or anecdotes, logical speculation, or many years of observation, as with ancient medical traditions.

Over the past twenty years CAM therapies have begun to be studied in more rigorous clinical trials with the result that some have been shown to be safe and effective and have therefore become part of standard practice. However, significant obstacles make it difficult to assess the value of CAM therapies. CAM practices may vary widely by practitioner, potentially influencing the effectiveness of an intervention in a clinical trial. Also, large numbers of people are needed to conduct most clinical trials, which is costly, so government agencies are highly selective in choosing what therapy trials to fund.

The more a treatment has been studied—and particularly the more

Scant evidence

Personal testimony

Theory and speculation

Test tube or petri dish (in vitro) lab tests

Animal studies

Small-group human studies
(Dozens of people)

Large-scale human study
(Hundreds of people)

Solid evidence

Large-scale double-blind human study
(Several thousands of people)

Large-scale double-blind human
studies reaching similar conclusions

9. Evidence Gauge.

it has been studied in large, randomly assigned clinical trials—the more assurance you can have that it does or does not work. (See chapter 2, "Clinical Trials.") Large, double-blind clinical studies can reveal whether a treatment has a therapeutic benefit for a certain percentage of people. If a treatment works for a large percentage of people with tumor classifications similar to yours, the odds are the treatment may work for you. Using medical search engines, you can even check those odds by looking up the published research results of many clinical trials. (See chapter 2, "Researching Your Disease and Treatment.") Most drugs receive FDA approval based on trials of approximately five thousand people. When smaller studies are conducted, less information is available to assess the likelihood a treatment may act on your body as it acted on those who were in the study. Personal testimony offers the least assurance that a treatment may work for you, and can be used, unfortunately, not only by well-meaning practitioners, but also by unscrupulous ones preying on people's hopes and fears. Personal testimonials and anecdotes, though often moving and hopeful, are not evidence that a therapy is effective.

Use the evidence gauge shown in figure 9 when considering the value and safety of any treatment.

Nature's Pharmacy in Cancer Treatment

Many patients who are concerned about using chemotherapy because it is "unnatural" are surprised to learn that a large number of drugs used in breast cancer treatment are derived from nature (5). Though modern medicines do not look natural since they come in bags of intravenous solutions, vials, or tablets, the majority of cancer chemotherapy drugs have their origins in naturally occurring substances, such as plants, fungi, marine creatures, and microorganisms.

One of the most effective breast cancer drugs, Adriamycin (doxorubicin), was discovered in 1962 by Italian scientists who were building on the discovery of penicillin from fungi (6, 7). Taxol (paclitaxel), perhaps the most famous of these naturally occurring anticancer drugs, is derived from the slow-growing Pacific yew tree (8). Initially the drug was isolated from the bark of the tree (9), but chemists found that it could be made from a more rapidly renewable resource: the needles of the yew tree (10). Today, improved relatives of Taxol are manufactured in a similar manner, such as Taxotere (docetaxel), which is also derived from the needles of the yew tree (11). Continually pharmaceuticals used to treat breast cancer are found in nature including combretastatin, an experimental anti-angiogenesis drug, derived from the bark of the African willow bush (12). You can learn more about approved and experimental cancer therapies that come from natural products in chapter 4.

A number of patients want to use natural remedies in advance of clinical trial outcomes. They ingest pills and capsules of various "natural" substances in hopes of attacking or preventing cancer, enhancing their immune system, or counteracting the side effects of cancer and cancer treatments. Supplementation is one of the most commonly used CAM therapies and one of the most controversial. Supplements may consist of substances found in food, such as vitamins and minerals. They may also contain synthesized extracts from nonedible plants, and some supplements are composed of more exotic ingredients, such as ground-up animal bone. Unfortunately, it is not possible to present a neat categorization system for the vast array of supplements. For example, a substance that could be classified as an herbal remedy could also be classified as an antioxidant and as a vitamin/mineral supplement. This chapter follows the NCCAM system in which supplements are grouped under "biologically based treatments." Before presenting a list of biologically based treatments, it is helpful to take a close look at a particularly popular category of supplementation, i.e., antioxidants, since ingesting antioxidants highlights the complexity of how substances can interact within the body. This discussion will illuminate the promise of supplementation along with revealing why precautions are necessary when considering taking them.

Antioxidants: Nature's Complexity

Antioxidants permeate our way of life as they occur naturally in foods, in our bodies, and are also manufactured, showing up on store shelves as vitamin, mineral, and herbal supplements. Vitamins C and E, beta-carotene, and lycopene are examples of antioxidants that people ingest in order to combat cancer. An antioxidant is a substance that protects cells from the damaging effects of oxidation. In other words, antioxidants can protect our bodies from the damaging "side effects" of normal life processes such as breathing and eating. Their need and use results from the yin and yang relationship that our bodies have with oxygen and (to a lesser extent) nitrogen for producing and using energy to live (13). Each of the cells of our body contains compartments of energy generators called mitochondria. Here chemical reactions take place between oxygen and nutrients to create energy. As a byproduct, a very small amount of oxygen is converted to reactive oxygen species (ROS), also called free radicals (14).

Free radicals can damage the DNA of cells, which in turn can give rise to cancer. The body already produces a number of its own antioxidant substances to keep the levels of free radicals in check, but deficiencies due to diet, disease, or environmental stresses can occur. Therefore, many scientists hypothesize that various dietary antioxidants may protect against cancer. While this hypothesis is supported by Petri dish and some animal studies, as yet no studies show that antioxidant supplements reduce cancer risk. Even more important, no human studies support the claims that antioxidant use can prevent recurrence of cancer or affect the course of cancer once it has returned. In fact, some clinical studies have revealed that antioxidants have, in some cases, increased the risk of cancer or tissue damage (15).

Free radicals also play a beneficial role in removing cells with mutated DNA through a process known as apoptosis, or programmed cell death. The contribution of free radicals to this process (16) may be another reason why cancer prevention studies with antioxidants that can eliminate free radicals have shown disappointing results. This very same process of apoptosis is often a common final mechanism shared by many anticancer drugs and radiation as they eradicate tumor cells from your body.

As a result, the use of antioxidants during chemotherapy or radiation therapy is controversial. Many naturopaths (and non-credentialed CAM practitioners) suggest that antioxidants will help protect normal cells while you undergo chemotherapy. However, most oncologists and researchers agree that using antioxidants during conventional treatment runs the risk of interfering with desired anti-tumor effects (17). The antioxidants may be protecting normal cells from damage but at the risk of protecting tumor cells as well. This remains one of the most hotly debated controversies among complementary and conventional medical practitioners because the potential danger to the patient is so great.

CAM practitioners, naturopaths in particular, point to cell culture and animal studies that show that antioxidant compounds like vitamin E enhance the effect of chemotherapy (18). These studies are provocative but deserve appropriate perspective. When given at doses much higher than in vitamin supplements, many antioxidant compounds actually suppress the cell growth cycle or cell survival pathways of cancer cells in a manner similar to some chemotherapeutic drugs; therefore, the antioxidants have the opportunity to work in concert with chemotherapy. However, these high-dose effects are likely to be distinct from normal-dose antioxidant effects (19). In essence, "antioxidant" is a poor term when referring to the potential anti-cancer effects of vitamin E alone or in combination with chemotherapeutic drugs like 5-fluorouracil because of the antioxidants' other growth-suppressing effects (18). These high-dose antioxidant effects are currently the subject of investigation by a number of cancer researchers, but the potential of this approach to aid chemotherapy has yet to be studied in a large, controlled clinical trial.

The complexity of how antioxidants operate in our bodies underlines the importance of informing your oncologist if you are participating in a CAM therapy. If you are a member of breast cancer support groups or read periodicals about alternative medicines, you will likely come across recommendations to experiment with a number of substances and bodily practices. Before you follow those recommendations, learn about the therapy that you are considering using. You will find brief descriptions of popular CAM therapies in the following sections. A number of them have been studied in clinical trials with results showing benefit, harm, or no effect. Links listed after certain therapies, as well as the links in the resource boxes throughout this chapter, will enable you to investigate specific modalities, often leading to results of ongoing studies.

Biologically Based Practices

The NCCAM's category of "biologically based practices" includes vitamin supplements; mineral supplements; diet regimens; hormonal, enzyme, and chemical supplements; complex natural products; and off-label use of prescription drugs, vaccines, and other biological interventions not yet accepted in mainstream medicine.

Vitamin Supplements

Potentially Beneficial

Vitamin D: Higher levels of vitamin D (in the form of 25-hydroxyvitamin D) have been linked to a lower risk of breast cancer (20). While not demonstrated yet in breast cancer, higher vitamin D levels have correlated with increased survival and decreased recurrence in colon cancer patients. In general, vitamin D can be obtained through sun exposure and dietary sources (such as vitamin D–fortified milk). Experts on vitamin D recommend taking a vitamin D supplement to attain the levels correlated with cancer protection. Vitamin D supplementation is safe as long as you do not have any risk factors for elevated calcium level (such as bone metastases or granulomatous disease such as sarcoidosis). Supplementation up to 2,000 iu a day is considered reasonable.

No Proven Benefit

B Vitamins: The family of B vitamins includes folate, B6, and B12. Dietary levels of B6 and B12 appear to have no effect once someone is diagnosed with breast cancer. Folate levels, however, may affect breast cancer risk (21). There are no clinical data examining the use of B vitamin supplements after a diagnosis of breast cancer.

Vitamin C: Vitamin C has long been of interest in cancer treatment. Research into vitamin C supplementation has shown that levels associated in Petri dishes with anti-cancer effects cannot be achieved by oral supplementation. In fact, at least one observational study has shown an increased risk of breast cancer with the use of oral vitamin C supplements (22). Studies are ongoing with intravenous vitamin C to determine whether there is a safe or effective dose in advanced cancer patients.

Potentially Harmful

Vitamin A: Beta-carotene (which can be converted to vitamin A) and vitamin A have been shown in epidemiological studies to be associated with reduced cancer risk (23). However, a clinical trial (known as CARET) that evaluated these compounds in men and women smokers revealed that beta-carotene and vitamin A supplementation increased their rates of lung cancer and death from all causes (24). There have been no studies evaluating the safety of vitamin A supplementation following a diagnosis of breast cancer.

Vitamin E: Alpha-tocopherol (vitamin E) has been shown in epidemiological studies to be associated with reduced cancer risk (23). However, vitamin E supplementation has not been shown to reduce breast cancer risk in prospective trials (25) and has been shown in multiple studies to increase risk of death due to all causes (26). Given no clear evidence of benefit, vitamin E supplementation is not recommended.

Mineral Supplements

Potentially Beneficial

Calcium: Calcium supplementation combined with vitamin D is recommended for women to maintain bone density. This may be particularly important for women who have had a chemically induced menopause and those taking aromatase inhibitors who may experience bone loss. Consult with your doctor about taking calcium supplements if you have bone metastases, as your calcium levels may already be high.

No Proven Benefit

Selenium: Selenium is a trace mineral found in food and available in supplements. Most experts agree that selenium has promising anti-cancer activity (27) but can be toxic at very high doses. The studies investigating selenium's capability to lower cancer risk in humans are mixed. No trials have yet addressed the use of selenium in breast cancer patients.

Diet Regimens

No Proven Benefit

Macrobiotic Diet: The standard macrobiotic diet in the United States consists of 50–60 percent organically grown whole grains; 20–25 percent locally and organically grown fruits and vegetables; and 5–10 percent soups made with vegetables, seaweed, grains, beans, and miso (a fermented soy product). The current form of the diet was popularized by Michio Kushi, based on a concept formulated by George Ohsawa. There is no evidence that adherence to a macrobiotic diet affects the course of breast cancer. Nutritionists caution about possible deficiencies in vitamins D and B12, iron, protein, and calcium, but these can be overcome with careful dietary planning. (Kushi Institute, PO Box 7, Beckett, Mass. 01223; 413-623-5741; http://www.kushiinstitute.org.)

Potentially Harmful

Gerson Diet: This is perhaps the most touted anti-cancer diet, in use since 1977. It was developed by Dr. Max Gerson, Albert Schweitzer's physician, and it is now overseen by Dr. Gerson's daughter, Charlotte. The diet is highly demanding. Patients begin by eating organic raw vegetables, with some cooked or animal foods added later. Freshly squeezed vegetable and fruit juices are drunk hourly. Two to three glasses of fresh calf's liver juice are also drunk daily. Frequent coffee enemas are used for detoxification, although "detoxification" is not defined clearly. The diet is not recommended by the National Cancer Institute, and no clinical trials are ongoing for its effectiveness in combating breast cancer. Deaths have been reported with its use due to electrolyte imbalances. (See http://www.cancer.gov/cancertopics/pdq/cam/gerson/patient.)

Budwig Diet: Proponents of this diet, originally designed by Dr. Johanna Budwig in 1951, claim that it prevents and cures cancer. The diet consists primarily of a combination of cottage cheese and flaxseed oil, along with numerous dietary prohibitions. Although widely touted on the Internet as a breast cancer "cure," no scientific animal or human studies have been published regarding this diet, and there is no evidence of its efficacy as a "cure."

Hormonal, Enzyme, and Chemical Supplements

Potentially Beneficial

Acetyl-L-Carnitine: Multiple small studies have shown that oral use of acetyl-L-carnitine can reduce painful peripheral neuropathy associated with Taxol and cisplatin use. Doses in these studies have ranged from 1 gram a day to 1 gram three times a day (28).

Coenzyme Q10 (CoQ10): CoQ10 is a substance that our bodies naturally produce in making energy. It is usually obtained from beef hearts for supplements. Cancer patients are known to sometimes have lower levels of this substance than those without cancer (29). CoQ10 has proven effective in protecting the heart against the toxic effects of chemotherapy drugs like Adriamycin (30). Nevertheless, there remain concerns that protection of normal tissues might also protect the cancer in some cases. More extensive studies are warranted. (See http://www.cancer.gov/cancer topics/pdq/cam/coenzymeQ10/HealthProfessional/page1.)

Melatonin: Melatonin is a hormone that affects our circadian cycle—our seasonal and daily rhythms, such as sleep and wakefulness. It may ameliorate the undesirable effects of chemotherapy and may fight cancer, but most of the clinical trials with this compound have been conducted by only one or two groups. It has been most commonly investigated for brain metastases. (See http://www.mskcc.org/mskcc/html/69298.cfm.)

No Proven Benefit

Immuno-Augmentative Therapy (IAT): IAT was developed by the late Lawrence Burton, PhD, who proposed that four specific immune proteins protect against cancer and that these must be in balance in order to allow antibodies to fight cancer. A patient's blood is tested for imbalances in the four proteins, then specific daily dosages of three of the proteins are prescribed to be administered by subcutaneous injections. A rigorous review of records of cancer patients treated with IAT showed no responses to therapy, though there were no acute adverse effects from the treatment (31).

Indole-3-Carbinol (I3C)/3′,3′-Diindolylmethane (DIM): Indole-3-carbinol and its metabolite, DIM, are derived from cruciferous vegetables. Both compounds show promising activity against breast cancer cells in Petri dishes, but as yet there is no clinical evidence that supplementation with either compound is beneficial in preventing or treating breast cancer.

Potentially Harmful

Antineoplastons: Antineoplastons are a mixture of amino acid derivatives, peptides, and amino acids found in human blood and urine. Dr. Stanislaw R. Burzynski reported in the early 1970s that these derivatives could reprogram cancer cells. The treatment, lasting nine months or more, is administered orally or through an IV infusion on an outpatient basis. Severe neurotoxic side effects have been reported. The NCI has concluded that there is insufficient evidence to support the use of antineoplastons in cancer due to small patient numbers in studies to date. (See http://www .cancer.gov/cancertopics/factsheet/Therapy/antineoplastons.)

Chelation Therapy: Disodium EDTA chelation therapy (oral or IV) has been proposed for many years as a cancer treatment. While IV chelation therapy is medically used for lead and mercury poisoning, uses in other situations have caused deaths due to lower than normal calcium levels in the blood. Renal failure and bone marrow toxicity have also resulted.

Dichloroacetate (or dichloroacetic acid, DCA): Dichloroacetate is a small molecule that has been used in patients with rare diseases of the mitochondria, the energy-producing organelle of our cells. In 2007 researchers at the University of Alberta showed that DCA could slow the growth of some tumors in rats (32). The press hype following their report noted that DCA was not patentable and therefore would not likely be sponsored for clinical trials by a pharmaceutical company. However, some Internet-based marketers are already selling DCA in the absence of human data. DCA is known to cause peripheral neuropathy, and its side effect profile in cancer patients is unknown. Additionally, DCA is listed as a probable human carcinogen by the U.S. Environmental Protection Agency (EPA). Therefore, it is unwise to self-medicate with DCA until more convincing data from human subjects become available. For updates on the clinical trials underway at the University of Alberta, use the following link: http://www.depmed .ualberta.ca/dca.

Hydrazine Sulfate: According to the National Cancer Institute's Physician Data Query (PDQ), hydrazine sulfate does not have anti-cancer activity in humans. The U.S. Department of Health and Human Services has classified it as a potential carcinogen. It may have potential to stave off cachexia (weight loss and wasting away), but the results are inconclusive. In the United States this product can be obtained legally only from a physician. (See http://www.cancer.gov/cancertopics/pdq/cam/hydrazinesulfate/HealthProfessional.)

Laetrile/Amygdalin: Laetrile is a purified form of the chemical amygdalin, found in many fruit pits. It can have toxic side effects similar to cyanide poisoning and is banned in the United States. According to the National Cancer Institute's PDQ, laetrile was found by mainstream clinical trials to be ineffective as a cancer treatment. (See http://www.cancer.gov/cancertopics/pdq/cam/laetrile.)

Complex Natural Products

This CAM category includes an assortment of plant samples (botanicals), extracts of crude natural substances, and unfractionated extracts from marine organisms. Many of the products listed as No Proven Benefit that have shown promising results in Petri dishes and in living organisms are undergoing further study.

Potentially Beneficial

Lactobacillus: A probiotic supplement that has been shown to reduce chemotherapy-induced diarrhea in clinical trials (33).

No Proven Benefit

Blue-Green Algae: Blue-green algae does not appear to offer more than plentiful vitamins and minerals. Possible toxicity and contamination have been associated with certain algae. The National Cancer Institute is funding research to study its potential anti-tumor effect. (See http://www.mskcc.org/mskcc/html/11571.cfm?RecordID=479&tab=HC.)

Curcumin or turmeric: Curcumin is a specific chemical component of turmeric (*Curcuma longa*) that has shown promising anti-cancer activity in Petri dish and animal studies. No human studies have been performed assessing its effect in patients with breast cancer (34).

Fermented Wheat Germ (Avemar): Fermented wheat germ extract has shown some promising anti-cancer properties in Petri dish studies. No human studies have been performed in women with breast cancer.

Flaxseed: A number of animal studies have shown promising effects of flax-seed in the adjunct treatment of breast cancer. To date, no human studies have been performed evaluating its safety or efficacy in breast cancer, although a study in men with prostate cancer indicates that it may have anti-cancer effects (35).

Ginger: Ginger taken in various forms has shown some promise in reducing chemotherapy-induced nausea, but clinical trials have had mixed results due to differences in trial design. There does not appear to be any adverse interaction between ginger and several forms of chemotherapy.

Ginseng: Some researchers are concerned that ginseng may have estrogenic effects and should not be taken by women with breast cancer. It may have a preventive effect, though. In one study that involved humans, 1,455 breast cancer patients who had used ginseng before their cancer diagnosis had reduced risk of death from breast cancer (36). (See http://www.mskcc.org/mskcc/html/11571.cfm?RecordID=501&tab=HC.)

Green and Black Teas/EGCG: Green and black teas come from the same plant, *Camellia sinensis*, which contains antioxidants called catechins. The most studied and marketed of these is epigallocatechin gallate (EGCG). Large amounts of EGCG — such as those present in green tea supplements — may have undesirable pro-oxidant effects in the body. As a result, most experts suggest getting your EGCG from teas. In order to get the highest level of catechins the tea needs to be steeped. Black tea has lower levels of catechins than green tea. However, black tea was found in test tube studies to be stronger than green tea in inhibiting aromatase, and it thus inhibits the body's production of potentially harmful estrogen. In 2005, the FDA concluded that there was little evidence that green tea protects against the development of breast cancer. (See http://www.fda.gov/bbs/topics/NEWS/2005/NEW01197.html.)

MGN-3/Biobran: MGN-3 is a modified arabinoxylan from rice bran; it has shown some promise in Petri dish studies against breast cancer. No animal or human studies have been performed.

Milk thistle: Milk thistle is the common name for *Silybum marianum*, an herb commonly used in Europe for liver toxicity. There are intriguing data in Petri dish and animal studies that milk thistle may have anti-breast-cancer properties; however, no human studies have been performed to date. The safety of milk thistle use during chemotherapy treatment has not been established.

Mistletoe Extract/Iscador/Helixor: This plant extract is used primarily in Europe and derives from anthroposophical medicine, a type of alternative medicine initiated in the 1920s in Switzerland. In Europe, two preparations are most often prescribed by physicians—Iscador (Weleda AG) and Helixor (Helixor Heilmittel). Iscador is sold in the United States as a homeopathic rather than "full strength" version. Laboratory studies have shown that the full-strength extracts kill cancer cells and can stimulate the immune system. Some human clinical trials conducted in Europe, including one on breast cancer patients, showed improved survival time for those taking the extract; however, the studies had flaws that made it difficult to draw firm conclusions. Though the extract has shown some potential in fighting cancer, the National Cancer Institute does not recommend taking it outside of clinical trials. An NCI clinical trial of Helixor A in combination with a standard chemotherapy in patients with advanced cancer has completed enrollment at the time of this writing, but results are not yet available. (See http://www.cancer.gov/cancertopics/pdq/cam/mistle toe/HealthProfessional.)

Noni Juice: Noni is the common name for the juice of *Morinda citrifolia*. While noni juice is purported to have cancer-healing properties, no scientific evidence supports this claim. A single clinical trial has been conducted in cancer patients, completed in 2006, with results not yet published as of 2009.

Shark and Bovine Cartilage (AE-941): Some lab, animal, and human studies have indicated that cartilage may inhibit the growth of blood vessels supplying nutrients and oxygen to tumors (anti-angiogenesis). Some of the purported active components of shark cartilage may be destroyed when taken orally, or they may simply be too large to be absorbed adequately. According to the National Cancer Institute's PDQ, although cartilage extracts have been studied for a few decades, their effectiveness in humans remains questionable. Few studies on humans have been reported in peer-reviewed journals; however, a number of clinical trials are underway. Results from the study of a proprietary shark cartilage product, AE-941, were released at the 2007 meeting of ASCO and showed that adding shark cartilage extract to treatment with standard chemotherapy and radiation therapy did not improve survival in patients with advanced non-small-

cell lung cancer. (See http://www.cancer.gov/cancertopics/pdq/cam/
cartilage/HealthProfessional/page7.)

Potentially Harmful

Essiac and Flor-Essence: Both Essiac and Flor-Essence are combinations
of several herbs, usually taken as a tea. Essiac was popularized in the
early 1920s by a Canadian nurse, Rene Caisse. No clinical studies have
been published on Essiac or Flor-Essence in breast cancer. *In vitro* studies
have shown that both Essiac and Flor-Essence stimulate breast cancer cell
growth. Surprisingly, both ER-positive and ER-negative cancer cells were
affected (37). (See http://cancer.gov/cancerinfo/pdq/cam/essiac.)

Hoxsey Herbal Therapy: Hoxsey therapy consists of herbal mixtures to be
used internally and externally as a salve. While the therapy is specifically
marketed as a cancer cure, there is no scientific evidence of any benefit.
The mixtures contain red clover, which is high in plant estrogens and may
cause breast cancer growth. (See http://www.cancer.org/docroot/ETO/
content/ETO_5_3X_Hoxsey_Herbal_Treatment.asp.)

Soy: Soy, which is made from soybeans, contains isoflavones, a subset of
plant phytoestrogens—compounds that may mimic the effects of estrogen. A study in mice showed that a soy isoflavone, genistein, interfered
with tamoxifen in reducing the growth of estrogen-receptor-positive
breast tumors (38). Most nutritionists who have studied soy effects are
currently of the opinion that it is reasonable to eat soy foods, but they
advise those with breast cancer against taking soy supplements and soy
milk since these concentrate the active chemicals to levels far greater than
in foods.

Whole Alternative Medical Systems

Whole alternative medical systems are built upon complete systems of
theory and practice. Often these systems have evolved apart from, and
earlier than, the conventional medical approach used in the United
States.

Potentially Beneficial

Acupuncture (Needles) and Acupressure/Shiatsu (Fingers on Pressure Points)

Acupuncture and acupressure are ancient Eastern medicines for tapping into what is described traditionally as the body's energy (qi) along meridians (lines) in an effort to restore healthy energy flow. There are no physiological correlates for these energies or meridians in evidence-based medicine. A number of studies have shown that acupuncture can help alleviate pain (39) and nausea (40). All but four states certify acupuncturists. Insist on disposable needles for acupuncture treatments. (American Academy of Medical Acupuncture: http://www.medicalacupuncture.org.)

No Proven Benefit

Homeopathy

Homeopathy is based on the use of medicine with similar side effects to those of the illness being treated but at extremely high dilutions, such that less than one molecule remains. There is no evidence that any homeopathic remedy has any benefit in cancer treatment, but there is also no evidence of harm.

Naturopathy

Naturopathy is the study and use of natural remedies for treatment. Individual components may be beneficial. Practitioners may vary widely in their training, with reputable naturopaths generally having the title Doctor of Naturopathy (ND). If you choose this modality, find a naturopath willing to work with standard medical specialists. Caution should be used when combining herbal mixtures with standard cancer therapies.

Traditional Chinese Medicine (TCM)

TCM is a very broad category, including methods of diagnosis and treatment practiced for over two thousand years. Individual components, including specific herbal supplements and acupuncture, have been tested and shown to be beneficial. Practitioners in the United States generally have a Doctorate of Oriental Medicine (DOM).

Potentially Harmful

Ayurveda

Ayurveda is an ancient system of health care native to India. The majority of treatment is herbal, but metals and minerals may be added. Specific herbal components show promise in preclinical studies, but Ayurveda alone has not been shown to affect cancer progression. Some imported Ayurvedic preparations have been shown to be contaminated with dangerous heavy metals, prompting FDA warnings regarding use.

Exercise and Manipulative Practices

Practices suggested by the NCCAM are based on manipulation and/or movement of one or more parts of the body. They may include exercise therapies, such as yoga asanas, tai chi, and other aerobic movement. They also encompass more Western manipulative practices, such as massage, chiropractic, and reflexology.

Exercise Therapies

Potentially Beneficial

Physical Activity: Many forms of physical activity involving aerobic exercise have shown benefit. The amount, frequency, and intensity of activity have varied in studies. Exercise has been shown to reduce chemotherapy-related fatigue and improve quality of life in women with breast cancer (41).

Yoga: Yoga encourages attention to your body and typically involves stretching and focus on breathing. It can promote flexibility, strength, balance, and good posture and aid in stress reduction. Among complementary therapies, yoga has been shown to be one of the most effective strategies in improving quality of life in cancer patients (42). Yoga of Awareness, a form of yoga developed specifically for cancer patients who may have decreased mobility, has shown great promise in the reduction of pain and improvement in well-being (43). Consult with your physician before engaging in any twisting or complex postures if you have bony metastases or osteoporosis to ensure that these are safe for you. (See International Association of Yoga Therapists: http://www.iayt.org.)

No Proven Benefit

Qigong/Tai Chi: Qi (Chi) is a term that refers to vital energy flow or the body's life force. However, there is no scientific evidence to support the existence of the forces described by these ancient terms. Qigong combines movement with postures and mindful breathing as a means to cultivate healthy energy (these movements are generally encompassed under the term "tai chi"). Qigong also has a spiritual basis and may also be classified in some cases as an energy therapy (see below). Available scientific evidence does not show that qigong is effective in treating cancer or any other disease; however, it may be useful to enhance quality of life.

Tai chi is a more commonly used part of Qigong. Research has found that tai chi can reduce stress and lower blood pressure. The slow movements may also be particularly well suited for cancer patients with decreased mobility or low energy. (See International Tai Chi Chuan Association: http://www.itcca.org.)

Manipulative Therapies

Potentially Beneficial

Massage: Massage therapy has many forms of practice, with Swedish, deep-tissue, sports, and trigger-point most commonly practiced in the United States. Scientific studies have demonstrated that massage can reduce nausea (specifically that caused by chemotherapy) and anxiety. Be sure that your massage therapist has experience in working with cancer patients, particularly if you have arm swelling (lymphedema) or cancer that has moved to the bone. Check with your doctor to be sure this is safe for you if you have osteoporosis or bone metastases. (See American Massage Therapy Association: http://www.amtamassage.org.)

No Proven Benefit

Chiropractic: Chiropractic is best known for manipulation of the spine and is generally safe; however, high-velocity manipulation is contraindicated in those that may have bone weakening due to cancer. Rarely cervical spine manipulation may result in adverse events. There have been no scientific studies performed to date regarding the safety or efficacy of chiropractic in cancer patients. Check with your doctor to be sure this is safe for you if you have osteoporosis or bone metastases.

Reflexology: Reflexology is the art of massaging specific spots on the hands and feet that are believed to correspond to the body's organs and systems in order to bring about better health. One trial has shown a short-lived positive effect of reflexology in lung cancer patients (44). (See Association of Reflexologists: http://www.reflexology.org.)

Mind-Body Interventions

Mind-body interventions seek to have effects on the body through mental practices. These interventions may include prayer, meditation, and guided imagery. Most beneficial practices appear to reduce stress responses in the body. It is complicated to measure and define stress, and the relationship between stress and a system as complex as the immune system makes studying their interaction difficult. Do not become overly concerned with stress, wrongly punishing yourself with thoughts that stressful events in your life caused your cancer and that you must not be stressed or depressed or your cancer will proliferate. A meta-analysis of scientific articles published over a thirty-year period led researchers to conclude that overall no association could be found between stress and breast cancer occurrence (45). Nonetheless, reducing harmful stress is advantageous for enjoying life.

Potentially Beneficial

Mindfulness-Based Meditation

Mindfulness meditation derives from the Hindu and Buddhist practices for developing a calm sense of awareness in a nonjudgmental manner; it is usually combined with a central focus on breathing. Most clinical trials have focused on mindfulness-based stress reduction (MBSR). MBSR is a combination of mindfulness meditation practices—being "in the moment"—and yoga practices. MBSR has been shown to have a number of beneficial effects in people with cancer, including reductions in mood disturbances, fatigue, stress, and blood pressure and reduction in sleep disturbances (46). (See Mindful Living Programs: http://www.mindfulliving programs.com/whatMBSR.php.)

Personal Prayer

Personal prayer or spiritual practice has been linked to improved quality of life measures and improved coping skills. (See http://www.cancer.gov/cancertopics/pdq/supportivecare/spirituality/HealthProfessional.)

Relaxation Training and Guided Imagery

Relaxation and guided imagery often are used to reduce stress and anxiety. In breast cancer patients, the practice has been shown in clinical trials to reduce anticipatory and post-chemotherapy nausea and vomiting (47), reduce cancer-related pain, reduce measures of stress, and improve multiple quality of life measures.

No Proven Benefit

Intercessory Prayer

Intercessory prayer involves another person or group of persons praying for the person who is sick. Studies have been performed evaluating the benefit of intercessory prayer in heart disease patients and have shown no benefit (patients did not know whether or not they were being prayed for). Cancer patients may find some comfort in knowing that others are praying for them, and there appears to be no evidence of harm in the practice.

Spiritual Healing

Spiritual healing may also be called laying on of hands. There have been no rigorous studies of its benefit, but it may provide comfort to those who engage in it. It should not be relied on in place of standard cancer therapy, as there is no evidence that it is effective in curing cancer.

Energy Therapies

Energy therapies involve the use of energy fields. There are two types, biofield therapies and electromagnetic-based therapies.

Biofield Therapies

Biofield therapies are intended to affect energy fields that purportedly surround and penetrate the human body. The existence of such fields has not been scientifically proven.

No Proven Benefit

Polarity Therapy: Polarity therapy was developed in the 1940s and is based on the concept that human disease is a result of body energies being out of balance. While not known to be harmful, no scientific studies have been conducted to show any efficacy of the practice.

Reiki: Reiki is an ancient form of therapeutic touch derived from Japanese traditions. Hands are systematically placed on the body by practitioners to do what is described traditionally as rechanneling the body's unhealthy energies. One study has shown a benefit of Reiki for cancer-related fatigue when compared with rest alone (48), but it was not possible to determine whether the effect was a result of people knowing that the treatment may reduce their stress since this was not a "blind" study in which participants did not know they were receiving a particular treatment. (See the International Center for Reiki Training: http://www.reiki.org.)

Electromagnetic-Based Therapies

These therapies involve the unconventional use of electromagnetic fields, such as pulsed fields, magnetic fields, or alternating current or direct current fields.

No Proven Benefit

Magnet Therapy: Practitioners place magnets of various sizes and strengths around the body in the belief that such treatment can treat pain and disease. No clinical trials support this belief. (See http://www.cancer.org/docroot/ETO/content/ETO_5_3X_Magnetic_Therapy.asp.)

Pulsed Electromagnetic Fields: Practitioners believe that human disease is caused by disruption or imbalance of natural energy fields and that the use of external devices can help bring these fields back into balance. Some of these devices carry claims that they can cure cancer, but no scientific evidence supports these claims. (See http://www.cancer.org/docroot/ ETO/content/ETO_5_3X_Electromagnetic_Therapy.asp.)

Considerations in Using a CAM Practice

Be aware that CAM practices are just beginning to be studied systematically, so much is still unknown. In the absence of studies it is hard to determine what constitutes a therapeutic dose, what combinations may influence the potency of the therapy, what substances may interact to create undesirable side effects, and when and how therapies should be administered.

Special Considerations Regarding Supplements

Consider Standard Treatment Periods a "Protected Zone"

Until more is known about specific substances, the most sensible approach is to eat a healthful diet and avoid additional supplementation while undergoing chemotherapy or radiation. In his book, *Complementary Cancer Therapies*, the highly regarded naturopathic physician Dr. Dan Labriola suggests that supplements be avoided during the period when standard cancer treatments do their work (49). Not only does he describe concerns about antioxidants' potential for interfering with anti-tumor medicine, but he also articulates concerns about creating potential complications such as bleeding and infections. The wisdom of this advice becomes apparent when you consider that years of research, based on thousands of patients, have produced the risk/benefit data that your oncologist uses in offering you treatment options. A potentially adverse variable, such as herbal or antioxidant supplementation, adds further uncertainty into the mix (50).

If you are taking an aromatase inhibitor or tamoxifen after chemotherapy, you might have a longer "protected zone," during which time it is best not to take remedies that have estrogenic effects, such as concentrated soy supplements. As some of these post-chemotherapy drugs are used for periods on the order of years, it is best to consult with a knowledgeable oncologist to know what supplements to avoid and for how long.

Once you are no longer in the protected zone, you may want to enjoy a no-pills, more carefree but healthful lifestyle, or you may want to be proactive and experiment with supplements. What you might try after chemotherapy, radiation, and hormonal therapy to prevent a recurrence could be different from what you might try to reduce the symptoms of metastatic cancer. With late-stage metastatic cancer you may be willing to take more risks. Whatever the stage of your disease, weigh the hazards, costs, and trouble of taking any supplement against its true, or hoped for, benefit.

Dietary Supplements Are Regulated as Foods, Not Medicine

In making your decisions, be aware of the striking differences in regulation between prescription and dietary supplements. Prescription medicines are government-approved, which to some extent assures their effectiveness, quality, and safety. Currently in the United States, the information on herbal and dietary supplements is not approved by any overseeing body; furthermore, the labels can be misleading. The FDA's authority over herbal manufacturers is limited to monitoring that manufacturers do not make direct disease treatment claims such as, "This product cures cancer," but a number of other claims can be made that can be misleading to those who are not informed about drug testing.

Effectiveness against Cancer in a Petri Dish Does Not Mean Effectiveness against Cancer in the Human Body

Manufacturers are permitted to cite scientific literature about supplements, and it is here that the breast cancer patient must be wary of the claims on labels or in literature. For example, a product may be purported to "boost the immune system," and advertising may even state that the product has been proven scientifically to stimulate natural killer cells, a type of circulating white blood cell. The manufacturer may provide an authoritative listing of scientific papers in impressive journals that would lead you to think that these claims are indeed true. However, a closer inspection of the articles often reveals that the cited experiments have not been done in humans; rather, they were performed on isolated cells in a Petri dish.

The results of these types of studies are a far cry from the results of studies in human beings. Many Petri dish–based experiments, often called *in vitro* or cell culture studies, use concentrations of a dietary supplement so high that these levels could not be realistically achieved in people. In fact, one of the major hurdles that a prescription drug must overcome is to prove that the recommended dose gets into the bloodstream at levels consistent with its proposed anti-cancer effect. Unfortunately for cancer patients, dietary supplements do not have to meet this standard, nor is advertising required to make this distinction.

Another related caution in looking at scientific citations on dietary supplements is that Petri dish studies are conducted in isolation from all of the other interacting processes of the body. While a product may seem to increase the "natural killer" activity of immune cells in a Petri dish, the immune cells in the body may not have the same unrestricted access to tumor cells as they do in culture. In rare cases, advertising may cite animal studies that meet a higher standard than *in vitro* studies. But again, the doses of a dietary supplement given to a mouse or rat that shrink tumors or stimulate immune cells are often likely to be orders of magnitude higher than those recommended for humans.

These cautions do not mean that all dietary supplement advertising is untrue or misleading. However, the studies cited in such advertising usually represent only the first step in a long process of investigating a cancer treatment that might ultimately be proposed for patients. Because herbal and other dietary supplements do not have to meet the high standards of proof required of prescription drugs, supplement claims made in advertising are most often premature. Many scientists view these claims as important starting points for continued study, in hopes that from among the thousands of marketed supplements, actual treatments might be selected and proven clinically useful. While this work progresses, the breast cancer patient should be wary and critical of CAM practices that claim to treat or cure cancer.

To aid the public and health-care practitioners in learning about supplements, in 1995 the National Institutes of Health established an Office of Dietary Supplements. For the most reliable information, investigate substances on government Web sites, such as the ones in the following resource box, and consult experts, particularly nutritionists and pharmacists, who can advise you on a supplement's quality and can recommend an effective, safe dosage.

AUTHORITATIVE SITES ON SUPPLEMENTS

- National Institutes of Health, Office of Dietary Supplements: Offers links to databases about supplements and general advice. There is a search engine in which you can type in "breast cancer" to link to the most recent studies, or type in the name of a particular supplement.

  http://ods.od.nih.gov/health_information/health_information.aspx

- National Institutes of Health, Office of Dietary Supplements Fact Sheets: Offers links to fact sheets written for the lay public about select complementary therapies, along with FDA warnings about contaminated or otherwise potentially dangerous supplements.

  http://ods.od.nih.gov/Health_Information/Information_About_
      Individual_Dietary_Supplements.aspx

- International Bibliographic Information on Dietary Supplements (IBIDS) Database: Allows you to search a database of citations and abstracts on published articles relating to supplements.

  http://ods.od.nih.gov/Health_Information/IBIDS.aspx

- Memorial Sloan-Kettering Cancer Center: Provides information on herbs, botanicals, and other products.

  http://www.mskcc.org/aboutherbs

- ConsumerLab.com: An independent supplement-testing organization that investigates specific formulations of herbal and nonherbal supplements for content and impurities; some information is free, but a subscription ($29.95/year) permits full access.

  http://www.consumerlab.com

Evidence of Effectiveness

Insurance companies may pay for some CAM supplements and therapies, and conventional hospitals and doctors may provide them, but these provisions are not always endorsements of their effectiveness. These institutions often are responding to consumer demand. U.S. federal agencies have begun funding large-scale clinical trials for complementary treatments and making the results public, and these results have become one of the most authoritative information sources. In 1998, the U.S. Congress established the NCCAM and the Office of Cancer Complementary and Alternative Medicine (OCCAM) specifically within the National Cancer Institute. As a result, promising complementary therapies are now being investigated with the same rigor as any promising new pharmaceutical medicine.

As discussed, establishing the effectiveness and safety of any substance or physical intervention is a long and painstaking process. Therapies that show promise in fighting cancer cells in a test tube become candidates for further study in animals, and those that are effective in animals are considered for small, then progressively larger human clinical trials. It is important to realize that most substances in the early, preclinical trial phases ultimately are not found to be effective in fighting cancers in humans.

On NCCAM and OCCAM Web sites you can obtain in-depth information, including what studies have been, and are being, conducted on particular supplements and therapies. Some select therapies have extensive information called Physician Data Query (PDQ), which offers the following information for a supplement or therapy:

An overview
General information
History
Laboratory/animal/preclinical studies
Human/clinical studies
Adverse effects
Overall level of evidence

The "overall level of evidence" can be especially helpful since, when possible, PDQ assigns a ranking to indicate the level of evidence available in support of the claims for a therapy. If a therapy is given a score, you can be assured that this therapy has some scientific evidence for what it purports to do. For access to PDQ and NCCAM information, use the sites noted in the resource box that follows.

Be wary of investigating a therapy by means of Internet blogs and listservs. Though these forums can be supportive and helpful, they are not monitored for accuracy. As a result, many forums are simply a collection of well-intentioned but anecdotal experiences. Many forum contributors post valuable information on treatments; however, the information may not always apply to your particular form of breast cancer or your bodily and emotional makeup. It is important to rely on your physician along with your own sound reasoning.

AUTHORITATIVE SITES ON CAM

- PDQ Summaries: Provide physicians and patients with information on cancer treatments, updated continually by the National Cancer Institute's Cancer Information Service, a section devoted to complementary therapies.

     http://www.cancer.gov/cancertopics/pdq/cam

- National Institutes of Health Resources: Allow you to look up a particular complementary therapy.

     http://nccam.nih.gov/health/bytreatment.htm

- National Center for Complementary and Alternative Medicine: Enables you to look up complementary therapies by disease.

     http://nccam.nih.gov/health/bydisease.htm

- NIH Clinical Trials: Show which complementary therapies are being studied by the NIH and indicate which clinical trials are possibly open for enrollment.

     http://nccam.nih.gov/clinicaltrials

- Office of Cancer Complementary and Alternative Medicine: Offers links to FDA alerts and clinical trials related to complementary medicines.

     http://www3.cancer.gov/occam/about.html

- National Standard: For a fee, provides extensive, current, evidence-based information on integrative therapies.

     http://www.naturalstandard.com

- *Integrative Cancer Therapies* Journal

     http://www.sagepub.com/journalsProdDesc.nav?prodId=
          Journa1201510

Selecting a Complementary Health-Care Practitioner

In addition to investigating CAM practices that interest you, carefully consider any therapist with whom you would like to work. Choosing a trained, credentialed practitioner will increase the chances that you will have a positive experience. Ask practitioners whom you are considering hiring where they received training and how long they have been practicing. Most states license acupuncturists and other complementary therapists. You can use the links under particular therapies in this chapter and the ones in the box below to contact national organizations that can help you locate an accredited practitioner.

NATIONAL ORGANIZATIONS FOR COMPLEMENTARY THERAPIES

- Council of Acupuncture and Oriental Medicine Associations
  http://www.acucouncil.org

- American Association of Naturopaths
  http://www.naturopathic.org

- American Holistic Medical Association
  2366 Eastlake Avenue East, Suite 322
  Seattle, WA 98102
  206-323-7610
  http://www.holisticmedicine.org

- National Center for Homeopathy
  801 N. Fairfax Street
  Alexandria, VA 22314
  703-548-7792
  http://www.homeopathic.org

- Ayurveda Institute
  http://www.ayurveda-nama.org/about_nama.php

resources

You likely will pay out of pocket for complementary therapies; it is a reason to be particularly cautious since no insurance company is overseeing the therapy or therapist to substantiate that the cost is worth the outcome. Before you agree to any treatment, a practitioner should be able to answer the following questions to your satisfaction.

Questions to Ask Your Complementary Care Practitioner

What is the aim of the treatment: to enhance the quality of life? to extend life? to fight cancer?

What evidence is there, outside of personal testimony, that this treatment is effective for improving quality of life or enhancing survival for late-stage breast cancer?

How many people have you treated with breast cancer and other cancers using this therapy, and what have been the results?

Can this treatment cause any harm, particularly while people are undergoing conventional treatment?

What benefits can I expect and how quickly?

What is the treatment schedule, and what are the side effects of the treatment?

What costs are involved?

Will you work with my primary oncologist to formulate a plan for me?

Be cautious when choosing your practitioner. Some well-meaning and not so well-meaning providers of CAM approaches are bounding with enthusiastic advice and "sure cures" that can cost you money, time, and energy without producing any result. The very wealthy, and even the not so wealthy, have chased after unconventional cures to little avail.

Be wary, too, of the dark side of complementary medicine. Avoid practitioners who are secretive, or who engage in expensive and implausible treatments. Avoid those who insinuate you are to blame for your disease, or who stridently assert that Western medicine is a conspiracy to take financial advantage of the ill rather than heal them, a claim that equally could be leveled at CAM practitioners. Insofar as possible, check out your practitioner, and trust your instincts.

Because misinformation and unchecked claims have been widespread in the field of complementary care, nonprofit organizations have been formed to combat fraud. Such organizations, and the American Cancer

Society, can inform you whether lawsuits have been filed against particular practitioners, and some organizations offer legal recourse if you have been cheated out of money or have been otherwise harmed.

CAM ANTI-FRAUD SITES

- National Council Against Health Fraud: A nonprofit organization that informs consumers about fraudulent health practices.
    http://www.ncahf.org

- Quackwatch Inc: A nonprofit corporation that, among other services, provides information on products and services, investigates questionable claims, and assists victims of quackery.
    http://www.quackwatch.org

    This section of Quackwatch specifically addresses cancer patients.
    http://www.quackwatch.org/00AboutQuackwatch/altseek.html

Integrative Cancer Centers

Many large cancer centers now offer complementary therapies—sometimes referred to as "integrative care"—and many hospitals offer select integrative support of various kinds such as dietary approaches, exercise/ touch therapies, meditation, and additional methods of psychological and spiritual support and healing. In mainstream medical settings, insurance may cover the costs of therapies. There are also a number of reputable complementary cancer centers that are not affiliated with conventional Western medical care. For a list of various kinds of centers, see appendix C.

The Bottom Line

Be certain to inform your oncologist if you use any CAM therapy. As noted, a number of supplements reduce the effectiveness of chemotherapy, hormonal drugs, and radiation, and some supplements can interact with conventional treatments in harmful ways.

Many current conventional cancer treatments have sprung from the natural world, and promising complementary medicines and lifestyle choices are currently under scientific study. Unfortunately, few popular complementary supplements and therapies so far have been found to fight cancer, though many offer comfort and enhance well-being. If you seek complementary care, be an educated consumer. Much remains mysterious about the connections of body, mind, and spirit. With a critical eye and an open mind, you may find ways that help you live a healthier, longer, and more fulfilling life.

Further Reading

American Cancer Society's Guide to Complementary and Alternative Cancer Methods. American Cancer Society, 2000.

Breast Cancer: Beyond Convention — The World's Foremost Authorities on Complementary and Alternative Medicine Offer Advice on Healing, by Isaac Cohen, Debu Tripathy, and Mary Tagliaferri. Atria Books, 2003.

Complementary Cancer Therapies: Combining Traditional and Alternative Approaches for the Best Possible Outcome, by Dan Labriola. Prima Lifestyles, 2000.

Choices in Healing: Integrating the Best of Conventional and Complementary Approaches to Cancer, by Michael Lerner. MIT Press, 1994.

Integrative Oncology, by Donald Abrams and Andrew Weil. Oxford University Press, 2009.

Integrative Oncology: Incorporating Complementary Medicine into Conventional Cancer Care, by Lorenzo Cohen and Maurie Markman. Humana Press, 2008.

Snake Oil Science: The Truth about Complementary and Alternative Medicine, by R. Barker Bausell, PhD. Oxford University Press, 2007.

CHAPTER 6

Managing Pain and Understanding the Dying Process

> Whatever our beliefs about death, it is a fact that
> there is such a thing as dying well, and that we can
> consciously work toward dying well the way pregnant
> mothers work toward birthing well and with the same
> uncertainty and absence of judgment about how we
> will actually fare in the event.
>
> —Michael Lerner, *Choices in Healing*

> My father's death forever changed my relationship to
> life. Sitting at his bedside when his breathing stopped,
> I was awed by the transformations in his body: the
> deep relaxation that smoothed his furrowed brow, the
> look of pained concentration that slowly changed to
> wonder, the pearly translucence that radiated softly
> around him. I felt that I was witnessing a sacred event,
> perhaps even a miracle.
>
> —Pythia Peay, *Common Boundary*

Two common fears of those with late-stage cancer are pain and death. Though an unwelcome sensation, pain is evidence of our aliveness. It focuses our awareness on our bodies' needs and guides doctors in treating illness. The therapies discussed in preceding chapters are often aimed at reducing pain. In conjunction with these therapies, you may be prescribed pain medications over many years throughout the course of your illness. This chapter opens with information about cancer pain and means for alleviating it. The remainder of the chapter addresses a different but related fear, the physical process of dying. People with serious illnesses naturally may wonder: How much pain might I experience near death? Will I be able to enjoy a fairly normal life until close to the time I die? Those who work with the dying say that each death is different—as unique as the life that was lived before it. There are, however, some commonalties about dying and common concerns expressed by those who are close to death. The latter section of this chapter addresses these concerns, beginning with a discussion of euthanasia and hospice, then moving on to describe typical physical processes of dying and the last moments of life, as far as observation allows us to know.

Pain from Metastatic Cancer

Individuals' tolerance to pain differs depending on a number of factors, including age, overall physical condition, cultural conditioning, and the type of treatment they are undergoing. Women who are premenopausal may be in greater pain during treatment as a result of undergoing aggressive therapies. Seniors, however, can be in greater pain since they are more likely to be taking a variety of drugs that can block or exacerbate the analgesic effects of pain medication, and they may be more sensitive to the effects of pain medication. Each person's pain is unique, depending upon body chemistry, as well as current and past circumstances. Be sure to acknowledge any pain that you might have and ask for care to reduce it to a tolerable level. Pain is often undertreated in the United States, possibly because Americans have an unfounded concern that taking painkillers will lead to addiction. Addiction, though, rarely occurs when opiates are being taken to relieve pain; rather, addiction occurs when pain medications are taken for recreational or escapist reasons.

Some people hesitate to talk about their pain for fear of complaining. Others do not want to admit to feeling pain for fear the cancer is progressing. Both fears can rob you of more quality time. Well-administered pain medication enables people to be more active and less dependent. A number of cancer patients also fear that pain medication will put them into a fog, robbing them of time to relate with their families or time to carry out their plans. Some people want to be conscious of the dying process and worry they will not experience this if given pain medication. Express your wishes since pain specialists can help you retain most of your awareness and function at a higher level than if you were not taking medication.

Your oncologist may or may not be highly knowledgeable about pain control. If you are not able to reduce your pain to an acceptable level working with your current doctor, ask to speak to someone who specializes in pain management. Specialists may be able to offer nerve blocks or pumps that infuse pain medication into your spinal fluid if management with oral and intravenous pain medications is not effective. Hospice organizations are knowledgeable about which doctors and nurses in your area offer specialized pain care. In the United States, the American Board of Medical Specialties recognizes Hospice and Palliative Medicine as a specialty, and many teaching hospitals have a palliative care team. Do not suffer needlessly; seek this help. Uncontrolled, severe pain is an emergency and needs to be addressed promptly.

Pain by Location of Metastasis

Depending on where you have a metastasis, your pain symptoms will be of various kinds, caused by different complications, and alleviated by different treatments. Below are common sources and symptoms of pain based on a metastasis's location.

Metastasis to the Bone

Initially pain may not be present when breast cancer metastasizes to the bone, unless the tumor causes a fracture. Pain from bone tumors is most often felt in the spine, hip, and ribs and usually manifests itself as a deep ache. If the bone tumor is pressing on a nerve, it can cause a shooting, burning pain. Sometimes bony metastasis causes high calcium levels in a person's blood that can lead to increased urination, abdominal pain, weakness, and confusion.

Metastasis to the Lungs and Pleura

Cancer invading the lining of the lungs causes difficulty or achiness in breathing and persistent coughing. This kind of metastasis does not always cause pain but can make one feel breathless, which can be distressing.

Metastasis to the Liver

Tumors in the liver can cause pain by stretching the capsule surrounding the liver. Some people experience discomfort and fluid accumulation in the upper right abdomen, and depending on whether the tumor is crowding the diaphragm, some experience shortness of breath and hiccups. When the liver begins to fail, it no longer is able to filter out harmful substances such as ammonia in our bodies. When the liver begins to malfunction, the ammonia that builds up in the bloodstream can lead to lethargy and confusion.

Metastasis to the Brain

Tumors in the brain can cause headaches and, if progressed, nausea. These tumors can also lead to increasing confusion and changes in personality.

Other Causes of Pain

Some cancer treatments themselves are sources of discomfort. Taxol, Navelbine, and carboplatin, among others, can injure nerves, leading to burning pain and numbness. Some people experience "tumor flare," an inflammation caused by chemotherapy. Though uncomfortable, this is temporary and usually is a sign of response to therapy.

Additional causes of discomfort can include dehydration and constipation, which commonly appear as cancer progresses. Lack of appetite (anorexia) and lack of thirst brought on by some treatments, or by many tumors, can lead to fatigue and loss of muscle mass (cachexia) from nutrient deficiency. Tumors take up much of the body's energy and nutrients. Before cancer has significantly progressed, weight maintenance and hydration may enhance a person's sense of well-being; however, near the time of death, forcing fluids and nutrients into the body can cause increased discomfort.

Describing and Evaluating Pain

In order for you to enjoy and participate in life, pain must be tolerable. Letting your health-care providers know that you are in pain is not complaining. Pain points to what needs to be addressed. Pain also offers information that is necessary for evaluating treatment. Not only does pain diminish the quality of life, but also the stress of pain on the body can be detrimental. Acknowledging pain, monitoring it, and reporting it are important to your physical and psychological welfare. Make this a high priority.

Keeping a Body Diary

You can help yourself and your caretakers better manage your discomfort if you monitor your pain in a diary. Keep a notebook or computer document handy, and on days when you have pain, jot down answers to the questions below.

> What day and time did the pain occur? Consider whether there is a pattern, such as the pain occurring regularly at a certain time of the day.
> Under what circumstances does the pain occur? Does it change when you reposition yourself, shortly after taking a drug, when you eat or engage in a certain activity, when you are under stress, etc.?
> Where in the body do you feel the pain?
> How would you describe this pain?
> How frequent is the pain, and how long does each occurrence usually last?
> To what extent is the pain interfering with your daily activities and pleasure in life?

A Vocabulary for Describing Pain

Drs. Ronald Melzack and Patrick Wall developed a set of categories to describe pain. They are listed below and are followed by a number of other descriptors that can help you when keeping a body diary and when speaking with health-care providers (1).

> Temporal: flickering, quivering, throbbing, beating
> Thermal: burning, scalding, searing
> Constrictive pressure: pinching, pressing, gnawing, cramping, crushing

The following descriptors are often used as well:

Sharp	Radiating
Dull	Achy
Steady	Sore to the touch
Prickly	Numb
Stabbing	Itchy
Shooting	Overall body malaise

The following prompts may offer ways to compare the pain to previous experiences:

> It is as if. . . .
> If this pain took a shape, it would be X wide, Y deep, and Z long.
> This pain is similar to the pain I had when I. . . .

Many times your physician will use a pain score to evaluate and follow your pain. The score is from 1 to 10, 1 being a very mild pain, 10 being the worst pain you ever experienced. While pain is different for different people (the pain you score as a four may be an eight for someone else), the score allows you and your doctor a shared reference to use in following your pain and response to treatments.

The Distinction between Acute and Chronic Pain

Acute pain is characterized by objective physical symptoms that appear even when a person is unconscious—for example, low blood pressure and erratic pulse. Acute pain is of short duration and is the body's natural response to trauma. Chronic pain lasts a long time, weeks or months. Although the autonomic system attempts to adapt to chronic pain, people's lifestyles and personality can be altered by long-term pain.

resources

CANCER PAIN

- Cancer-Pain.org: An extensive site on cancer pain.
  http://www.cancer-pain.org

- American Pain Foundation: An extensive site on how to cope with all kinds of pain.
  http://www.painfoundation.org

- World Health Organization *Cancer Pain Release*: A World Health Organization publication to improve the control of cancer pain.
  http://whocancerpain.bcg.wisc.edu/old_site/index.html

Attacking the Causes and Symptoms of Pain

Pain is treated differently depending on its source. The major causes of pain are bone fractures, pressure on nerves, and organ malfunction. Health-care professionals consider administering the gentlest means possible to alleviate the pain, such as lifestyle changes or pills. Pills can deliver the same level of medication to the bloodstream as injections, though an injection can provide faster relief. Also, some liquids can provide quick relief. When necessary, increasingly invasive treatments are considered to alleviate pain, such as nerve blocks that can deaden or kill nerves. Frequently the source of the pain is targeted; for example, tumors may be irradiated to reduce their size and keep them from pressing on other parts of the body. Sometimes surgery is called for to insert hip pins to stabilize a hip fracture to prevent pain.

Pain treatment is highly individualized. What works for one person may not for another. It requires trial and error along with patience to see whether a treatment will be effective, whether an individual experiences particular side effects, and whether those side effects diminish as the body adjusts to a specific drug. Keep in mind that you may find yourself particularly tired when you first begin taking painkillers. This tiredness is often the result of your body resting after fighting pain for a prolonged time, and your need for rest will diminish over time. Your body also needs some time to adapt to the drug, after which you will become more alert.

Monitor the side effects and effectiveness of your pain medication. When taking pain medication for a prolonged time, people can build up a resistance to the sedation without building up a resistance to pain relief. If a drug is not effective, the dose can be altered, or another of many pain medications can be tried that may have fewer side effects and offer better results. Early pain intervention is key in practically any treatment because drugs for pain work best if taken immediately after pain surfaces. Once neurons repeatedly fire pain signals, the neurons are harder to shut down. Last, pain medication is best taken on a consistent, round-the-clock basis if the pain is constant.

Painkilling Drugs

Non-Steroidal Anti-Inflammatory Drugs (NSAIDs)

Mild pain can be alleviated with over-the-counter anti-inflammatory medicine such as aspirin, ibuprofen, and naproxen sodium. Check with your physician to make sure these drugs are appropriate for you, and take care not to exceed the recommended dosage since some of these drugs can cause gastrointestinal sores or kidney and liver damage. For more intense pain other prescription NSAIDs are used, often in combination with opioids.

Opioids

Drugs such as morphine (MSContin, Oramorph, MSIR, Roxanol, and others); codeine; Dilaudid (hydromorphone); methadone (Methadose); oxycodone (OxyContin, OxyIR, Roxicodone, and others); and fentanyl (Duragesic, Actiq, and others) are in a class of drugs known as opioids. The major side effects of opioids include constipation, lethargy, and nausea, though these side effects can often be managed by starting with lower doses and adding laxatives to the regime. They can be administered orally, rectally, nasally, through a skin patch, intravenously by pump, and even directly into the spinal fluid by pump. Pain specialists rarely administer intramuscular shots since the amount of medication is not easy to keep constant and the shot can hurt. After as little as three days of opioids, a person can be more alert than before having taken the drug. Developing a tolerance to opioids is common, meaning that you will eventually require more powerful doses for the same effect. If one is taking medicine to relieve pain, the need for higher doses should not be confused with addiction, which rarely occurs.

Drugs to Enhance the Effects of Opioids

Corticosteroids (Steroids): These drugs can reduce inflammation/swelling, elevate mood, and stimulate appetite. Side effects can include blurred vision, weight gain, and restlessness. They can also worsen diabetes.

Anticonvulsants: These drugs, such as carbamazepine (Tegretol), gabapentin (Neurontin), and pregabalin (Lyrica), are used to control shooting and burning pain from nerve damage.

Tricylic Antidepressants: These drugs, such as amitriptyline, can sometimes reduce the side effects of nerve damage. The benefits are usually not felt for one to two weeks and peak at about four to six weeks. In addition to reducing pain, these drugs can help combat insomnia and depression. Side effects can include dry mouth, constipation, and urinary retention.

Neuroleptic Agents: These drugs, developed originally as anti-psychotics, can be used for pain reduction, as well as the reduction of stress and delirium.

Lorazepam (Ativan): This drug reduces anxiety associated with pain and breathlessness.

Hydroxyzine: This drug is an antihistamine that quells anxiety. It also helps with itching that can sometimes occur with some pain medications or with cancers that affect the liver.

Bisphosphonates and Calcitonin: These drugs can strengthen bone and sometimes inhibit processes that produce bone pain.

LOOKING UP DRUG INFORMATION

* RxList: Allows you to search for a drug by name and offers plentiful information about dosage, uses, and side effects.
    http://www.rxlist.com

* MedlinePlus Drug Database: A service of the U.S. Library of Medicine and the National Institutes of Health that provides information about drugs through questions and answers.
    http://www.nlm.nih.gov/medlineplus/druginformation.html

Additional Methods to Alleviate Pain

Transcutaneous Electrical Nerve Stimulation (TENS)

This treatment is sometimes used to control spasmodic pain. Electrodes are placed on the skin in the area of pain, and the patient has a battery pack to send low voltage to that area to block pain.

Marijuana

As of this writing, marijuana is legal in the United States for medical purposes in fourteen states. It can reduce nausea, relieve anxiety, and increase appetite, though it usually does not directly reduce pain. It works best with people who have had previous exposure. Marinol, which consists of tetrahydrocannabinol or THC (one of the active substances in marijuana), is approved for medical use for nausea by the FDA. Marinol does not contain the many other cannabinoids that, according to patients' reports, may be needed to produce full beneficial effects.

Exercise

Strengthening muscles and moving joints can decrease discomfort and stiffness and restore balance, coordination, and circulation. Exercise can stimulate appetite, improve sleep, and promote feelings of well-being. Swimming can alleviate depression and keep joints flexible. Even if confined to bed, people report that repositioning themselves and doing flexibility exercises relieve discomfort. Exercise is helpful until the last moments of life, but it is important to slow down or discontinue motions that cause sharp pain or dizziness.

Acupuncture

Some studies have shown that acupuncture can be effective in reducing certain types of pain, though other controlled studies have yielded inconclusive results (2).

Application of Heat and Cold

Cold and hot packs and moist heat can alter sensations and relieve tense muscles.

Hypnosis

Studies have shown that people who are able to be hypnotized can be relieved of their pain through this method. Many countries have nonprofit organizations that train and certify hypnotherapists that you can consult; one such organization is the American Society of Clinical Hypnosis (3).

Pampering

Some people's discomfort responds to a bit of pampering. For example, you may want to indulge yourself by taking mineral or bubble baths, getting a massage, putting on aromatic lotions, enjoying fragrant teas and coffees, eating favorite foods, surrounding yourself with pleasant-smelling incense and candles, or having someone brush your hair.

Creative Endeavors

Some evidence points to creativity reducing pain. Try giving your pain "a voice" on paper, in song, in drawing, or in other artwork. Transform pain into something else, like an oyster takes an irritating piece of sand and produces a pearl.

Visualization/Imagery/Meditation

A number of studies have confirmed that meditation can reduce pain (4). Many cancer clinics have integrative or complementary programs that offer meditation instruction, or you may want to try meditation on your own by listening to a meditation tape. Often imagery is used so that you can envision healing taking place in your body. Sometimes people picture a serene scene. You can focus on your breath, count, or repeat a phrase of your choosing, such as "Pain is a sensation," or "Live fully." You can focus on sensory input in the here and now (sights, smells, bodily sensations, sounds, tastes). You do not need to be overly concerned with what you select as your focus since the benefit is the concentration itself.

Distinguishing Pain from Suffering

Though all beings experience pain as a part of living, humans experience not only pain, but also suffering. It is helpful to make a distinction between the two, pain being a sensation and suffering our interpretation of it—that is, our thoughts and feelings about the pain. By focusing on physical pain, rather than suppressing it, some people can sort the pain sensation from their emotional response to the sensation. In doing so, they can face the fear or anger that leads to their suffering, and both the sensation and the angst are diminished.

resources

END-OF-LIFE CONCERNS

- American College of Physicians: Offers a home-care guide for advanced cancer.
  http://www.acponline.org/patients_families/end_of_life_issues

- Dr. Ira Byock's Site: Offers resources for people facing terminal illness, with plentiful links.
  http://www.dyingwell.org

- Growth House, Inc.: Offers plentiful information on end-of-life care.
  http://www.growthhouse.org

- On Our Own Terms: Offers information about the PBS series of the same name.
  http://www.pbs.org/wnet/onourownterms/final/index.html

Rest assured that it is possible to die peacefully from breast cancer and that many people are fairly active close to their final days. A relatively painless death may be the result of an individual's tolerance to physical discomfort, effective pain management, and/or metastases in locations that produce few debilitating effects or that have few nerve endings. Most people, though—roughly 80 percent—do experience pain in the final stages of cancer, the most prevalent kind being bone pain (5). Still, with proper care, nearly all pain can be relieved. The exceptions are not a result of some specific condition but are tied to the many factors that influence a person's physical and psychological experience of pain.

Euthanasia and Suicide

If pain is not well controlled and becomes intolerable, or fears about the dying process become overwhelming, some people consider suicide or consider asking others to assist in hastening their death. Before we delve into motivations for and concerns about euthanasia, a discussion of types of euthanasia will aid further discussion.

Active Suicide

Active suicide involves purposefully taking one's own life using external means, such as by inhaling large amounts of carbon monoxide or by taking an overdose of narcotics. The Hemlock Society's Web site and the book *Final Exit* detail ways to kill oneself.

Passive Suicide

This type of euthanasia is sometimes thought of as allowing death to take its course by not prolonging life through interventions. At the patient's directive, life-sustaining medications such as antibiotics, life-sustaining procedures such as resuscitation, and life-supporting machines such as respirators can be withheld or stopped. Somewhat less passively, one can die by purposely stopping activities that maintain life, such as by refusing to eat. Starvation can be an unpleasant and fatiguing death, but many people report euphoria near the time of dying.

Doctor-Assisted Suicide

This type of suicide can be indirect, such as when a doctor provides a patient with the means to end her life by prescribing deadly drugs or gases, or it can be direct, such as when a doctor ends a patient's life by administering a fatal injection. Doctor-assisted suicide is legal in a few European countries. In the United States, Oregon, Washington, and Montana legally sanction doctor-assisted euthanasia.

Some consider the debate over physician-assisted suicide a false one to an extent. Heavy doses of opiate drugs, which are often given by health-care providers at the patient's request to control pain or ease difficulty in breathing, slow respiration and hasten death. In a 1997 U.S. Supreme Court opinion, Justice Sandra Day O'Connor stated, "A patient who is suffering from a terminal illness and who is experiencing great pain has no legal barriers to obtaining medication from qualified physicians, even to the point of causing unconsciousness and hastening death" (6).

Other-Assisted Suicide

When someone other than a doctor assists in a suicide, it is termed other-assisted suicide. The ethics and legality of this must be carefully considered. Betty Rollins wrote a positive account of assisting in her mother's suicide in her book *Last Wish*.

Motivations and Considerations Concerning Euthanasia

Physical Pain

If you are considering euthanasia because you fear pain or because you are in unbearable pain, seek help from a pain specialist. Nearly all pain can be made tolerable. Find a pain expert and give various methods a chance to alleviate your physical suffering before deciding to end your life as a result of great physical pain.

Depression

Feelings of despair are common in people who are dying. Sometimes these feelings are present because of inadequate pain control. Still, everyone facing death is grieving, in some way, the loss of her or his life. Depression can be temporary, often a part of the dying process that gives way to the acceptance of death. Like pain, depression has gone undertreated in the terminally ill. If you are depressed, be fearless in telling your health-care providers and/or loved ones. Many avenues are possible for transforming these feelings, such as allowing time for the depression to pass, talking with a good listener, attending support groups, talking with counselors or spiritual advisers, taking antidepressant drugs, reading inspirational material, or engaging in meaningful activities.

Concerns about Being a Burden

Many cancer patients worry about becoming an emotional or financial liability to those close to them. Quite the contrary is often the case. The emotional and spiritual growth for the dying, and those caring for the dying, can alter their lives for the better. Loved ones can become closer, and many people resolve unhealed emotional issues. Positive outcomes such as these may be enhanced with the guidance of clergy, counselors, or hospice personnel. Social workers can also lead you to sources of funding if you are in need. You can reduce, and possibly eliminate, financial burdens on your loved ones by making use of the information and resources mentioned in this book in the chapter about practical matters.

Nonetheless, the expenditure of time and energy for those caring for someone who is unable to care for herself can be taxing. It is unwise to expect a few family members or friends to shoulder your care without a wider circle of assistance, and that assistance is available. If others offer to help, give them some ideas about how they could do so. You might want to suggest a range of possibilities, from small gestures to more involved tasks, letting them choose their level of contribution. Their helping you can help them as well.

Concerns about an "Undignified" End

It is usually possible to avoid dying a horribly dependent, painful, confused death, so be certain you are not rushing into euthanasia when what you fear will happen is simply that: a fear. If you are concerned that you will be kept in a highly dependent, prolonged state of unconsciousness with the use of hospital technology, this concern can be addressed through legal instruments that make clear your wishes not to continue your life through artificial means. (See chapter 7.)

The anxiety about becoming unsightly and problematic is a highly emotional issue. One way to explore this worry is to think of someone you love. If that person became dependent and confused and no longer acted like herself or himself, would you love that person less? How would you feel if this person were to end her life? Keep in mind that your concern for an undignified death may be the last vestiges of your feeling unloved in life, and this may be a time for you to acknowledge the love of others over your own fear of not being loved.

Religious/Spiritual Considerations

Many major religions, such as Christianity, Judaism, and Islam, take the position that only God has the right to end life. Some Eastern religions, such as Tibetan Buddhism, believe life is a preparation for the moment of death; furthermore, the way that you meet that moment determines your next state. Religious leaders from many traditions have noted that the dying process can reveal important spiritual and emotional insights for the dying and those who assist the dying. It is not unusual that your final partings with others, and their witnessing the dying process, will affect their lives in meaningful ways.

Considering the Feelings of Loved Ones

Just as your dying a natural death has consequences for your loved ones, so would your death at your own or others' hands. Since dying is a process, you may find that as days pass and your disease progresses, you may be more or less inclined to consider euthanasia. The decision is only final, of course, if you carry it out; otherwise, to the extent your values allow it, euthanasia is always an option. If you contemplate it, do so considering the above information and the material in links that follow.

resources

EUTHANASIA

- bbc.co.uk: Offers diverse and comprehensive information about euthanasia.
  http://www.bbc.co.uk/religion/ethics/euthanasia

- Compassion and Choices: Advocates for euthanasia in the United States.
  http://www.compassionandchoices.org

- EUTHANASIA.com: Advocates for natural death and against euthanasia.
  http://www.euthanasia.com

- *Final Exit: The Practicalities of Self-Deliverance and Assisted Suicide for the Dying*, by Derek Humphry.

- *Last Wish*, by Betty Rollins: A daughter's account of assisting her mother in hastening death.

Choices in Dying

If you had a choice, where would you like to die: at home? in a hospital? at some special location? How natural or how high-tech would you like your death to be? Most likely, unless you clearly state otherwise or are in hospice care, when you are near death, you will be brought to a hospital. If you would like "do-everything" measures, you will get these in a hospital. If your desire is to die elsewhere and to die without modern technology brought to bear to keep you alive longer, you will need to have an advance directive, a "Do Not Resuscitate" order, and family members who will advocate for your wishes. Without advocates, sometimes advance directives and orders not to resuscitate can be overlooked.

Whether you do, and especially if you do not, want life-prolonging technology, be sure to designate someone who can check that you receive adequate pain medication. If you choose to die outside of a hospital, you can best assure that you have access to pain medication through hospice, though your doctor(s) may work with you directly as well. You can also ask those who are caring for you to make the passage from life to death peaceful and meaningful for you. You may want to consider in advance who you hope can be with you near the time of your death. Might you like to hear certain music? Would you like a certain picture or object close at hand? Would certain smells or clothes possibly comfort you? Would you like to be outside? It is perhaps hard to imagine what will matter to you, if anything, in your last days and moments, but you could speculate and make your wishes known.

Hospice

When medical science can no longer add more days to life,
hospice adds more life to every day.

Dr. Cicely Saunders, a British physician, began modern-day hospice care at St. Christopher's Hospital in England during the 1960s, spurring a world-wide movement. In 1974 the National Cancer Institute founded the first hospice in the United States in Connecticut. Now thousands of hospices can be found in the United States, and millions of people in developed countries around the globe benefit from hospices as well.

Hospice's philosophy is neither to prolong life nor to hasten death; rather, it is to enhance the quality of life. Hospice supports the patient and those closest to the patient near the time of death. It aims to keep the dying person in charge. In concert with the dying person's wishes, hospice personnel follow the directives of the lead physician. They provide information and make suggestions. They offer physical, emotional, practical, and spiritual assistance at life's end. Hospice supports your caretakers not only while you are alive, but also after you have passed away.

Hospices are not all alike. Some are nonprofit; others are for profit. Some require that you stop certain kinds of treatment, even clinical trials, before they will provide care. If there is more than one hospice organization in your area, ask to see each of their policies and what they offer.

Generally hospice workers teach family members how to tend to your needs, along with making available a team of professionals, including the following:

> Skilled nurses who assist with medical procedures.
>
> Nursing assistants who provide personal care such as bathing, changing dressings, and assisting with personal hygiene.
>
> Social workers who provide information about, and referrals for, community services like Meals on Wheels.
>
> Clergy and counselors who address spiritual issues and offer support.
>
> Trained volunteers who run errands, do housework, and provide companionship so that your family and friends can tend to their life concerns.
>
> Bereavement counselors to help the primary caregiver for thirteen months following a loved one's death.

Some hospices also offer physical, occupational, or speech therapy; nutritional counseling; medical equipment; support groups; and inpatient care facilities. If your loved ones are not able to care for you at home, many hospices have a hospice home, a section of a hospital, or a nursing home where you can receive help.

You become eligible for pre-hospice care if a doctor estimates that you could die from your illness within the next eighteen months. You are eligible for full hospice care if your primary doctor, along with the hospice medical director, believes your disease may take your life in the next six months. The majority of health insurance providers cover hospice expenses. Hospice is Medicare-approved, and in forty-one states, Medicaid-approved as well. Some hospices and some care provided by religious orders, such as the Sisters of Mercy, rely on charitable contributions and ask for little or no money for their services.

You may be reluctant to accept help from anyone but those closest to you, but keep in mind that most of those who make use of hospice care report that their assistance was invaluable. You and your loved ones may hesitate to discuss or contact hospice, fearing that to do so means that you are giving up on life. Even physicians often fail to recommend it because of the delicacy of speaking directly to someone about dying. Unfortunately, the reluctance to consider hospice results in people missing out on much-needed assistance. Most people die within two to three weeks of enrollment in hospice. Clearly, most people wait too long to make contact (7).

If you would like information about hospice in your area or if you would like to use hospice services, you, your doctor, or a loved can call your local hospice. You can use the links below to find the one closest to you. Even if you think it may be some time before you need hospice services, consider making contact. The earlier you are in touch with hospice, the better. Early contact provides you and those who will care for you with an opportunity to develop a relationship with the hospice staff. Talking about hospice may be the first step in acknowledging that you will die at some point, and though such acknowledgment is difficult, keep in mind that involving hospice is not a death sentence. A number of people receive hospice care and their health improves so that they no longer need these services.

HOSPICE AND CARING FOR THE DYING

- Hospice Net
    http://www.hospicenet.org/index.html

- National Hospice and Palliative Care Organization (NHPCO)
    800-658-8898
    http://www.nhpco.org

- Caring Connections
    http://www.caringinfo.org

- Americans for Better Care of the Dying (a grassroots group)
    202-895-9485
    http://www.abcd-caring.org

How We Die

But is death as horrible a thing as it is commonly asserted to be?

—Phaedrus

Birth and death are inextricably joined and natural. At our birth our cells hold the genetic plans that will eventually stop the functioning of those very cells. Even if we do not die an accidental death or die from a particular disease, our death will inevitably arrive. Throughout our life at various points we may come close to dying but live on. This is true for some cancer patients who vastly outlive their prognosis or who appear near death, perhaps being bedridden and unable to care for themselves; then their cancers go into remission, and for a time they lead nearly normal lives.

Unpredictability applies to death, like it does to life. Each person's death is different. Some people who are dying from cancer are debilitated for many months; others may appear to be about to die one day, then rally the next in a seesaw fashion; others live a near-normal life until the day they die. What a cancer patient may physically feel leading up to death depends, in part, on what organ is primarily affected. As the disease progresses, usually more organs become cancerous. Very close to the moment of death, the organ that is most damaged may trigger other organ systems to shut down. Respiration eventually ceases, and ultimately we die because the brain does not receive enough oxygen. Below are explanations of how death may come depending upon the organ that is most afflicted with metastases.

Bone Metastasis

Bone metastases do not lead directly to death; however, the tumors can lead to elevated calcium levels that, if not responsive to treatment, can lead to delirium, followed by a coma and death. This would be like drifting off into a dream, and it is not a painful way to die.

Lung Metastasis

When cancer spreads to the lungs, breathing becomes difficult. Oxygen does not fill the lungs and get into the body as it did before the appearance of tumors. Sometimes fluid develops in the lungs as well. When people become breathless, narcotics, barbiturates, and anti-anxiety drugs can help relieve this distressing sensation. As the tumor progresses, patients get weaker, increasingly less responsive, and then pass away.

Liver Metastasis

When the liver can no longer function in cleansing blood, it manufactures a toxic metabolite of ammonia that kills the neurons in the brainstem that control heartbeat and respiration. As the ammonia level builds in the body, people become more confused and then begin to lose consciousness. As the ammonia continues to increase, people drift into a coma and pass away. This is not painful.

Brain Metastasis

With the progression of brain tumors, family members will notice changes in their loved one's personality and weakness in their arms and legs. Sometimes people will have difficulty communicating with words and/or difficulty understanding language. Some brain tumors can be associated with seizures; however, these can usually be controlled with medication. As tumors progress, people will become less interactive and weaker until they pass away.

Commonalities in Dying from Cancer

The following dying process is seen in many people, and the description that follows is loosely based on hospice nurse Barbara Karnes's booklet *Gone from My Sight: The Dying Experience* (8). What is described below is not a certain path. You may experience many, or hardly any, of the feelings and physical signs that are often a part of the dying process, and the process may take place over an appreciably longer or shorter time than is described in the timetable that follows. The last moments of life depend on the cause of death and the individual. What follows is, at best, a rough guide.

One to Three Months Prior to Death

Most cancer patients experience cachexia. This is a condition that causes weight loss and is still poorly understood: tumors secrete various proteins into the blood, such as tumor necrosis factor, that appear to contribute to the condition. People with cachexia usually complain of decreased appetite and increased fatigue. Many times family members will try to convince their dying loved one to eat. As mentioned earlier in this chapter, such urging may be fine in early disease stages, but as tumors progress, the increased nutrition feeds the tumor as well. Eating a lot will not change the course of the disease, and people should be allowed to eat only if it brings them comfort.

As the patient, you may sense you are dying. Often people begin to withdraw from the outer world, sleeping more, having less interest in on-going events or in seeing anyone but those closest to them. You may not care to talk as much as you used to, simply preferring someone's touch or someone's presence. You may lose your appetite. Usually people first stop eating meats, then vegetables, eventually eating only soft foods. Last of all, people stop drinking liquids.

All of these conditions are part of the natural progression of dying. It is fine to detach from the world, as this is part of the process. Your body will let you know whether you can tolerate solid foods or liquids. Instead of dehydration being uncomfortable, it can in fact lessen pain. Let your loved ones know in advance that this may happen so that they are not unduly alarmed and so that they can more easily follow your lead.

Those caring for you can help you. You might ask them to maintain a quiet environment, perhaps limiting visits to a few close people. They can refresh you by giving you a popsicle or ice chips to wet your mouth. They can put balm on your lips and moisturizing lotion on your skin. They can hold your hand and let you rest or sleep. They can help by not expecting you to expend your energy on trying to act in ways you do not feel up to. Let them know, though, that you will be aware of what they say and that you can appreciate their presence.

One to Two Weeks Prior to Death

Generally people at this time become increasingly clear that they are near-ing death. You may be sleeping most of the day now. You may become con-fused, calling out and talking with people who are not physically present, recalling and imagining times and places as in dreaming. The lack of oxy-gen to your brain may also cause you to become restless so that you tug on bedsheets and make repetitive movements. You may begin to lose control of your bladder and bowels. Your desire to urinate might decrease, and the urine itself may become the color of dark brown tea, a result of decreased liquids and poor circulation through the kidneys.

Certain physical changes signal that your body is shutting down; vari-ous life functions are destabilizing. You may have low blood pressure; your pulse may vary from nearly zero to up to one hundred fifty beats per minute. Your breathing may range from as few as six breaths a minute to upwards of fifty. You may moan as you exhale, not out of distress but because your vocal cords are relaxed as the air passes over them. During sleep or deep rest, breathing may completely stop, then resume.

Fluids can accumulate in the throat and lungs that can lead to loud gurgling sounds. You may cough, but no fluids will be brought up. Your temperature may fluctuate from hot to cold. Your skin may become flushed when you are hot, bluish when cold, and clammy from perspiration. Your skin may also settle into a pale yellowish color, though this is not jaundice. Poor circulation can cause your nails, hands, feet, or joints to become pale or blue.

Family members may now realize that you are dying and not want to let you go. In advance of this time you could inform your loved ones that these changes are normal and that the changes may come and go. Let them know that you may become disoriented, and ask them to accept and listen reassuringly to what you might say without contradicting you. Ask them to listen to you as if you were telling them about your dreams. They could comfort you by elevating your head or by turning you on your side should you become congested. You might also find it soothing if they gently wipe your mouth or skin with a warm, moist cloth.

One to Two Days to Hours before Dying

Hospice workers and medical personnel report that many people display death awareness at this point. You may know assuredly that you will die soon, and you may have some control over the time you let go of this life. Some people have been able to stay alive for a special occasion that is about to happen. Some people attempt to stay alive to say goodbye to a loved one. Some people prefer to die without others present. Many parents will die when their children are not in the room.

It can be a great gift to you if those who love you let you know they will be all right after you die and let you follow your inclinations to leave this life. Depending on how you view death and depending on your physical and emotional circumstances, you may or may not resist death when it comes close to you. Some people die peacefully, and others struggle against death to the end.

Shortly before death people often experience a surge of energy. You may get out of bed, want to talk with certain people, possibly request a favorite meal. Then, right before the time of death, your breathing and heartbeat will become irregular; disorientation and congestion will become more pronounced. Your breathing may become fast and raspy. You may develop what sounds like a rattle as air passes over a thin buildup of fluid in your vocal cords. You will not be choking, nor likely be troubled by this, but the sound can be distressing to loved ones if they do not under-stand you are not suffering.

As circulation begins to cease, your skin will become blotchy and ashen-colored. As your body relaxes, you may release the contents of your bowels and bladder. Often your eyes will be open, or semi-open, and sometimes will tear, but you will not appear to be seeing. Eventually you will become nonresponsive. Your breathing can lapse into short quick breaths in the last minutes before dying. You may appear to take a last breath, then two long spaced breaths. Your pupils will dilate, remain fixed and glassy. You will have left this life.

Brooke Daniels, one of the authors of this book, recounts an incident from her experience as a hospice physician:

> I had the honor of taking care of a woman dying from breast cancer. She was staying in our inpatient hospice unit for better pain man-agement during the last days of her life. While she was there, her supportive family would come to visit with her daily. In particular, one of her uncles would come, bringing a warm smile and stories of their lives together in the past. He would also sit by her bedside and tell her about the everyday news of the family. When she was tired, he would just be a presence at the bedside, so she knew she was not alone. As time passed, she slipped into a coma. Her uncle's visits continued, and he persisted in sitting at her bedside, sharing stories with her and the staff. On her last day of life he was an hour late coming to her room. When he arrived, although she was uncon-scious, she lifted her arm, waved, and then peacefully passed away. Her uncle then looked at me with tears in his eyes and said, "You know, I don't know if she was waving goodbye or hello."

Further Reading

The Cancer Pain Sourcebook, by Roger Cicala. McGraw-Hill, 2001.

Dying at Home: A Family Guide for Caregiving, by Andrea Sankar. Johns Hopkins University Press, 1991.

Dying Well, by Ira Byock. Riverhead Trade, 1998.

The Final Act of Living, by Barbara Karnes. Barbara Karnes Books, 2003.

Final Gifts: Understanding the Special Awareness, Needs, and Communications of the Dying, by Maggie Callanan and Patricia Kelley. Bantam, 1997.

Final Journeys: A Practical Guide for Bringing Care and Comfort at the End of Life, by Maggie Callanan. Bantam, 2008.

Final Victory: Taking Charge of the Last Stages of Life, Facing Death on Your Own Terms, by Thomas A. Preston, MD. Prima Lifestyles, 2000.

Grave Matters: A Journey through the Modern Funeral Industry to a Natural Way of Burial, by Mark Harris. Scribner, 2008.

The Hospice Choice: In Pursuit of a Peaceful Death, by Marcia Lattanzi-Licht, Galen W. Miller, and John J. Mahoney. Fireside, 1998.

Last Rights: Rescuing the End of Life from the Medical System, by Stephen P. Kiernan. St. Martin's Griffin, 2007.

The Needs of the Dying: A Guide for Bringing Hope, Comfort, and Love to Life's Final Chapter, by David Kessler. Harper Collins, 2000.

CHAPTER 7

Practical Matters

The avoidance of death is the avoidance of life. . . .
The sooner we can embrace death, the more time
we have to live completely and live in reality.
—Joan Halifax, *The Great Matter of Life and Death*

Don't waste life in doubts and fears; spend
yourself on the work before you, well assured
that the right performance of this hour's duties
will be the best preparation for the hours or ages
that follow it.
—Ralph Waldo Emerson, *Immortality*

Financial and legal matters are inescapable when dealing with a prolonged
and life-threatening illness. It is beneficial to familiarize yourself with
relevant laws and options for managing practical matters such as work
leave, medical insurance, and wills. This chapter provides helpful information on medical rights, medical expenses, and final arrangements. In
educating yourself on these matters, you will be prepared for a host of
situations that may arise. You can save time and money and hopefully
protect yourself and your family from legal problems. You can also best
assure that you will receive the care you would like in your final days and
leave a pleasing legacy.

Medical Rights

Medical injustice for the seriously ill can take various forms, from one's
being denied access to medical records to being fired. In the United States
federal laws guarantee a number of rights; for instance, you are protected
against certain kinds of medical discrimination from employers and insurance companies. Many people are not aware of the benefits and pro-

tections they are afforded under the federal acts listed below. In addition to the federal laws mentioned in this chapter, many states offer additional safeguards and rights. State and federal laws are continually being passed, modified, or revoked. No doubt many of these policies and laws will be long-standing, but just as certainly many will change. Be certain to consult the Web links and organizations listed in the resource boxes to obtain current information.

Americans with Disabilities Act of 1990

This act protects those who are disabled from employment discrimination. A disabled individual who is qualified for a job cannot be denied applying for, securing, being fairly compensated for, or advancing in a job or be denied other standard conditions of employment because of a disability. Disabilities are defined as physical or mental impairments that substantially limit one or more major life activities. Employers must make reasonable accommodations to help qualified employees carry out their work unless making an accommodation creates undue hardship on the employer's business and/or lowers the quality of service or the standard of production. Employers are not required to provide personal items for a disabled employee, such as a lymphedema sleeve; however, they are required to provide accommodations such as job restructuring, modified work schedules, and modified equipment.

If you feel that your employer is treating you unfairly or that your workplace is hostile to you because you have cancer, contact the Equal Employment Opportunity Commission (EEOC). For most workplaces you must file a complaint within 180 days of the time a discriminatory incident occurred and within 45 days if you work for the federal government. You do not have to have a lawyer. An investigator at EEOC will determine whether or not your complaint falls under the commission's purview, and if so, your complaint will be investigated and EEOC will speak on your behalf.

Family and Medical Leave Act of 1993

The Family and Medical Leave Act of 1993 (FMLA) guarantees unpaid medical leave for most working Americans. Those who qualify can take up to twelve weeks of unpaid work leave during any twelve-month period because they are ill or because they need to care for an ill family member and doing so prevents them from working. The family member must be directly related to the person who is taking a leave; not even a parent-in-law qualifies. An employee can request that this leave be intermittent rather than a single block of time.

Your employer must abide by this act if you work for a public organization or company—that is, one funded by local, state, or federal taxes—or if you work for a private company that has fifty or more employees. In addition to working for an employer that meets these stipulations, you must have been employed at this workplace for at least twelve months and have worked no less than 1,250 hours over that twelve-month period.

You and your employer must follow guidelines to obtain what is referred to as an FMLA leave. You need to provide medical certification, and possibly your employer will ask you to obtain a second medical opinion; if so, your employer must pay the bill. Under certain conditions you or your employer may choose to use your paid accumulated leave time to cover part or all of your leave. Neither you nor your employer can designate a paid leave as an FMLA leave after the leave has been taken. When possible, you should request an FMLA leave at least thirty days in advance. You must try to schedule your leave so as not to disrupt your place of employment but not at the expense of your care.

Legitimate reasons for requesting an FMLA leave include receiving and recovering from cancer treatments and tests; overnight stays in a hospice, hospital, or medical care facility; and incapacitating mental illness. During your leave, though your employer is not required to pay you, your employer must continue your health-care benefits. Be aware, however, that under some conditions, your employer may recover health-care premiums the company paid if you do not return to work, possibly making you liable for those expenses. On your return to work your employer must offer you the same job that you held when you took your leave or an equivalent job with equivalent pay and benefits.

If you are among the 10 percent highest-paid employees in your company, you could be considered a "key" employee under the FMLA. If so, your employer could prevent you from resuming your job if it were shown that reinstating you would cause grievous harm to the company. To prevent your reinstatement your employer has to let you know that you are a "key" employee when you make known your intent to take FMLA leave, has to make clear to you that the company does not want to reinstate you and why, and has to give you a reasonable opportunity to return to work after your leave, and if you request reinstatement, your employer has to make the final decision to deny you your previous job at the end of the leave. For further information on the FMLA, look under U.S. Government, Department of Labor, Employment Standard Administration, in your phone book, and contact the nearest office of the Wage and Hour Division.

U.S. DEPARTMENT OF LABOR: FAMILY AND MEDICAL LEAVE ACT

http://www.dol.gov/esa/whd/fmla

Consolidated Omnibus Budget Reconciliation Act of 1985

The Consolidated Omnibus Budget Reconciliation Act of 1985 (COBRA) protects those who leave or lose jobs from losing access to group insurance rates. If you or your spouse leave or lose a job at a place of employment where at least twenty people are enrolled in the company's health insurance plan, you can maintain access to the group health insurance benefits for up to three years. To do so you must apply within 60 days of leaving your job and pay the full insurance costs and administrative fees yourself that your employer was previously paying for you. The group rate likely, but not assuredly, offers more coverage for less money than any individual insurance plan. By federal law your employer should provide you with instructions for enrolling in COBRA. If you work at a place of employment with less than twenty employees, check your state Department of Health and Human Services to see if your state may have created a mini-COBRA for employees leaving smaller business.

U.S. DEPARTMENT OF LABOR: CONSOLIDATED OMNIBUS BUDGET RECONCILIATION ACT

http://www.dol.gov/dol/topic/health-plans/cobra.htm

The Health Insurance Portability and Accountability Act

The Health Insurance Portability and Accountability Act (HIPAA) offers insurance protection for those looking for work and medical privacy protections. Some insurance plans have no "preexisting conditions" clauses that limit when you can start receiving insurance coverage as a new enrollee. However, if your new plan does have such clauses, under this federal act you cannot be denied health insurance coverage for a preexisting condition unless you had medical advice, diagnosis, care, or treatment for it within six months before enrolling in the new health insurance plan. Also, any genetic information cannot be considered a preexisting condition. If you did receive medical advice or care for a preexisting condition within six months of enrolling in your current policy, you can be denied health-care coverage for this condition for a maximum of twelve months.

If you were employed for a year or more and covered under another insurance policy and have not been without insurance for more than sixty-three days of enrolling in your new policy, you do not have to wait to be covered for a preexisting condition. This act also assures that you cannot be dropped from your group health insurance policy because you have a particular illness, nor be charged more than others who have similar illnesses. If you seek new employment, remember that it is unlawful for employers to ask questions about your medical history in a pre-offer interview. At this time you do not have to reveal that you have cancer.

HIPAA also protects your medical privacy. As a result of this act, medical institutions must have your permission before they can send your medical information to others, such as an insurance company or employer. Furthermore, this act requires institutions to show you your medical records at your request. When your health-care provider presents you with a waiver asking you to give permission to release your medical data, keep in mind that in order for you to receive good care many medical professionals need quick and easy access to your records. You can, however, tailor a waiver restricting where your medical records can be sent and/or specifying a time frame for sending them.

U.S. DEPARTMENT OF HEALTH AND HUMAN SERVICES: HEALTH INSURANCE PORTABILITY AND ACCOUNTABILITY ACT

http://www.hhs.gov/ocr/hipaa

Protecting Your Privacy

Increasingly medical records are being recorded digitally into what is called an Electronic Medical Record (EMR), which can be transferred with a click of a computer key. This is a significant health-care advancement as well as a possible privacy concern. In addition to the privacy protections for your medical records afforded by HIPAA, you can ensure your privacy in other ways. It is a good idea to review your medical file periodically to check its accuracy. If you have a large medical record, you may want to request a summary of the file to make copying and reading it more manageable. If you see medical information in your patient record that could harm you if it were released, ask to tailor your permission waiver to eliminate the problematic section, or ask to add your own comments to the medical file, being sure to designate them as yours.

Ask, too, to see who has requested your medical record. You can write a note to be put in your file stating that you would like to be notified when requests are made for your record. In addition to protecting your medical record, to further ensure your privacy ask your pharmacy if it releases information about prescription orders to marketers. Your health information is a salable commodity. Ask the companies or banks that hold your credit and debit cards to whom they release information about your buying habits. Be mindful of accepting cookies from Web sites that enable your Internet habits to be tracked, and be careful when responding to surveys or warranties. Much of the information you give about yourself to others is necessary to complete transactions and is ultimately helpful to you, but be aware that many companies are interested in having this information for other financial purposes.

Be mindful not to sign away your rights when signing medical forms and waivers. Though some forms will improve your care, some are in the health-care provider's best interests, not yours. It is likely that you will be asked to sign a form agreeing that you are responsible for payment for the medical expenses that are provided and, further, that it is ultimately your responsibility to pay for unpaid/disputed claims. This form may require you to pay the doctor, clinic, or hospital up front if you have a disputed claim and may put you in the position of being reimbursed by your insurance provider rather than the health-care provider's having to work with your insurance provider to get paid. Further, signing this form may take away your right to sue your provider with regard to billing matters.

Signing some forms could also restrict your access to view your medical information or your ability to sue your provider for malpractice. As best you are able, do not allow yourself to be rushed or intimidated when you are asked to sign a form. Take a moment to read it over and ask questions. If you feel any hesitation, ask if you can take the form with you to read over and sign later. If not, ask if you will be denied treatment if you do not sign. If you are told that you will be so denied and you still want to go ahead, put a note by your signature that you are signing under protest or duress because you were told by "[name of informant]" that you would be denied treatment if you did not sign.

PRIVACY CONCERNS

- Health Privacy Project: Offers information about individual states' privacy laws.

    http://www.healthprivacy.org

- Medical Information Bureau: Enables you to check if your medical records are on file with this agency, which releases information to health insurance companies.

    http://www.mib.com

- Privacy Rights Clearinghouse: Advocates consumers' rights to privacy.

    http://www.privacyrights.org

Patients' Bills of Rights

A number of times federal legislators have proposed sweeping legislation, known as patients' bills of rights, to protect the medical rights of American citizens. None, as yet, has become law. The most current proposal is the Patients' Bill of Rights Act of 2005, which offers protections for individuals with private health-care insurance and protections for their employers. This bill would put the following safeguards in place if passed by Congress and signed into law:

> It would ensure that patients had independent, timely, and binding external appeals when denied coverage.
> It would ensure that insurance companies were held accountable for denying benefits, while it would protect employers from lawsuits.
> It would require that insurers provide basic, important information to clients about their medical coverage, outlawing gag clauses and practices.

A different patients' bill of rights was adopted by the U.S. Advisory Commission on Consumer Protection and Quality in the Health Care Industry in 1998. The content of this bill of rights overlaps some with the Patients' Bill of Rights Act of 2005 in that it states what rights an individual has with respect to a health insurer; however, the 1998 bill is broader in scope in that it mentions protections individuals should be afforded with respect to health-care providers, such as medical personnel and hospitals. It addresses various rights, including respectful care, nondiscrimination, and confidentiality, that are not a part of the 2005 congressional bill. Though this 1998 document, like the congressional bill, is not law, it has been voluntarily adopted by a number of insurers and providers.

Yet another patients' bill of rights was created by the American Hospital Association; it focuses on the kind of care you should receive from hospitals. You can see all three of these patients' bills of rights using the links in the following resource box. Since most people will have numerous dealings with health insurers and providers, it is wise to look over these bills. You could use these documents for making a case for what is considered reasonable care if you find you need to register a complaint or pursue legal action.

PATIENTS' BILLS OF RIGHTS

• Patients' Bill of Rights Act of 2005 Summary: Lists protections for patients who have private health insurance.
   http://energycommerce.house.gov/index.php?option=com_content&
      task=view&id=1328

(Resources, continued)

• Patients' Bill of Rights Act of 2005: Allows you to track the bill's progress.
    http://www.govtrack.us/congress/bill.xpd?bill=s109–1012

• Patients' Bill of Rights Adopted by the U.S. Advisory Commission on
  Consumer Protection and Quality in the Health Care Industry
    http://www.cancer.org/docroot/MIT/content/MIT_3_2_Patients_Bill_
      Of_Rights.asp?

• American Hospital Association Patients' Bill of Rights
    http://www.library.dal.ca/kellogg/Bioethics/codes/rights.htm

Paying for and Managing Medical Expenses

Problems with medical expenses can seem especially cruel combined with
the stress of dealing with cancer, and unfortunately, they are not uncommon. Millions of Americans have no, or inadequate, medical insurance
and mistakenly believe that the United States has a "safety net" assuring
that anyone can get care without a severe blow to one's economic well-
being. Under the current system, those who are uninsured or underinsured are best off if their income is considerably below the poverty line
and they have few or no assets. In this case people are given some medical
services without charge, and if they seek medical aid, they can qualify for
many programs. Those under sixty-five years old who have little or no
health insurance are the worst off since they sometimes have to declare
bankruptcy and surrender their assets in order to qualify for economic
aid. Ironically, those who can least afford to pay have the highest medical
bills since they are charged the fees the hospital and providers set, rather
than the lower fees that the insurance industry negotiates with hospitals
and providers. Even those who have good health insurance can discover
that it may not cover the costs of certain kinds of care or may not have an
annual cap for out-of-pocket expenses. Also, when people can no longer
work, they can lose their current insurance or have to pay a considerable
amount of money to keep it.

In this section we offer general guidelines for helping you cover your
medical expenses, followed by brief descriptions of government-sponsored

health-care programs; means for getting extra help for medical services (particularly if you have limited resources); and information about handling denied claims, managing the influx of bills, avoiding damaged credit, and handling insurance company denials for treatment. Recognize that what follows is basic information. Programs have changing deadlines, qualifications, and costs. It is imperative to use the links provided to get complete and updated information and to get assistance before you make any major decisions.

General Guidelines for Covering Medical Expenses

The first step for everyone who has health insurance coverage of any kind is to learn what medical care is and is not covered in the plan. Your physician cannot know what every patient's insurance covers, so you need to familiarize yourself with your plan.

If you have private insurance, ask for a copy of a simple, straightforward brief document of coverage, co-payments (or "co-pays," the costs to you for using the insurance), and limits, and then ask for the more extensive written information. Highlight all the areas that you think could be relevant for you, and keep your plan information handy, even bringing it to appointments. Keep handy as well the phone numbers you need in order to call to ask questions about pre-certification, claims, and the hours the insurance offices are open. Checking in advance that you are covered for procedures, treatments, or surgeries will ward off unwelcome news that you are not covered and owe money on a claim.

If you are employed, find out who in your human resources/personnel department can help you with questions or concerns about health-care coverage and workplace policy regarding illness and disability. Read the free copy of "What Cancer Survivors Need to Know about Health Insurance," which you can download or order from the first link in the next resource box, and become familiar with what help you can get from the patient advocate foundations also mentioned in that resource box.

Second step: keep excellent records. Have a notebook or a computer available to write notes when you speak with those advising you about what is and is not covered and why. Do not forget to write down the date and the name of the person with whom you are speaking. Also, from day one keep all bills and receipts of payments. If you have any doubt about a piece of paper, keep it rather than throw it away.

Third step: be prepared for possible frustration and disappointments.

Getting the financial aid you need or a bill straightened out can require great perseverance. Be firm, polite, and persistent. Filing appeals can pay off.

Fourth step: do not hesitate to get help in order to understand medical financial matters. This is crucial if you are looking for financial aid. Most health-care providers can direct you to a savvy social worker who advises people with serious illnesses. If they cannot, look in the phone book for your county's department of social services and ask the department to direct you to such a person. Obtaining the best financial aid is complicated and fraught with hurdles. The requirements and benefits change often, such as each time new legislators are voted in, and programs differ by state, county, and city. You need a professional social worker to know what assistance is available. Many states have Medicare premium assistance programs for which people do not realize they qualify. Local social workers also may be able to direct you to aid programs at specific hospitals, churches, or free clinics and special grants for people with particular illnesses or particular circumstances. The patient advocate organizations listed in the following resource box can also lead you to assistance and can help you decipher programs and forms. If you are in financial need, it is unlikely that you can discover all that is available to you, and it is unlikely that you can handle the bureaucracy without the guidance of a social worker and/or advocate.

Fifth step: if you have financial concerns, talk with your doctor and other health-care providers. Tell them you want the best care, but when possible, you want less expensive substitutions. Ask them to be careful not to order unnecessary or duplicate tests and to let you know when a particular test or procedure they are ordering will be particularly expensive and is uncertain to provide meaningful results. When ordering drugs, you may want to have your health-care plan's preferred drug list with you, and ask to have drugs ordered that will reduce out-of-pocket costs or have handy Wal-Mart's list of generic drugs, which are extremely low-cost. You can obtain this list at a Wal-Mart pharmacy or download it using the Wal-Mart link in the resource box in this chapter titled "Financial Assistance for Cancer Patients."

Finally, do not rush into treatment; become an informed medical consumer. When necessary, weigh the costs of "heroic" medical measures against the likely outcome. It is easy to get swept up in the medical system, the mentality of which is often "try anything at any price." It is a harsh reality that medical care can be expensive and that someone has to pay for it, either people in an insurance pool, the larger society, you, and/ or sometimes your family. Family members may be reluctant to bring up the expenses of unfruitful procedures and treatment near the end of life that drive some households into bankruptcy. Take time to think over the trade-offs of costly care, perhaps with a trusted counselor or social worker. One cannot put a price on life, but a price will be paid for prolonging life, and medical decisions sometimes need to be considered in light of the financial consequences for many lives.

LEGAL ASSISTANCE REGARDING MEDICAL RIGHTS

- Cancer Care: Offers "The Challenge of Cancer in the Workplace: How to Communicate with Your Employer."
  800-813-HOPE or 212-221-3300 for recording
  http://www.cancercare.org

- National Employment Lawyers Association: Advocates for employee rights.
  http://www.nela.org

- National Coalition for Cancer Survivorship: Offers "Working It Out: Your Employment Rights as a Cancer Survivor."
  http://www.canceradvocacy.org/resources/publications/
    employment.pdf

- National Coalition for Cancer Survivorship: Offers information on current laws and policies to ensure that all Americans have access to quality cancer care.
  http://www.canceradvocacy.org/get-involved/cancer-advocacy-
    and-policy

- National Coalition for Cancer Survivorship: Provides a free copy of "What Cancer Survivors Need to Know about Health Insurance," which explains Medicare, Medicaid, and Medigap programs in clear language.
  http://www.canceradvocacy.org/resources/publications/insurance.pdf

- U.S. Department of Health and Human Services: Provides the latest information on federal laws related to health care, Medicare, Medicaid, and Caregivers and provides statistics.
  http://www.hhs.gov/aging/index.shtml

resources

(Resources, continued)

- Breast Cancer Legal Project: Offers "Surviving the Legal Challenges: A Resource Guide for Women with Breast Cancer"; free for breast cancer survivors in California, $10 for out of state.
  888-774-5200 or 213-637-9900 for publication
  http://www.cwlc.org

- Georgetown University Health Policy Institute: Offers consumer guides for each state and the District of Columbia that discuss legal rights with regard to getting and keeping health insurance.
  http://www.healthinsuranceinfo.net

- American Bar Association: Lists some breast cancer legal services in selected areas of the country for those with low incomes.
  http://www.abanet.org/women/probono.html

- LambLawOffice.com: Allows you to look up by state the legal amount one can be charged to obtain medical records.
  http://www.lamblawoffice.com/medical-records-copying-charges.html

- Cancer Legal Resource Center: Provides free advice on legal matters related to cancer.
  http://www.disabilityrightslegalcenter.org/about/
    cancerlegalresource.cfm

- Patient Advocate Foundation: Offers assistance in dealing with employment discrimination, denial of insurance coverage, and government assistance programs.
  http://www.patientadvocate.org

- National Patient Advocate Foundation: Provides information and supports access to health care.
  http://www.npaf.org/about-npaf/index.html

- Center for Patient Partnerships: Provides an application process to obtain an advocate who once was a patient to help you with medical, legal, and financial matters. Komen advocates are available to aid breast cancer patients.
  http://patientpartnerships.krambs.com

U.S. Government–Sponsored Health Care
and Cost Coverage for the Uninsured

Medicare

Medicare is federally funded health insurance for people who are sixty-five years old and older and for those under sixty-five who have been receiving social security disability benefits for twenty-four months. There are different kinds of Medicare coverage (A, B, C, D), all of which usually require you to pay out-of-pocket expenses for various kinds of care to varying degrees. You can learn the current cost for premiums (the cost to you for having this insurance) and the deductibles and co-pays by going to the first Web site in the next resource box and looking on the site for "Medicare and You." Although Medicare is a federally funded program, coverage is administered through individual states; therefore, some treatments are covered in some states and not in others.

Because Medicare does not have a cap on out-of-pocket expenses and does not cover all types of medical expenses, many people have additional private coverage. Below are brief descriptions of the different kinds of Medicare coverage. Because of their complexity, we advise you to familiarize yourself with further information using the Web links in the next resource box, including the link leading to your Senior Health Insurance Information Program (SHIIP). Wikipedia has reader-friendly information on Medicare as well.

Medicare Part A: Hospital Costs: Medicare A helps pay for hospital costs, skilled nursing facilities, hospice, and chemotherapy drugs when they are administered in a medical facility, and expenses associated with clinical trials such as tests and checkups, but it does not pay for the experimental drugs themselves, which are usually covered by the pharmaceutical company producing them. Part A covers overnight stays in the hospital and convalescence in a skilled nursing facility if certain criteria are met. If the criteria are met, the first twenty days in a skilled nursing facility are paid for in full. After that period Medicare requires a co-payment that in 2009 was $133.50 per day. Medicare's hospice benefit covers services related to terminal illness with minimal co-payments for drugs and respite care. Medicare does not cover the cost of room and board at a residential hospice.

Medicare Part B: Medical Insurance: Medicare B pays for 80 percent of approved medical expenses, which can include doctors' services, outpatient hospital care, medical tests, physical and mental therapists, and some medical supplies. It covers all chemotherapy drugs that are administered through an IV and the same drugs in pill form if they are available, along with certain anti-nausea drugs. Medicare does not cover private-duty nursing or personal care services such as help with bathing, eating, running errands, or cleaning house, though Medicaid may help with those services. The premium for Medicare B is determined by your income. In 2009 the standard premium was $96.40 a month, with a $135 annual deductible. Those whose income is below 135 percent of the federal poverty line and who have limited assets are eligible for additional subsidies through the Medicare savings programs.

Medicare Advantage (Previously Called Medicare Choice or Medicare Part C): Medicare Advantage represents private insurers who have contracted with the government to provide your Medicare benefits. The coverage is unique in that these insurers must enroll participants regardless of their age or health status, but they can restrict the doctors and hospitals to which you can go. Sometimes even if your doctor and hospital are in an insurer's "network"—meaning that the insurer will help cover the costs if you obtain your care from the providers in the network—the plan will not pay for services that are traditionally covered under Medicare. Once you sign up for a plan, you cannot change or cancel your plan for one year, though there is an appeal process. You can compare plans using links in the Web sites in the following resource box. We advise you not to sign up for a plan without speaking first to a social worker or patient advocate since comparing plans is complicated, and it is not always beneficial to enroll in Medicare Advantage. Be advised that it is not legal in any state for companies to solicit you to join any Medicare plans or Medicare supplemental plans by phoning or going door to door; so do not respond to such requests.

Medicare Part D—Prescription Drug Coverage: Medicare D represents private insurers who help cover certain prescription costs. If you do not have other drug coverage, be sure you look into Medicare D near the time you turn sixty-five since there is a financial penalty for enrolling after you are eligible. If you have few resources, see if you qualify for Medicare Part D Low Income Assistance through the Social Security Administration; such assistance significantly reduces out-of-pocket costs. If you have private health insurance, your current prescription benefits may be better than those offered by insurers through Medicare D, and by law your current insurer must let you know if this is indeed the case. Any prescription coverage as good as or better than Medicare's is called creditable coverage. You need to carefully consider whether you should enroll in this coverage and compare various insurers' plans. Nearly all plans require monthly premiums and co-payments. Certain plans do, however, significantly reduce costs for some people.

Which drugs are covered varies from plan to plan in Medicare D. Some of the drugs you may need could already be covered under Medicare A and B, so you want to be sure that a plan will help you further cover those costs or the costs of other uncovered drugs that you will be taking. You can get free information about a plan by calling Medicare or SHIIP, or you can also speak to a social worker or a patient advocate. Once you sign up, you cannot change or cancel your plan for one year, but there is an appeal process if you discover your medications are not covered. Do not end a program for which you have signed up unless you are sure you qualify for other kinds of assistance.

Medicare Supplemental Insurance (Also Called Medigap Insurance): Medicare Supplemental Insurance refers to private insurance from companies that are regulated by, but do not contract with, the government. If you are sixty-five or older and purchase one of these supplemental insurance policies within six months of enrolling in Medicare Part B, you cannot be denied coverage, regardless of your medical condition. These policies do not cover prescription costs, but they may help with other medical expenses not covered, or not fully covered, by Medicare. For this supplemental coverage to benefit you, you must be familiar with what coverage you currently have, then carefully compare that with what Medicare Supplemental Insurance plans offer, considering the premiums, deductibles, and co-pays. Once again it is best to speak with those who are knowledgeable about Medicare programs before you enroll in any of these plans.

MEDICARE ASSISTANCE

- Medicare and Medigap: An extensive site that includes information on enrollment and services covered and allows you to compare health and prescription drug plans.

    800-633-4227

    http://www.medicare.gov

(Resources, continued)

• State Health Insurance Assistance Program (SHIP): An independent source of information that helps people sort through confusing Medicare information by state of residence.
  http://www.shiptalk.org/Public/home.aspx?ReturnUrl=%2fdefault.aspx

• Medicare Rights Center: An independent source of health care that assists people with Medicare.
  http://www.medicarerights.org

Medicaid

Medicaid helps cover medical expenses for people with few resources and low incomes. The federal and state governments share in providing these funds to individuals, so the specifics for Medicaid eligibility and coverage vary from state to state. If you do not meet the criteria for benefits, it may be possible for you to pay off medical bills each month and/or reduce your income by purchasing other approved items and services, then count these payments as a means for reducing your monthly income to the level that would qualify you for Medicaid assistance. You may not meet the criteria for benefits if you recently immigrated to the United States. Most states require that you live in the country a minimum of five years before being eligible for Medicaid.

It can take 45–90 days to enroll in Medicaid. A social worker or a patient advocate from your doctor's office may be able to speed the process by speaking with a Medicaid case manager. If your prognosis is to live less than six months, an expedited review can be requested. Call your county department of social services to learn how to start the application process for Medicaid as soon as possible. You will likely need to supply the names, addresses, and phone numbers of the physicians who will treat you, as well as copies of personal information such as tax records, bank statements, vehicle and property taxes, and your Social Security card. From the beginning, keep receipts of all medical expenses, including equipment, supplies, over-the-counter medications, and transportation costs to medical appointments. Reimbursement for expenses is retroactive up to three months once your Medicaid application is approved. Be aware that not all doctors will see Medicaid patients, and the physicians that do usually limit the number of Medicaid patients they see since Medicaid often reimburses them less than what they typically charge for their services.

Learn more about your state's program through the Web link in the resource box below or by contacting your state's department of social services and/or health. The phone number should be listed in the government pages of your local phone book.

U.S. GOVERNMENT MEDICAID

http://www.cms.hhs.gov/home/medicaid.asp

State Insurance Plans for High-Risk Applicants

If you do not qualify for government programs such as Medicare, Medicaid, and COBRA, you may be able to reduce costs for private insurance premiums if your state has a state insurance plan for high-risk applicants. Contact your state insurance commission for further information, and investigate the state risk pools using the link in the next resource box.

STATE INSURANCE PLANS

* National Association of State Comprehensive Health Insurance Plans: Lists states with high-risk pools, including Web sites and phone numbers.
  http://www.naschip.org/states_pools.htm

Breast and Cervical Cancer Treatment and Prevention Act

Even if you do not qualify for Medicaid because your income is above your state's eligibility level, you may still qualify for medical assistance through the Breast and Cervical Cancer Treatment and Prevention Act. In order to enroll you must get screened for cancer at a Centers for Disease Control and Prevention (CDC) site. This act provides the following services to low-income or uninsured women:

Clinical breast examinations	Referrals to treatment
Mammograms	Diagnostic testing for women
Pap tests	whose screening outcome
Surgical consultation	is abnormal

You can learn more about qualifying for this assistance and find out if there is a CDC site near you by using the link in the following resource box.

BREAST AND CERVICAL CANCER TREATMENT AND PREVENTION ACT

• Centers for Disease Control and Prevention: To learn more about the Breast and Cervical Cancer Treatment and Prevention Act and locate a screening site nearest you.

888-842-6355

http://www.cdc.gov/cancer/nbccedp/about.htm

Workplace Disability Benefits

If you become disabled while employed, contact your workplace's human resource office to learn whether you are covered by a company disability policy and what the qualifications and benefits are.

Social Security Disability Benefits

If you have paid into Social Security for a number of years, you, and possibly members of your family, can qualify for disability benefits. You must meet the government's definition of disability and be completely unable to work. The benefits begin after the sixth month of your disability and are based on your average earnings covered by Social Security.

Approval for Social Security disability takes 120 days. If you are denied, appeal. You can learn about the qualifications and apply for disability using the first link in the following resource box.

Supplemental Security Income

If you become disabled and have few financial resources, you may be eligible for supplemental security income to help cover costs for basic needs such as food, clothing, and shelter. You can learn if you are eligible for benefits and how to apply using the first link in the resource box below.

SOCIAL SECURITY DISABILITY PROGRAMS AND ADMINISTRATION

- Social Security Online
  http://www.ssa.gov/disability

- Social Security Administration: Apply and learn where to find your local Social Security office.
  800-772-1213
  http://www.ssa.gov

Veterans' Benefits

Veterans are entitled to certain free or low-cost health care at veterans' hospitals or, in some cases, at private hospitals if no Veterans' Administration (VA) hospital is within driving distance. The type and level of care is determined by various factors, including a veteran's type of discharge, length of service, extent of service-connected disability, and financial need. If the veteran's service took place after 1980, he or she must have served a minimum of two years. Spouses and children of veterans may be entitled to some health care at a VA hospital and to grants that cover some expenses. To learn more, explore the link in the resource box below and contact a social worker at a VA facility near you. You can learn where the nearest facility is, learn about health-care eligibility, and apply for care at the link below or by calling the VA.

VETERANS' BENEFITS ADMINISTRATION

877-222-8387
http://www.vba.va.gov

Income Tax Deductions

If you itemize when paying federal taxes, you can deduct medical expenses that exceed 7.5 percent of your adjusted gross income if you are not in a high tax bracket. Keep all receipts for all out-of-pocket expenses, including such costs as co-pays, prescriptions, wigs, transportation to medical appointments, and dental expenses. Also, check whether or not your state has medical tax deductions.

INCOME TAX DEDUCTIONS

• Internal Revenue Service, U.S. Department of the Treasury
   800-829-1040 for information
   800-829-3676 for publications
   http://www.irs.gov

Cafeteria and Flexible Benefit Plans

If your employer offers a cafeteria plan, also referred to as a flexible benefits plan or health-care savings account (HSA), you can designate that a portion of your salary be set aside to cover medical services during a given year. The money set aside is not taxable, reducing your taxable income. Be careful, though. You can lose all or some of the money that was set aside if you overestimate your medical expenses. In the case of overestimation the money is not returned to you but goes to your employer and the company managing the plan.

Hill-Burton Act of 1946

Even if you have assets, if you have a low income, you may be able to get inexpensive treatment at hospitals that receive federal funding under the Hill-Burton Act. You do not need to be a U.S. citizen, but you must have resided in the country for a minimum of three months to qualify. Hospitals choose which particular treatments they will provide to the needy, so you need to check what services under this act are provided at a hospital near you. Funds are limited and can run out quickly, so it is best to apply early each new year. To find hospitals near you, contact the closest department of health and human services, or call the hotline listed in the following resource box.

resources

TREATMENT PROVISIONS UNDER THE HILL-BURTON ACT

• U.S. Department of Health and Human Services, Health Resources and Services Administration: Lists the steps for applying for Hill-Burton free or reduced-cost care.

  http://www.hrsa.gov/hillburton

• Hill-Burton Hotline
  800-683-0742
  800-492-0359 in Maryland

Hospital Charges for the Uninsured

All hospitals, whether they are public, private nonprofit, or private for profit, are obligated to save people's lives in an emergency, regardless of whether an individual has insurance; however, only public hospitals are under obligation to offer continued care. All hospitals will charge you for the fees associated with their services. If you have absolutely no resources, these charges may be written off, but if you have a few resources, your assets will be tapped for payment. For those with few resources there are sometimes programs, like the ones mentioned in this section, that may offer help, so it is important to speak to a social worker affiliated with the hospital or one who is knowledgeable about local resources to assist you in lowering the hospital charges.

Obtaining Health Care Abroad

If you have assets that you fear will be severely depleted by medical bills, you could look into getting your medical care abroad. Increasingly Americans are making this choice. When selecting a medical facility, look into whether it is accredited by the Joint Commission on Accreditation of Healthcare Organizations International, using the Web site in the next resource box. You would, of course, need to compare the total costs of your medical bills in the United States with the costs of your medical bills abroad, including travel and lodging costs. Some services, such as Med-Retreat, have sprung up to do that for you and to make arrangements for your care.

If you live near the Canadian or Mexican border, you could also look

Practical Matters   233

into the current laws about purchasing your pharmaceuticals from those countries. Be highly suspicious of any pharmacy that does not require a prescription; however, some drugs that require a prescription in the United States do not in other countries.

If your parent(s) or grandparent(s) are from another country that has nationalized health care, you may be able to become a citizen of that country and be covered under that country's health-care plan. You could start by contacting that country's consulate in the United States to learn about citizenship criteria.

OBTAINING HEALTH CARE OUTSIDE OF THE UNITED STATES

- Joint Commission on Accreditation of Healthcare Organizations International: Lists accredited health organizations worldwide.
  http://www.jointcommissioninternational.com

- U.S. Department of State: Offers a link to the foreign consulate organizations in the United States.
  http://www.state.gov/s/cpr/rls/fco

- MedRetreat: Explains the process of going abroad for health care and lists surgeries and tests offered through MedRetreat.
  http://www.medretreat.com/index.html

- PharmacyChecker: Allows you to select reputable domestic and international pharmacies to obtain the best prices on specific medicines.
  http://pharmacychecker.com

resources

Nonprofit, Private, and Grassroots Assistance

State and local health and human service social workers are aware of private funding and other types of assistance for those with cancer. Many organizations and charities offer free or sliding-scale rates for services such as counseling, advocacy, support groups, and practical in-home assistance (shopping, cleaning, meals, and companionship). For example, the American Cancer Society often provides transportation to appointments, educational pamphlets, and contact with others who have advanced breast cancer, along with helpful goods such as wigs, hats, cosmetics, and breast prostheses. Also, national and local religious orders and churches, such as

Catholic Charities, often provide help for those with serious illnesses. In addition to exploring local resources, check the cancer Web sites listed in the following resource box. Last, some people have found that their own, or their family and friends', grassroots fund-raising helped them manage difficult financial times. People have successfully held benefits or spaghetti dinners or have sent out a call over e-mail or a Web site to raise money to help someone unable to pay for a medical procedure or treatment. It takes considerable effort and persistence, but when people ask for and seek the assistance they need, many times they find helping hands.

FINANCIAL ASSISTANCE FOR CANCER PATIENTS

- Linking ARMS: CancerCare and Susan G. Komen Breast Cancer Foundation offer grants for women with breast cancer who are underserved, uninsured, and underinsured.

  http://www.komen.org/intradoc-cgi/idc_cgi_isapi.dll?IdcService=SS_
  GET_PAGE&ssDocName=LinkingARMS

- American Cancer Society: Offers comprehensive information with links to financial support.

  800-227-2345

  http://www.cancer.org

- National Breast Cancer Coalition: Provides updates on legislation that affects access to health care.

  http://www.natlbcc.org

- Cancer Care Inc.: Publishes *A Helping Hand: The Resource Directory for People with Cancer* and manages the AVONCares Program for Medically Underserved Women, which helps women regardless of citizenship.

  800-813-4673 or 212-712-8367

  http://www.cancercare.org/services.html

- YWCA ENCOREplus Program: Offers a variety of help to support women who are medically underserved.

  800-953-7587

  http://www.ywca.org/site/pp.asp?c=djISI6PIKpG&b=297532

(Resources, continued)

- National Council on the Aging, BenefitsCheckUp: Provides ways to connect to government programs to help with health-care costs and other benefits for older people.
    http://www.benefitscheckup.org

- National Association of Hospital Hospitality Houses: Helps with housing for those needing treatment away from home.
    800-542-9730
    http://www.nahhh.org

- National Association of Healthcare Transport Management: Helps patients cover costs for airline travel for treatment.
    800-296-1217
    http://www.nahtm.org

- Corporate Angel Network: Arranges free transportation for cancer patients using empty seats on corporate jets.
    http://www.corpangelnetwork.org

- The Wellness Community: Offers social services.
    888-793-WELL
    http://www.thewellnesscommunity.org

PRESCRIPTION ASSISTANCE

For help in paying for prescription drugs, contact the company that makes the drug you need, and ask if it has a compassionate care or indigent patient program. Many pharmaceutical companies do. If so, find out the requirements for participation. Also try the following organizations.

- Department of Health and Human Services: Put "prescription drug assistance" into the search engine to learn what federal and state programs are available.
    http://www.hhs.gov

(Resources, continued)

- Pharmaceutical Research and Manufactures of America: Helps match people to prescription aid using an online questionnaire.
  https://www.pparx.org/Intro.php

- Cancer Supportive Care Programs National and International Drug Assistance Programs: Lists numerous programs offered by pharmaceutical companies.
  http://www.cancersupportivecare.com/drug_assistance.html

- NeedyMeds.com: Offers general information about how to cover pharmaceutical costs.
  http://www.needymeds.com

- Together-Rx.com: Offers a prescriptions savings program to eligible Medicare enrollees.
  http://www.togetherrxaccess.com

- The Medicine Program: Offers some options for obtaining lower-cost prescription drugs.
  http://www.themedicineprogram.com

- Wal-Mart: Offers over three hundred different drugs at very low cost— under $10 per prescription fill or refill (up to a thirty-day supply); includes antibiotic, antidepressant, anti-inflammatory, and anxiety medicines. The list can be viewed on the site. The program is available at all Wal-Mart, Sam's Club, and Neighborhood Market pharmacies (except in North Dakota, where Wal-Mart does not operate its own pharmacies but instead leases space to third-party providers). Some other large box stores are offering programs as well.
  http://www.walmart.com/catalog/catalog.do?cat=546834
  http://www.walmart.com/catalog/catalog.gsp?cat=487805

Tapping into Assets

In addition to obtaining outside funding to cover your medical expenses, you likely can, if necessary, liquidate assets. This section lists possible assets you own and can tap into. Withdrawing money early out of insurance and saving plans nearly always diminishes their current and future worth. Even so, cashing in assets may subsidize a treatment or give you the chance of a lifetime to fulfill a longed-for wish.

IRAs and Annuities

Generally, people are penalized 20–40 percent on any money that is withdrawn early from an IRA or an annuity, with the highest penalty levied on those less than 59.5 years old. However, there is no penalty if you qualify for a hardship exception. To be eligible you must have few assets, your medical expenses must amount to 7.5 percent or more of your gross adjusted income, and you must show that you will use the money from your IRA in order to cover your medical expenses.

Life Insurance

Life insurance policies often have provisions for you to obtain your benefits before you die. Check with your agent and/or employee human resources service representative. It may be possible for you to receive accelerated benefits on your insurance or take out loans against your insurance if doctors estimate you have fewer than twelve months to live.

Reverse Mortgages

If you are sixty-two years old or older and have nearly paid off your home mortgage or if you own your home outright, you can see if you qualify for a reverse mortgage. People often consider this option if they are "cash poor but house rich." A reverse mortgage is a loan against your home. The money you receive is the equity you have paid to own your home. You retain ownership of your home, and you continue to maintain the property and pay property taxes. You can opt to have the loan money paid to you in a variety of ways, including a lump sum, monthly payments, a line of credit, or a combination of these. The money from the loan is tax-free and does not affect your Medicare or Social Security eligibility, but it can impact your eligibility for Medicaid and supplemental Social Security benefits.

You will pay an interest fee on the loan and closing costs that are similar to fees for buying a house; both interest rates and closing costs differ by lender. When the loan comes due because you either move out of your house, sell it, or die, the loan is paid off with the equity in your home, reducing or eliminating the money that would come to you or your heirs. It can be costly to refinance or pay off a reverse loan before it comes due. Reverse mortgages are a complicated type of loan with many options, so it is important to educate yourself about them before having a mandatory talk with a counselor, or before you talk with a lender, so that you can ask pointed questions. Be wary of information on commercial Web sites. You can begin your investigation using the links in the following resource box.

REVERSE MORTGAGES

- Federal Trade Commission Facts for Consumers: Reverse Mortgages, Get the Facts before Cashing in on Your Home's Equity
  http://www.ftc.gov/bcp/edu/pubs/consumer/homes/rea13.shtm

- U.S. Department of Housing and Urban Development: Lists "Top Ten Things to Know If You're Interested in a Reverse Mortgage."
  http://www.hud.gov/offices/hsg/sfh/hecm/rmtopten.cfm

- AARP: Reverse mortgages.
  http://www.aarp.org/money/revmort

- YMCA: Retirement Fund, Reverse Mortgages.
  http://www.yretirement.org/content.aspx?tag=pf_mor1

Viaticals

A relatively new, potentially risky way to obtain insurance monies is a "viatical." You can sell your insurance policy to another company, giving the new company rights to the full value for the policy at the time of your death. You may be able to sell the policy for anywhere from 55 to 80 percent of its value. You do not have to pay taxes on the settlement if you provide evidence that doctors believe you have fewer than two years to live. The longer you are expected to live, the less the viatical company will offer for your policy.

Recently some states have begun to regulate these companies, and though viaticals can be a blessing, many people have been cheated out of money. Before considering a viatical, talk first with your insurance company to see whether your policy allows for accelerated benefits. You might also consider borrowing money from family and friends, drawing up a legal agreement that they would be beneficiaries of your insurance at the time of your death, thereby giving the insurance benefits to them as opposed to a company.

If you proceed with viaticals, be aware that you lose your medical privacy to some extent since the company must monitor your condition. Get bids from more than one company, and check state laws for minimum payments for insurance policies. If you have a whole-life policy, get the complete cash value. Currently, federal law states that you do not have to pay taxes on settlements if you have less than two years to live, but check into the current status of both state and federal tax laws on settlements. Also check whether the settlement would disqualify you from Medicaid benefits. Beware of unethical practices and investigate the company with which you plan to work. At one time the industry had trade groups that followed a code of ethics but it is largely unregulated.

VIATICALS

- Gloria Wolk's Guide: *Cash for the Final Days*, from Bialkin Books.
    http://www.viatical-expert.net

Selling Your Assets

You can liquidate your belongings to raise cash using tried-and-true methods—for example, by placing ads to sell items in your local newspaper or on Web sites such as eBay or Craig's List; by pawning items; by bringing clothes to consignment shops; or by having a garage sale.

Paying for Bills and Avoiding Damaged Credit

When you see a health-care provider (doctor, clinic, hospital), your insurance information will be requested, and you will likely need to cover the costs of a co-pay. If you do not have insurance, you will be asked to pay for services on the day of service or within a reasonable time frame. It is essential to keep all receipts for payment in case of billing disputes and/ or in case you have, or learn you can get, supplemental aid. With health insurance or Medicare, the first statement that you will likely receive in the mail will not be a bill but an explanation of benefits (EOB) from your insurer or a summary notice if you use Medicare. Though these are not bills, save them. The EOB and summary statements let you know which expenses your insurer or the government has paid and will let you know what you owe your health-care provider. The bills from health-care providers will come periodically, and some unpaid expenses may be in process. For example, expenses may be listed on a bill that your insurer has not as yet paid. Your health-care providers and your insurance company or Medicare will not sort out your expenses and give you one final bill. You need a system to keep track of the statements sent by your insurer and the bills sent by your health-care providers.

Keeping track of what you owe is not easy, even for people in the health-care industry. You can get on top of the situation by putting all bills and insurance statements in a three-ring notebook and/or maintaining computer files or spreadsheets using a system that makes sense to you. A good way to organize your billing is by the date of service (the dates that your lab tests, procedures, doctor's visits, etc. took place). One possibility is to keep separate files for your insurer's statements and for your providers' bills, arranged in chronological order. When you get a bill from your provider, look at the date of service for each charge and note what you or your insurance company paid for that service; then note any remaining money that you owe, including co-pays. If you agree with what your insurer says you owe, send that amount to your health-care provider promptly.

If your insurance is slow to pay a charge listed on your health-care provider's bill, call the provider. A charge from your health-care provider is referred to as a claim. When talking about a claim, you need to refer to the date you received the service. When talking with your provider, have the claim handy and take notes. Jot down the date and time you are calling, as well as the name(s) of those with whom you speak. Ask for the date the health-care provider submitted the charge/claim in question to your insurer. It is not uncommon for claims to be lost, so you may need to ask the provider to resubmit that claim, then ask the billing department to give you more time to pay since the insurer did not get the claim. Next, call your insurer and ask if they received the claim in question from your provider. If so, ask on what specific date the claim was received, why it is taking a long time to process the claim, and when the processing will be complete. Again, write down the date, time, and names of people with whom you talk and take notes when people answer your questions, using their terminology when possible. If you discover your insurance company is not paying your provider in a timely manner or is refusing to pay for treatment, ask the provider to send you a written explanation. Call back your health-care providers, letting them know the situation, and ask them to put a hold on that charge while you work to get it paid.

Do not let months pass by in the expectation that eventually your insurer and health-care provider will settle overdue bills. They might, but health-care providers may eventually send overdue charges to collection agencies, even without your knowing it. To your dismay you could receive a letter from an agency threatening to damage your credit unless you pay immediately. If your bills are turned over to a collection agency, call the health-care provider and ask which claims were handed over to the agency. Refer to your records to see if a mistake has been made. You may need to call your insurer, and then talk again to your health-care provider. You may get support in urging the insurer to pay for a claim through the human resources department at your workplace. You may also want to familiarize yourself with your federal and state medical rights and consult patient advocate resources such as the ones listed in the preceding section of this chapter.

To check whether the collection agency has reported damaging information about your credit to a credit bureau, obtain a free copy of your credit report from one of the major credit reporting agents listed below, though you would be wise not to do this repeatedly since repeated requests may negatively impact your credit score. If you spot a charge that is in dispute, contact the credit report company, and both verbally and in writing ask that the disputed charge be removed until it is resolved.

CREDIT REPORT AGENCIES

- AnnualCreditReport.com: Provides a free annual credit report.
  877-322-8228
    https://www.annualcreditreport.com

- Equifax: www.equifax.com
    800-685-1111

- Experian: www.experian.com
    888-397-3742

- Trans-Union: www.transunion.com
    800-888-4213

(Resources, continued)

- myFICO.com: Offers one-stop services to obtain credit reports from all three agencies and quarterly or monthly monitoring for credit problems.
  http://www.myfico.com

Avoiding Overcharges and Billing Errors

As mentioned at the opening of this section, if you have insurance, know what your insurer does and does not cover. Keep a copy of this information in the notebook where you keep your medical records. Pay particular attention to the declarations or standard information page and the sections on exceptions and exclusions. If you have Medicare, ask for the current year's summary of benefits (call 800-633-4227 or go to www.medicare .gov). If time allows, when your doctor prescribes a treatment or surgery, ask the doctor's office to call your insurance company to check to what extent the care (procedures, medicine, etc.) will be covered; this is referred to as pre-authorization or pre-certification. Before going to a new doctor or facility, call your insurer to learn to what extent your policy will cover expenses charged to you under the new provider's care.

If you are paying yourself, or if you want to be sure you are not overcharged, whenever possible ask in advance what the estimated costs will be for the care your doctor recommends. You can also call a clinic or hospital billing department to learn what a room costs per night and what you yourself can bring to cut expenses (medicines, tissues, etc.). If you want to be sure you are not overcharged, keep a record, or have someone with you keep a record, of what is given to you when you are receiving medical treatment so that you can check later that you are not being charged for services or time you did not receive, though some care is not observable — for example, pathologists examining tissue samples.

Once your bills arrive, you may be able to reduce expenses by uncovering errors and padded costs. A large credit-reporting agency, Equifax Services, estimates that the average hospital patient pays more for hospital bills than necessary. Even if you are well insured, you may want to try to reduce costs since many insurance policies have a lifetime cap for medical expenses.

Decoding hospital bills can be daunting. If something on your bills looks suspicious, call the billing office of your health-care provider and ask for an itemized bill, which should be provided at no cost. If the clerks in the billing office are not cooperative, remind them that the American Hospital Association's "A Patient's Bill of Rights" states that patients have the right to know what they are being charged for.

A detailed bill may or may not reveal common overcharges, such as duplicate tests or charges on the date of a hospital discharge. If you see charges that you do not understand, ask the billing office for a clearer explanation in lay terms. Also, check with other health-care professionals or medical suppliers to learn the customary cost for the service or item in question. This requires polite inquiry and vigilance on your part. Since it is in your insurer's interest not to be unnecessarily charged, the company may help you understand your bill and investigate possible overcharges. You can also enlist aid from agencies that will investigate your bills for a percentage (usually half) of any fees they recover; one such agency is listed in the following resource box.

If you uncover an error, notify your health-care provider and your insurer in writing right away, and keep a copy of your letter or e-mail. As already suggested, keep notes, including dates and names of all the people with whom you talk about the complaint. If the error is not taken care of, contact your state's consumer protection agency or attorney general's office.

TROUBLESHOOTING MEDICAL BILLS

- Medical Billing Advocates of America: Helps you uncover overbilling errors.
  http://www.billadvocates.com

- National Association of Attorneys General: Offers information for contacting your state's consumer protection agency or attorney general's office.
  http://www.naag.org

- *The Medical Bill Survival Guide,* by Pat Palmer: Lists agencies state by state that can help you uncover overbilling.

resources

What to Do If Your Insurer Will Not
Cover a Treatment or Procedure

An unfortunate complaint of those with a life-threatening illness is that one's insurer can deny a claim—in other words, refuse to cover the cost of a treatment or procedure. If your insurance company has denied a claim, first check whether or not your health-care provider will appeal the claim. Ask if you can aid your doctor's office in that process since some offices are understaffed and reluctant to take on more responsibilities. If staff members are not willing to do so, keep on good terms with them so that they are more willing to give you advice and assistance in appealing the claim yourself. You may want to contact an advocacy agency for help, such as the ones listed in the resource box at the end of this section.

To prepare an appeal yourself start by contacting your insurer for a copy of the company's appeal process. Also contact your doctor's office and request a copy of the chart notes and/or diagnostic information that explains your need for the treatment or procedure that was denied. To make a stronger case, use the links in the resource box in chapter 2 titled "Authoritative Sources for Breast Cancer Research" to learn what studies show that this treatment can be beneficial for those in your circumstances. Make copies of these studies to include in your appeal.

Remind your insurer of the Patients' Bill of Rights Act of 2005, which states that you are entitled to speedy independent review if your appeal is denied a second time. This act is not law but is well respected and upheld by a number of insurers. If your insurer will not conduct an independent review, you can seek one yourself. Independent reviewers will investigate how other insurers have responded to requests for the particular kind of care you are seeking. If it is commonly covered, the reviewers can put pressure on your insurer to pay for that treatment.

If your request for a treatment is denied even after an independent claim review, you could hire a lawyer, but at this time, under the Employee Retirement Income Security Act of 1974, you can sue only for the cost of the treatment, not other damages. The time involved for formal legal proceedings can be substantial since even a "quick case" can take a year to be heard in court. If your options run out, look into alternative means for funding your treatment, such those mentioned above in "U.S. Government–Sponsored Health Care and Cost Coverage for the Uninsured" and "Tapping into Assets."

INSURANCE-RELATED CONCERNS

- National Coalition for Cancer Survivorship: Provides a free copy of *What Cancer Survivors Need to Know about Health Insurance*.
    http://www.canceradvocacy.org
    http://www.canceradvocacy.org/resources/publications/insurance.pdf

- Alliance of Claims Assistance Professionals: Provides assistance in getting insurance companies to pay for denied treatment.
    877-275-8765 (toll free)
    http://www.claims.org

- National Insurance Consumer Helpline: Offers assistance for insurance problems.
    800-942-4242

- Georgetown University Health Policy Institute: Offers consumer guides for getting and keeping health insurance for each state and the District of Columbia.
    http://www.healthinsuranceinfo.net

- American Bar Association: Offers advice to breast cancer patients for fighting denied claims.
    http://www.abanet.org/women/tensteps.html

In closing this section about medical laws and government health-care programs, we want to again caution you that laws and policies may have changed since the publication of this book, so we urge you to use the links in the resource boxes to learn the most current information. With the United States undergoing healthcare reform as of this writing, there is hope that in the future all citizens will have access to good care and that no one will suffer financial hardship because of illness.

Final Arrangements: Will, Durable Power of Attorney, Advance Directive, Memorial Service

We live in a culture that does not readily acknowledge death. As a result, some people wait until the last minute or never get around to responsibly managing their end-of-life affairs. Tending to these matters better assures that your final days and your legacy will be as you wish. Completing arrangements offers peace of mind, especially when considering the good that can result.

Putting your wishes in writing can be a creative process. Consider how your final arrangements might make a personal statement, possibly settling resentments or making loving gestures. Preparing a will and an advance directive in themselves are loving gestures since those who care about you will be saved considerable trouble, unnecessary expense, and possible conflict. Carrying out your wishes can also give your family and friends satisfaction and peace, reminding them of you, knowing you spared them uncomfortable decisions. It is best to start making plans early on in your disease and to confer with and inform all those who have a stake in the process.

Including your loved ones in your decision making may be a turning point in your family dynamics. Doing so publicly acknowledges, though does not hasten, death. You may notice others are uncomfortable when talking with you about wills, advance directives, and memorial services. Planning may be the beginning of their grieving, and initiating the discussion will help them handle their heartache when you someday do die. Loved ones usually take their cue from the person who is not well. Most likely you need to muster the courage to break your own, and their, silence. Discussing these sometimes difficult issues together has the potential to resolve conflicts and foster intimacy.

Keep in mind that no matter how well you prepare for death, unpredictable issues can arise. Buried desires and old resentments may surface. When making decisions on issues such as how to distribute assets, resist being caught up in current feelings that may change rapidly. Think back over the length of your life to who and what matters most to you.

Listed below is a standard checklist of practical and legal documents to prepare and copy for significant people. Store the originals in a secure place that is known to your loved ones and/or executor.

Checklist of Documents

Will	Bank and credit card accounts
Durable power of attorney	Real estate papers
Advance directive (living will)	Tax records
Financial papers	Automobile title
Insurance papers	Loans

Investments	Birth certificate
Work and retirement benefits	Social Security card
Funeral arrangements	Military Service papers

Wills and the Distribution of Assets

A will is a legal instrument instructing the person whom you name as an executor how you would like your possessions and financial assets distributed after your death. You can name an attorney or a financial adviser as the executor to save a loved one the time or trouble in carrying out the directives in your will. This choice is especially wise if you have considerable assets. You can save money, however, if you chose someone to whom you are close and whom you trust explicitly. Name an alternative executor in case the person you name first is unable to carry out the duties. Naming co-executors can make decisions and paper signing more cumbersome, but it allows for shared control. Also, consider the location of your executor. Handling matters from a distance can be difficult. Discuss openly with your loved ones whom you would like to be executor. Find out who is willing and able to execute a will. The executor is usually responsible for the following:

> Probating the will, when the court legally sanctions the document.
> Establishing, managing, or completing financial and legal commitments, including work matters, investments, and trusts.
> Filing state and federal tax documents.
> Paying remaining debts.
> Distributing remaining assets.

DUTIES OF AN EXECUTOR

- USAA Education Foundation Nonprofit Organization, Duties of an Executor: Offers information about the typical duties of an executor, including a checklist.
  http://www.usaaedfoundation.org/family/cp07.asp

resources

The earlier in the disease process that you create or update your will, the less likely your wishes can be called into question. A will can be nullified if it can be proven it was written under significant stress or heavy medications, such as morphine and chemotherapy. If you are looking and feeling well at the time of the execution of your will, consider videotaping the proceedings so that the video can be used as evidence if the will is contested. Once it is written, give copies of your will to all who are mentioned or may have a stake in your assets. Without a will your assets will be distributed according to the laws in your state. The costs for carrying out this process are charged to the estate, and the assets will take more time to be distributed than if there was a will.

Legal services for preparing a will are relatively inexpensive, ranging anywhere from $100 to $2,000, depending on how many provisions you put in. If you have more than one piece of property and numerous investments, or you have estranged children, or you have had more than one marriage with children, it is wise to seek the counsel of an attorney. If you have few and simple assets and few people to whom you will leave them, you may be able to write a legal will yourself. You must follow the laws of your state. You can save money and trouble if you give away some items before your death. You could also put names on the bottoms of objects to let your loved ones know what you would like to be distributed to whom, though this does not assure that your wishes will be carried out. If you would like more certainty in how your assets are distributed but have few resources, ask your county or state bar associations if they offer pro bono (free) services.

WILLS

- USlegalforms.com: Offers state-specific forms for wills online.
  http://www.uslegalforms.com

- Internet Legal Research Group: Has an archive of free legal forms that includes estate planning.
  http://www.ilrg.com

- Estate Planning for Pets Foundation: A nonprofit corporation that provides information for how to prepare for your pet's future after you die or if you become incapacitated.
  http://www.estateplanningforpets.org

(Resources, continued)

- Quicken Willmaker Plus: Uses an interview-style approach to create wills and other provisions; can provide a starting place even when you ultimately use the services of an attorney.
     http://www.nolo.com/resource.cfm/catID/FD1795A9-8049-422C
        -9087838F86A2BC2B/309

Trusts

There are a number of different kinds of trusts, such as charitable trusts or educational trusts, but all are a means to protect assets to aid beneficiaries. You can create a trust fund by drawing up a legal document using the laws of your state. A trustee oversees the assets until the time of your death or later, depending on what you stipulate (for example, a trustee can oversee assets until a beneficiary reaches legal age).

Living trusts are a particular kind of trust in which you can place assets such as real estate holdings, bank accounts, and securities. You appoint a successor to distribute these assets at the time of your death, and until that time, you can be your own trustee and run the trust. You no longer legally own these assets, so they will not go through probate like a will does, and often you can reduce the amount of tax your beneficiaries will have to pay on inheriting the assets. Some families have lost significant monies from badly drawn trusts, so you would be wise to consult with a lawyer or financial planner who has expertise in writing trusts if you have significant assets or have a number of stipulations you want followed with regard to distributing them.

TRUSTS

- Federal Trade Commission, Living Trusts: Offers advisory information on living trusts.
     http://www.ftc.gov/bcp/edu/pubs/consumer/products/pr008.shtm
- USlegalforms.com: Provides living trust forms by state.
     http://www.uslegalforms.com/livingtrusts

Insurance or Pension Monies

In writing your will, remember that you may have insurance money that will be distributed to your loved ones. Even if you have not personally arranged for life insurance, your loved ones may still be entitled to funds from your workplace or the government. If you have paid Social Security taxes over a long period, your spouse or children could collect considerable money. Check as well into veterans' benefits if applicable.

If you have a life insurance policy, talk with your agent about the value of the policy and what can be done, if anything, to increase its monetary worth. Ask, too, how to expedite the paperwork. Your loved ones may be entitled to money from other sources as well. Check your credit card companies and the human resources departments at your or your spouse's workplace for possible death benefits. Inquire whether you are entitled to money for accrued sick leave and vacation time or disability compensation that you can leave to a beneficiary.

Bequests and Memorial Donations

In writing your will, you might consider organizations or causes you could help. Think about what ways you wish the world were different. For example, would you like your contribution to benefit children, women, animals, the environment, poverty, injustice, intolerance, a particular mental or physical illness? Is there a church, school, institution, or organization that has made a difference in your life? Do you want to make a gift at the local, regional, national, or global level? Where might your contribution have influence, even if mostly to encourage those who share your vision?

A donation does not necessarily require money. Bequests can be objects, possibly ideas, like a poem. You may want to donate an item to some institution that can help it carry out its work. This is an opportunity for you to take action on what you care about and make a difference.

It may surprise you to learn that organizations can be wary of gifts, fearing legal disputes with heirs or fearing that the conditions of the gift could burden them. Many educational, religious, and other nonprofit organizations will happily supply you with guidelines for making contributions that will assist you, and the organizations, in carrying out your desires. At the same time you may want to inquire about the organizations' policies for setting up a memorial fund to which family and friends can contribute in your name as a remembrance.

Durable Power of Attorney

The laws regarding durable power of attorney differ by state. Durable power of attorney is a document that designates someone as your "agent." The agent manages your financial affairs while you are alive if you can no longer do so yourself, as opposed to the executor of a will, who manages your legal and financial affairs once you are deceased. Consider setting up a durable power of attorney since a simple power of attorney restricts the agent's ability to sign papers. With a durable power of attorney your agent can legally act on your behalf in all transactions. Your agent will have the lawful right to pay your bills and oversee estate expenditures from your trust. In other words, this person will assume your financial decision making.

Without a power of attorney if you became unable to manage your affairs, your family would have to go to court to have someone appointed to manage your finances. Your family would have to pay the legal costs for making this appointment, and important financial matters are often left untended. Pick someone as power of attorney who is reliable, trustworthy, and knowledgeable in managing finances. This person will also need the confidence, respect, and trust of your family and loved ones.

DURABLE POWER OF ATTORNEY

- Medlawplus: Offers information on power of attorney and a form for your state for a small fee.
  www.medlawplus.com/library/legal/durablepowerofattorney.htm

Advance Medical Directives and Health-Care Proxy

An advance medical directive, sometimes referred to as a living will, tells your physician what medical procedures and drugs you want to have administered, or what procedures and drugs you do not want to have administered, in the event you are not able to communicate your wishes. A health-care proxy is the person you designate to talk with medical personnel about those wishes. In most states, when you cannot speak for yourself, doctors will turn to your health-care proxy when life-prolonging decisions arise.

The role of health-care proxy is different from that of durable power of attorney. You may or may not want the same person to do both. An attorney can serve in either or both roles, which possibly saves loved ones from making difficult decisions and provides you with a legal advocate as well. However, your loved ones may want to be more in control, may be more readily available, and knowing you better, may be clearer on what you would want.

Imagine you are no longer thinking coherently or are unconscious and close to dying. Would you like measures to prolong your life? Some of those measures include cardiopulmonary resuscitation, such as drugs, electric shock, and respiratory devices to restore a heartbeat and breathing. Consider whether you would like a respirator to artificially maintain your breathing and other life-prolonging measures such as intravenous nutrition and/or hydration given through a tube placed in your vein; kidney dialysis to remove waste from your blood if your kidneys fail; surgery; or pain medication that may hasten death. If you are uncertain, talk with medical and hospice personnel about their experience with these procedures. Consider the physical pain and financial costs and the point at which you would want to refuse these procedures or end them, depending on your chances of recovery. Your religious beliefs and the wishes of your loved ones may influence your decisions as well.

After weighing the possibilities, follow your desires. You do not want to be vague in this document; rather than saying that you do not want "heroic measures," state specifically what you do or do not want—for example, you do not want to be put on a ventilator or you do want to be artificially resuscitated. Some of the Web sites in this chapter offer decision tools to help you consider these choices. Whatever you decide and whomever you select as your health-care proxy, check your state laws by contacting the state attorney general's office. You can talk to an attorney knowledgeable about these documents and/or use the resources in the next resource box. Some states require specific legal forms, and some do not recognize personally drawn-up forms as legal documents.

The Patient Self-Determination Act (PSDA) requires that any medical institution receiving federal money for Medicare or Medicaid ask you if you have an advance directive, and if not, it must provide you with information about composing one. According to this federal law, the institution should also provide you with a statement about your state's rights in determining your health-care decisions and that institution's philosophy about such decisions.

Give copies of your advance directive to your loved ones, doctors, hospital, and attorney. Still, if you were to lose the ability to proclaim your wishes, in some states and under some circumstances, your family's wishes may take precedence over your advance directive and health-care proxy, so as best you can, be sure your family understands your desires.

If you do not want life-prolonging procedures, to further assure you are not resuscitated, obtain a MedicAlert bracelet with DNR (Do Not Resuscitate) inscribed on the back. If you anticipate being hospitalized at an institution, ask your doctor to write and sign a DNR order that is honored by that hospital, and get copies for yourself and your loved ones.

END-OF-LIFE DOCUMENTS

- American Bar Association: Provides resources for legal concerns at end of life.
    http://www.abanet.org/aging

- Caring Connections: Provides a host of end-of-life information, including information on advanced directives.
    800-658-8898
    http://www.caringinfo.org

- NOLO: Provides "do-it-yourself" legal advice.
    http://www.nolo.com

- U.S. Living Will Registry: Provides a commercial registry for advance directives.
    http://www.uslivingwillregistry.com

- Aging with Dignity: Provides advice and legal tools for end-of-life concerns.
    http://www.agingwithdignity.org

- MedicAlert Foundation: Provides 24-hour accessible information to medical personnel including Do Not Resuscitate orders.
    888-633-4298
    http://www.medicalert.org

Memorial Services

Regardless of the place of your death, a doctor must sign a death certificate. Should you die in a hospital, a funeral director may be called or may appear. In lieu of a for-profit agency, a loved one or a religious group can act as a funeral director. In this case, the designated person must obtain a Permit for Disposition and file a burial or cremation certificate. Outside of the death certificate and the Permit for Disposition, you have a number of options for memorial services and for what you would like done with your body.

Commercial "Complete Service" Funerals and Cemetery Burials

At the time of your death your loved ones are particularly vulnerable. Often they are overcome by grief and may not think clearly when approached by a funeral director. As kindly and holy as funeral directors may appear, they are involved in a commercial venture, so it is important to research your options and choose wisely. Thinking ahead is the best way to assure that your funeral service is the way you want it and that any inheritance you may leave is not unduly diminished to cover a funeral expense.

Some in the funeral industry target people who have traditionally religious beliefs or burial rituals, such as Catholics, Baptists, Southerners, Hispanics, African-Americans, and Asians. If you are a member of a religious community, your community may direct you to a preferred funeral director who may have connections to chain funeral services. Increasingly, churches and synagogues form affiliations with one of the three big chain funeral companies: Service Corporation International, Alderwoods Group, and Stewart. The biggest sellers of caskets are York and Batesville. Caskets usually account for up to half the price of a funeral and can be priced many times more than wholesale cost.

Charges for paperwork, preparation of the body, transportation, plots, burial markers, etc. can be highly marked up. Funeral homes have been known to add unexpected pricy charges for small amenities. It is possible that the same casket and services at a locally owned funeral parlor may cost less than half of what a chain may charge. Using the resources below, you can investigate whether or not the charges of any recommended funeral director are reasonable and whether a director in your area could provide equivalent services for significantly less. If you do not make arrangements beforehand, or if your family is not savvy about unfair and hidden costs, you could pay significantly more than necessary.

When meeting with a funeral director or planner, do not indicate your financial status. Do not prepay or sign over an insurance policy to mortuaries if your death is not imminent. Often funeral plans change after a plot is purchased, or the funeral company may be bought out or go out of business. In these circumstances you could lose all or a considerable amount of your money. Prepaid plots can have hidden charges and restrictions that end up costing your loved ones more than if you or they made arrangements nearer the time of your death. If you want to be sure you have money to cover funeral expenses, designate a certificate of deposit or life insurance policy to cover the expense, or open a joint savings account for this purpose with a family member.

According to the National Funeral Directors Association's Web site, the average cost of a funeral in 2006 was $7,323, excluding cemetery costs, though the figure can be higher or lower depending on where you live (1). Before handing over money or signing any papers, ask for an itemized statement of all costs, including any standard costs after the burial, which sometimes are unreasonably high. People have unknowingly signed papers that resulted in their paying hundreds of dollars for the tending of a gravesite. The U.S. Federal Trade Commission requires that funeral homes provide an itemized statement. If a funeral director or counselor states that an expense is required by law, you can ask to be shown that law.

If you would like a religious service, learn from the funeral parlor and your religious leader what the standard service is like, and consider what options you have to tailor the arrangements and ceremony to your liking. Plan your service as you would any big event, or draw parameters and let your loved ones decide how to honor you. Keep in mind, however, that lack of clarity may cause squabbles or difficult choices for those left making these decisions.

If you have not made arrangements before the time of your death, the best advice to your loved ones is that they should take their time and avoid the inclination to make decisions out of grief and guilt that could end up benefiting the funeral provider rather than honoring your or their desires. Your family can leave your body at the hospital or at home and quickly do some investigating in order to obtain unbiased advice, which they are unlikely to get if they make decisions with an appointed grief counselor or funeral director who may have ties with particular providers.

If you are a veteran, the government will provide a headstone or marker, and you, and usually your spouse, can be buried in a national cemetery or in the columbarium at Arlington National Cemetery. A flag will be presented to your family. You may also qualify for a few hundred dollars to cover burial expenses.

FUNERAL INFORMATION

- Funeral Consumers Alliance: A federation of nonprofit consumer information societies protecting and helping individuals plan dignified, affordable funerals; offers extensive links and resources.
  http://www.funerals.org

- Funeral Help Program
  http://www.funeral-help.com/index.html

- Funerals Consumers Alliance: Offers advice on obtaining reasonably priced caskets and urns.
  http://www.funerals.org/frequently-asked-questions/casketretailers

- Aurora Casket Company: Offers help in planning traditional funerals.
  http://www.funeralplan.com

- Veterans' Benefits Administration: To learn if you qualify for burial and memorials benefits.
  800-827-1000
  http://www.cem.va.gov

Cremation

Approximately one-quarter of all Americans choose to be cremated rather than buried, and this figure is rising rapidly. By the year 2010 it is estimated that 38 percent of Americans will be cremated (2). People choose cremation for various reasons. They may not want their body to decompose in the ground or to take up land space, though there are environmentally sound burial alternatives. Cremation also can cut costs and allow for more simple or creative burials. In cremation the clothed or unclothed body is burned in intense heat, usually for an hour, until it is nearly consumed. Any metal parts are then removed, and the remaining bone fragments, which usually weigh about seven pounds, are carefully swept into a container. Laws require that crematories carefully tag bodies so that loved ones are sure to receive the correct remains, but a small amount of a person's remains may be left in the burning chamber, and a very small amount of remains from previous cremations may be swept into future containers.

Once in the container, the remains, which resemble crushed seashells, can then be transferred to a permanent urn or scattered in a variety of places and ways, depending on state laws. Though ashes pose no environmental hazard, some states do not allow you to scatter the remains of loved ones on certain public and private property since future owners or visitors may object. A number of creative possibilities for scattering ashes are mentioned in the next section.

The typical cost of a cremation is significantly lower than that of traditional burials. You can enlist a funeral parlor for traditional services, such as embalming and viewing, but this is not required in most states. Since mortuaries carry out cremations, the costs, such as those for an urn or transportation of the body, are subject to high markups. You can protect yourself from unreasonable expenses by checking the sites listed in the preceding and following resource boxes.

CREMATION

- Cremation.com: Provides information on cremation and locates services in Canada and the United States.
  http://www.cremation.com

- The Internet Cremation Society: Provides a search engine to learn of a local cremation society. Societies typically cost less than funeral parlors.
  http://www.cremation.org

- Ontario Consultants on Religious Tolerance: Discusses Jewish and Christian beliefs on cremation and burial.
  www.religioustolerance.org/crematio.htm

Donating Your Body to Science

To learn what conditions must be met for you to donate your body to science you can contact the nearest medical school. Organs from people dying from cancer are not used for transplantation, and sometimes medical schools prefer bodies with organs less damaged by cancer. If your body is accepted, it will probably be used in anatomical laboratories for training future doctors. After signing the papers, you will likely be issued a card with a number your loved ones can call twenty-four hours a day to arrange for the medical facility to pick up your body. Medical schools usually transport your body immediately, precluding the option that your body could be laid out. Loved ones who are not present at the time of your death do not see the dead body, a concern for some people. Making this arrangement will likely eliminate all funeral costs other than a memorial service. Future physicians are grateful for such a gift and first-year students at most medical schools conduct annual memorial services to recognize and celebrate the donors and their families.

BODY DONATION

- MedCure: Offers information on body donation.
    http://www.medcure.org

- Biogift: Facilitates body donation.
    http://www.biogift.org

- FlatRock.com: Offers articles on body donation.
    http://www.flatrock.org.nz/topics/older_and_under/death_wish.htm

Specialized and Distinctive Arrangements

Since the law does not require that anyone be embalmed or have a wake or a funeral, you can tailor your final arrangements and create a memorial service that suits you. Cultures, religions, governments, families, and individuals have acknowledged death in a variety of ways, from the wild and lavish to the subdued and austere. Costs and arrangements, of course, differ considerably. You can use the list below as a means to consider possibilities.

Place: Church, home, park, beach, restaurant, rented hall.
Music: Live or recorded, with or without singing.
Visual images: Photos, PowerPoint, artwork.
Mementos: Flowers, candles, incense, funeral programs, prayer cards, personal or symbolic objects.
Readings: Liturgical, prayer, poetry; quotes; speeches by loved ones; sharing circles.
Special events: Parade, potluck, after-service meal, symbolic gestures.

In Britain and the United States some people are returning to the ways of yesteryear by arranging to die at home, including having loved ones care for their body at death, having noncommercial memorial services, and having their body either cremated or buried on personal property or in a nature preserve. People opt for these types of arrangements for a number of reasons: to have more control over their last moments, to have more environmentally friendly funerals, and to avoid unnecessary expense.

With some preplanning using the resources in the next resource box, you and your loved ones can learn how to arrange for the certificate of death and the Permit for Disposition required by law and learn simple procedures for caring for a deceased person's body. Embalming, which adds toxic chemicals to the environment, is not essential if the body is kept fairly cool and then buried or cremated in a few days. Having filled out the proper forms, a family member or the person you designate with power of attorney can transport your body for cremation or burial.

Your local board of supervisors can tell you about the laws regarding burial on private land. Through the following links you can also learn if there is a collectively owned cemetery near you or any nearby nature preserve/woodland where you could be buried. You or your family can order an earth-friendly cardboard or pre-made biodegradable casket, which you can decorate if you wish. Often in nature preserves a nonintrusive boulder or tree will mark the site of your burial, and your site will be noted in a public record on the preserve.

Another unique burial, which is advertised as costing the same as a conventional funeral, is to send your cremated remains on a rocket launch into outer space. A portion of your cremated remains is put in a capsule, and then depending on your preference, your remains are released into earth orbit, lunar orbit, or deep space. Your remains do not contribute to space or earth pollution. Other possibilities include having a star named for you or having your remains added to the formation of ocean reefs.

UNIQUE FUNERAL ARRANGEMENTS

- Final Passages: Offers advice for home- or family-managed funerals.
    http://www.finalpassages.org

- Crossings: Offers advice for home- or family-managed funerals.
    http://www.crossings.net

- Green Burial Council: Advocates a green burial.
    http://www.ethicalburial.org

resources

(Resources, continued)

- Forest of Memories: Offers information on green burial in North America.
  http://www.forestofmemories.org

- Eternal Reefs: Offers information on having cremated remains form sea reefs.
  http://www.eternalreefs.com

- Space Services, Inc.: Offers information on sending cremated remains into space.
  http://www.memorialspaceflights.com

Obituaries, Markers, Epitaphs, Final Good-Byes

You need not leave the writing of your obituary to others. You can get an idea of what is customary for your community by reading obituaries in your local newspaper, then write your own in advance of your passing. Call for your paper's specifications before doing so. You also may want to write an epitaph for a headstone or for a notice on a social networking site. To stir your imagination, use the links below to read epitaphs and learn about symbols that have been used for centuries to commemorate and celebrate people's lives. Your loved ones may want to have a commemorative marker or a special spot as a means to remember you. A tombstone, a plaque, a tree, a bush, or an inscription and photo in a mausoleum are all possibilities. Last, you may want to leave your history, wisdom, or messages as a final remembrance. You could create a memoir in words or images or have an e-mail sent to your loved ones after you die. Whatever you choose, the best remembrance of all will be the happy memories you leave behind.

REMEMBRANCES

- Ethicalwill.com: Offers guidance in passing along meaningful messages to loved ones.
  http://ethicalwill.com

(Resources, continued)

- Association of Personal Historians: Offers guidance for preserving your personal history.
    http://personalhistorians.org

- Modern Memoirs Publishing: Specializes in personal memoirs of all types.
    http://www.modernmemoirs.com

- myLastEmail.com: Provides a service for leaving messages after your death.
    http://mylastemail.com

Further Reading

The Affordable Funeral: Going in Style, Not in Debt, by R. E. Markin. Flaming Hooker Press, 1996.

Be Prepared: The Complete Financial, Legal, and Practical Guide for Living with a Life-Challenging Condition, by David S. Landay. St. Martin's Press, 1998.

Final Victory: Taking Charge of the Last Stages of Life, Facing Death on Your Own Terms, by Thomas A. Preston, MD. Prima Lifestyles, 2000.

Talking about Death, by Virginia Morris. Algonquin Books, 2004.

CHAPTER 8

Emotional and Spiritual Well-Being

> In this well-ordered universe, the perfect
> vehicle for our spiritual growth and
> unfoldment is exactly our present situation.
> —Sevakram, *Interchange*

> All things are impermanent, with the nature
> to arise and pass away. One who lives in this
> truth achieves harmony and happiness with
> all that is.
> —Buddhist chant

Death is the end of all sensation, thought, and experience in this life and begins a transition into the unfathomable. Being keenly aware of your mortality places you in the midst of an extraordinary time, likely the most challenging time of your life and the one most rife with the potential for profound understandings. In learning you have an incurable disease, you experience the loss of much of what you had hoped and expected would come to pass. Uncertainty, though always present, is now inescapably evident. Changes taking place in your body cause the end or alteration of your usual roles. The loss of control is ever present while you wait for test results and when you find yourself incapable of doing what was once routine. The pressure of making major decisions about treatment, finances, work, relationships, and priorities at times can be unbearable. At this moment, however, you are alive, and for the time to come, even given the great challenge of having a terminal illness, there is much that you can do to live with hope, joy, and peace. This chapter is designed to help you live to the fullest extent while facing your mortality. It opens by relating common responses to loss, then discusses issues that can arise when interrelating with others, and concludes with ways of approaching death.

Responding to Loss

All we can do is be who we are with all of our imperfections and warts, and allow
death to take us as it will. What is important is letting go of our ideas about how we
should be and surrendering to the fullness of our humanity.

—Rodney Smith, *Lessons from the Dying*

Each of us responds to dying in an individual manner; however, most
people identify, to varying degrees, with the stages of loss described by
Dr. Elizabeth Kubler-Ross and her team of researchers. Kubler-Ross's
groundbreaking book, *On Death and Dying*, was directed to doctors but
is very accessible to lay people. After interviewing numerous terminally
ill patients in the 1960s, Kubler-Ross and her team observed that many
people experience the following five stages when facing death: denial and
isolation, anger, bargaining, depression, and acceptance. These stages did
not necessarily occur in a lock-step sequence; they frequently overlapped
or reoccurred, and some did not occur at all. As evidence for the existence
of each stage, Kubler-Ross provided excerpts and examples from the many
personal interviews her team recorded and analyzed. Although we use
our own examples and have paraphrased definitions of these stages, this
section uses Kubler-Ross's work as a framework. We hope you find the
stages a helpful means for exploring common feelings and thoughts that
people have and behaviors in which they may engage when faced with a
terminal illness.

Denial

Resisting change is like holding on to the wheel of a moving oxcart.
Sooner or later we get run over.

—Buddha

Denial is not accepting reality. At times the reality can be totally masked
from a person's awareness, and at other times it may reside just below
conscious thought. Sometimes people behave in ways that show that at
some level they know the reality of a situation, but they may not be willing or able to acknowledge its existence openly, such as when talking with
others. This defense mechanism can be a necessary and useful means for
protecting ourselves from a devastating truth until we have the resources
to contend with it. Refusing to accept something can allow us the time

needed to absorb the shock of a life-altering situation and to prepare for what needs to be done next. When people become stuck in denial, though, they can cause harm to themselves and to those around them. At different points in the progression of an illness denial can keep them from taking necessary actions and may prompt them into taking unnecessary or detrimental actions. Denial can be what keeps someone from scheduling appointments, tests, surgery, or treatment. It can be why someone seeks numerous "second" opinions or goes to extreme lengths to try unorthodox treatments. It is often why people avoid writing wills, contacting hospice, and making funeral plans.

Denial can surface when people who are employed and very ill need to consider when to stop working. Though a few people are able to work, at least in some capacity, until near the time of death, most people will reach a point when it is to their and their workplace's benefit for them to relinquish their professional responsibilities. Such a point can be emotionally painful since work can be a large part of people's identity and daily life, engendering feelings of worthiness and normalcy. If you plan in advance for this time, you can leave your job with recognition and pleasure, rather than with embarrassment or discontentment. Consider being proactive rather than reactive. Ask your doctor what she or he anticipates is the probable trajectory of your illness. It could be helpful to ask a colleague whose judgment is sound to assess how well you are performing your duties. At some point you will need to have a frank talk with your employer, but before doing so, be sure you have looked over your contract and workplace policies to learn about your benefits, especially those related to sick leave, vacation time, workers' compensation, and health and life insurance.

Perhaps you can work out a graduated plan for reducing your workload, possibly checking back periodically with your supervisor to determine when you need to transfer your responsibilities to others. If you own your own business, you will need to draw up a plan for turning it over to someone or closing it down. Picking a stopping date, perhaps when you finish a particular project, and a date when you will say good-bye may ease others' concerns and your own. You may find a way to phase out of your work role into a new role, such as that of an adviser, and depart your professional obligations in a gracious manner that acknowledges your contributions. Consider, too, how you want to complete home and personal projects. It may help to plot out a timeline, breaking down the work and assigning due dates. Perhaps a project can be left uncompleted. Whatever we have done will continue to evolve and have impact. In one sense, everything we do is unfinished and ever changing. The reward can be the work itself.

Denial often surfaces as well when patients and physicians need to consider when to stop treatment. Even after many treatments have failed, some patients and doctors have difficulty turning to pain management as the primary objective of medical care. Some fear that if they stop treatment, they are giving in to death. Such an idea causes many people to depart life in a manner that is not to their liking, such as dying while undergoing harsh treatments that compromise their remaining time, finances, and quality of life, or dying at the hospital after a decision has been made to withdraw them from life support when their preference was to die more naturally at home.

Perhaps the most pernicious consequence of prolonged denial is that it robs people of intimacy with others. People who do not acknowledge that they are dying forfeit the chance for reconciliations, acts of forgiveness, and farewells. Not to accept the reality of death could keep you from talking with others about dying and receiving comfort for the most significant of all life's events: its end. It could be unnecessarily, tragically lonesome.

Anger

Let us not look back in anger, nor forward in fear, but around in awareness.
— James Thurber

When life does not go according to our desires and expectations, we frequently react with anger. The anger that stems from coping with a deadly disease can be more intense than what people experience in more ordinary circumstances and can surface in unexpected ways at surprising times. A terminal disease naturally spawns a host of disappointments. You may feel singled out from others who have been cured of cancer or who are in remission. You may be upset that so many others appear to be in good health and look to be long-lived. The hand you have been dealt could seem unfair, and you may ask, "Why me?"

You may be mad, too, about the troublesome and limiting side effects caused by treatment and the cancer's progression. You may be irritated by the time, trouble, and expense required to take care of yourself and become exasperated in having to take many medications and having to tolerate frequent blood draws, scans, and appointments. You may feel short-tempered around others who do not understand, or seem not to care about, what you are experiencing, including loved ones and health-care providers. Perhaps, too, you resent media reports proclaiming that breast cancer is highly curable.

Your anger may also be directed unfairly at yourself. You may be infuriated and remorseful believing that you caused your own cancer. If you experience such thoughts, keep in mind that others engaged in, or did not engage in, the same activities that you did, and they did not all get cancer. Outside of rare instances when people inherit a breast cancer gene that carries a high probability of malfunctioning and causing cancer early in life, your cancer is the result of multiple factors, including the natural aging process. Furthermore, the body of scientific studies has not conclusively shown that breast cancer is linked to any particular personality type, painful life event, or emotional state. The worry that you brought about your own demise is likely ill founded, as is the notion that you could cure your illness if you "straightened out your act" or were not depressed. Even if you did do something that contributed to your plight, remember that you were doing the best you could at that time and would likely do things differently if you could have seen into the future.

All this anger is human, reasonable, and should not be denied; rather it would be helpful for it to be expressed when possible in a manner that is not harmful to you or others. Sometimes anger is the result of not being proactive and needing to assert oneself. If this is the case, it may subside when you take more control of decisions in your life, even in small ways, like choosing when you want to do something, or in big ways, such as in deciding what you think is best for your treatment rather than deferring to others. You may understand and better control outbursts if you write about your anger in a journal. You can possibly transform your fury through creative endeavors such as drawing or molding in clay a likeness of your anger or in expressing it through dance or movement. Depending on the situation, you could discharge your anger in a number of ways, from squeezing a ball in your hand, to screaming or yelling, to physically exerting yourself, such as in ripping magazines or throwing pillows around. The act of expressing your feelings safely is what is most important.

Anger can creep up or break loose out of the blue. You may find yourself furious over a trivial matter, or you might burst out crying unexpectedly. Be wary of displacing your anger onto someone who is not to blame. People suffering great loss can find themselves in the position of needing to apologize for treating others unfairly. Forgive yourself if this occurs since this is not unusual, and you are in unusual circumstances. Anger can be like a storm that passes and clears the air, but if you find that yours is habitual and harmful, try some of the activities above, examine the links in the resource box below, and/or talk with a counselor.

CREATIVE ARTS THERAPY

- Confronting Cancer through Art: Displays the artwork of those confronting cancer.
  http://www.upenn.edu/ARG/archive/ccta/intro.html

- Literature, Arts, and Medicine Database: Offers a keyword search engine that leads to art, film, and literature related to cancer and dying.
  http://litmed.med.nyu.edu/Main?action=new

- National Coalition of Creative Arts Therapies Associations: Leads to information about therapy through art, dance, movement, drama, music, and poetry.
  http://www.nccata.org

- The Creative Center: Offers workshops and bedside programs in New York City and provides nationwide exhibits of artwork done by those touched by cancer.
  http://www.thecreativecenterarts.org/2008/03/artists-in-residence
  .html

- *Writing Out the Storm: Reading and Writing Your Way through Serious Illness or Injury,* by Barbara Abercrombie.

Bargaining

There is no medicine like hope, no incentive so great, and no tonic
so powerful as the expectation of something better tomorrow.
—Orison Swett Marden

It is basic human behavior to try to make life more to our liking, and one way we attempt to do so is to offer something in hopes of getting our desire. You may find yourself making deals with God, or with yourself, that you will do something you believe you should do and in return be granted the fulfillment of some wish. Some people perform good deeds with the thought that in doing so, they might be graced with the time they need to take a longed-for trip or attend a special occasion. Or some may decide to eat in a more healthful manner as a pact with God that for their doing so, God will put their cancer into remission. Taking action can give people a feeling of empowerment. Actions may have other benefits as well; for instance, eating well may help an individual develop more energy. Bargaining can be motivating and can offer hope. It causes no harm as long as you are not crestfallen if your wish is not granted. It is important to realize that some outcomes are not in our hands.

Depression

The darkest hour is just before the dawn.

—Proverb

Depression is a natural response to certain physical and emotional conditions, not a weakness or a character flaw. It can be the result of various factors. When one faces death, one suffers great losses, including the anticipation of the ultimate loss, life itself. Also, people with late-stage cancer can be in pain, be highly restricted, and possibly feel isolated, which makes them susceptible to despair. Even with a fine quality of life, unwelcome changes and great discomfort can accumulate and lead to depression. You are not alone if you are experiencing continual sadness and apathy.

Direct physical causes of depression can include pain caused by cancer and cancer treatment affecting bodily functions. Studies have found that people in pain, quite reasonably, are more likely to be depressed (1). Most problematic physical sensations can be relieved by pain medication, thereby sometimes alleviating depression. Another direct physical cause for depression can be steroids used for cancer treatment, such as Decadron and prednisone; if these are causing depression, perhaps other medicines can be tried. It is important, though, not to withdraw too quickly from steroidal drugs such as these since withdrawal can also trigger feelings of gloom.

Other causes of depression are circumstantial. As sociologist Kathy Charmaz says, "Living with a serious illness takes effort and devours time. It also means overcoming stigmatizing judgments, intrusive questions, and feelings of diminished worth." Charmaz identifies stages of illness, including the interruption of life, the intrusion upon daily activities, and, last, the immersion into symptoms and treatments (2). If the disruption of normalcy, power, and roles is causing you distress, try setting a new routine or cultivating a new role or project. If you are feeling depersonalized, take some action to restore your identity; for example, if you will be staying in the hospital or at a hospice home, bring photos or other personal mementos. Similarly, a break from the norm can be restorative. If you are able, go on a balloon ride, skinny dip, get a professional massage, or plan a small adventure to a favorite spot. Spend time in nature to uplift your spirits. Getting into water or sitting beside a lake or the ocean can ease depression. Something as simple as going for a walk can break a negative chain of thought, as can engaging in creative endeavors that require concentration, such as writing, gardening, cooking, or making something with your hands.

Those with cancer must deal with much uncertainty, which for some leads to unhappiness. One moment you can be confident about planning into the future, and the next you wonder if you are able to visit someone that afternoon. Serious illness ushers in a multitude of anxieties, including worrying about test results, finances, and death itself. Look for ways to reduce uncertainties when possible; for example: request a walk-through for a medical procedure; ask when to expect test results and tell your doctor when a decision is riding on the outcome. Do not stop making plans, but let others know they are tentative and cancel if necessary.

To address the fear and sorrow of dying it may help you to talk about your anxiety, to engage in uplifting activities, and to connect with your faith or the values that guide and give meaning to your life. It can be excruciatingly lonely if you cannot express your panic and sadness to someone. Having the opportunity to express oneself fully can ease depression and bring peace. Choose someone who is capable of letting you be free and real. It may help to seek a counselor, particularly one who specializes in end-of-life issues, or a spiritual adviser such as a pastor, rabbi, priest, religious leader, or someone whose insight and wisdom you admire. Reading passages from scriptures and other inspirational literature, including the reflections on death following this chapter, may quell your apprehension. You can try praying, saying affirmations, and meditating to reduce anxiety. Most faiths have a prayer that can be said in times of distress, or you could select or create one that is meaningful to you. Similarly, you can find or create an affirmation such as, "I will be gentle with myself and others." You can use any brief statement that grounds and affirms a belief that you would like to nurture, repeating it at regular intervals during the day.

Cultivate appreciation. Each day write down one marvelous thing that you never noticed before or one thing for which you are grateful. Reflect on the many others who have faced, or are facing, limitations and a shortened life. Seeing the universality of suffering can open your heart to compassion for yourself and others. Many young people with life-threatening diseases are devoid of self-pity, having few expectations about what life should be. Look to the lack of self-pity in children and animals. In addition to these suggestions for reducing anxiety and depression, your doctor may think it is wise to prescribe medications that can enable you to live more normally and interact more fully with others. If you find yourself unhappily isolated, take action. Reach out to others as suggested later in this chapter. We are not meant to be islands, particularly in time of great need.

Some people can tell they are despondent, but not everyone can. When scholar Eve Kosofsky-Sedgwick dealt with breast cancer, she created her own set of questions to assess whether or not she was depressed. In considering her questions, we can see the extent to which depression can compromise one's quality of life and capacity to experience joy:

> Can I laugh? Do I? Can I laugh out loud?
> After I cry, can I let go of the sadness for a while?
> Do other people's stories interest me?
> Do I brood for a long time when a caretaker acts thoughtlessly?
> Do I have the energy to squawk when my pain meds aren't doing the trick?
> Is anyone home when beauty, love, or enlightenment knock on the door? (3)

A more formal list of symptoms of depression is put forth by the National Institute of Mental Health. If you have experienced one or more of these indicators of depression for more than a week, you should take action to attempt to reduce the symptoms and/or seek a professional who treats depression. If you are having suicidal thoughts, seek immediate aid!

> Persistent sad, anxious, or "empty" mood
> Feelings of hopelessness, pessimism
> Feelings of guilt, worthlessness, helplessness
> Loss of interest or pleasure in hobbies and activities that were once enjoyed, including sex
> Decreased energy, fatigue, being "slowed down"
> Difficulty concentrating, remembering, making decisions

> Insomnia, early-morning awakening, or oversleeping
> Appetite and/or weight loss or overeating and weight gain
> Thoughts of death or suicide; suicide attempts
> Restlessness, irritability
> Persistent physical symptoms that do not respond to treatment,
>   such as headaches, digestive disorders, and chronic pain (4)

If you suspect you are depressed, take swift action to address your condition since people become increasingly lethargic and apathetic as hopelessness takes hold. Depression, like other kinds of pain, is best nipped in the bud. Most hospitals have chaplains, counselors, and support groups. A mental health professional can work with you to try to determine the precise source of your depression, and then together you can target means to alleviate it.

Like physical pain, depression is underdiagnosed and undertreated in the United States. One study found that nearly half of all cancer patients met the psychiatric criteria for depression, and the incidence increases as the disease progresses (5). Do not expect that your doctor will necessarily notice your failing mood. Not all health-care professionals know how to recognize and treat depression. Your oncologist may be so focused on treating your disease that she or he will not be considering all the collateral consequences of your illness, especially if you do not report how you are feeling.

Acceptance

The world is ruled by letting things take their course.
—Lao-Tzu

In people with incurable diseases, the acceptance of death is not characterized as a state of euphoria; rather, it is typified by the absence of struggle. That is not to say that people do not want to live. Acceptance can coexist with trying to live as long as possible. For example, many people put their illness in God's hands, believing God will inspire and guide nurses and doctors to help them live longer. Dying peacefully may come easier to those who have prepared for letting go of life and/or to some who have deeply spiritual beliefs. In her book, Kubler-Ross states that the passage of time and help from others can aid someone in the acceptance of death. Most people with breast cancer have that time. However, not everyone at the end of life accepts death. Some, as the poet Dylan Thomas advocated, "do not go gentle into that good night." But for those that do, perhaps it is because they sense, or believe, they are moving beyond this life, surrendering who they are now to something else, something greater.

Last, though not a stage in itself, Kubler-Ross and her team discovered that hope perennially surfaced throughout all the stages. There are many kinds of hope—hope for forgiveness or reconciliation or greater joy. There is the hope of living longer and of dying peacefully. Hope can be as simple as wishing for a moment of relief or for grace to show itself on any given day.

Interrelating with Others: Those You See Occasionally

To look directly into the face of humanity and not turn away is perhaps

the greatest gift we can give to one another.

—Camus

It is often our relationships with others that create and define our happiness. In fact, your emotional health may be more closely tied to how you feel about your relationships than how you feel about the course of your disease. You may be unusually blessed with equanimity and be surrounded with thoughtful, loving people. Even so, particularly in times of crisis, interactions with others can sometimes be strained. What follows are some common difficulties that can arise when interacting with others and how to prepare for them.

Health-Care Professionals

Because you are dealing with the most important of matters—your survival—interactions with your doctors and other health-care providers can be emotionally charged. It is easy to idealize and/or demonize those caring for you. They may appear to be queens or knights riding in on medical steeds to rescue you. Patients can easily develop attachments to their doctors, sometimes resulting in romantic feelings. Doctors are in positions of seeming power, dedicated to helping you with issues of life and death that are intimate by their very nature. If you find yourself idealizing a health-care provider, be careful not to expect too much of him or her since such expectations could set you up for an emotional tumble.

Keep in mind that like everyone, health-care professionals experience significant demands in their workplace and personal lives and need to attend to matters other than their medical practice. Still, you have the right to a reasonable amount of their attention. It may help you to determine what is reasonable by talking with other patients, or when you feel you are not getting enough consideration, talk with your doctor to see if she or he could offer you more. As much as health-care providers are surrounded by illness, it may be hard for them to fully imagine what it is like to be a seriously ill patient. Realizing this may keep you from personalizing a behavior or remark that strikes you as insensitive. However, do not accept mistreatment. Speak up if a health-care provider says or does something that upsets you.

The time when treatments stop working ushers in a sometimes difficult transition for a patient and doctor. Once your medical care becomes primarily pain management, your contact with your oncologist likely will be reduced. She or he will need to direct more attention to other patients. You may want to talk with your doctor in advance of this juncture to find ways to ward off the feelings of desertion that patients often experience. It might be possible to arrange for periodic contact, such as brief e-mails, or perhaps you can organize other support to lessen feelings of abandonment.

Clergy and Counselors

Similar to health-care professionals, clergy and counselors are in positions to help you, and the same feelings of admiration and affection, as well as disappointment and anger, can emerge. Clergy and counselors will be imperfect, as everyone is. They will have worked through their own issues concerning illness and death to varying degrees. If you are not finding the help and comfort you hoped for, request from them what you would like; for instance, perhaps you would like a pastor to call you, or to pray for you, or to provide you with a deeper understanding of a religious text. Do not hesitate to look elsewhere to get your needs met if you believe the person you are seeing cannot offer you wise counsel.

Others with Cancer

When one has an imminently life-threatening cancer, it could be disturbing to be with others whose cancer has not progressed. You may find it difficult to go to support groups with members whose prognoses are not immediately life-threatening or who are already long-term "survivors." You might even hate the word "survivor," feeling as though you have been barred from a desirable club. Those with early-stage or curable cancers may be more light-hearted than you find yourself capable of being, and if they are more demoralized about their cancer than you are about yours, that too can be troubling. It also may be disconcerting to learn that others who were recently diagnosed are getting newer, more effective treatments that were not available when you had earlier-stage breast cancer. It is hard not to think, "If only I had had that." But the reality is that treatment is ever changing, and someone may have been thinking a similar thought about the treatment you were given. You may sense that a number of others with cancer fear they will be the next person to have a recurrence, or find yourself the recipient of unwished-for sympathy. We mention these feelings so that you know you are not alone in having them. However, even if you experience some of these unsettling emotions, you may also find that those with cancer, whatever stage they are in, are able to empathize to some extent with your situation and could well be among your greatest supporters.

Acquaintances Who Are Well

A number of your acquaintances may act as if nothing is different when they see you. They might remark how good you look or say they are sure you will be fine. Such comments may strike you as dismissive. On the other hand, to have acquaintances continually acknowledge that your life is in danger can be anxiety-provoking. Acquaintances frequently do not know what to say, though they may sincerely care how you are. Sometimes their comments stem from ignorance about the progression of cancer; thoughtless remarks can also be a result of their inability to cope with, or their inexperience with, grave illness and death. Rarely do people intend to be hurtful. Such an understanding on your part may make it easier for you when people are socially clumsy or trivialize what you are experiencing.

More problematic are comments that stem from others' righteousness and deep fear. You may encounter people who, without being asked, will advise you what to do, and what not to do, to cure yourself. Some people might insinuate that you have done something that caused your disease. As scholar Susan Sontag noted in her book *Illness as Metaphor*, "Any disease whose causality is murky, and for which treatment is ineffectual, tends to be awash in significance" (6). Some may ascribe your illness to a cause with little evidence, or to a cause that may reassure them that they will not be in your shoes. Do not hesitate to cut conversations such as these short, and if someone persists in making you uncomfortable, tell the individual what topics are off limits. If necessary, avoid her or him.

Interrelating with Those Closest to You

It is the same with your wealth, your possessions, and your family—they are all yours only in name; they don't really belong to you, they belong to nature.
—Ajahn Chah Subatto, *Our Real Home*

A serious illness affects not only the person who is ill; its impact radiates out from the ill person across the network of interrelationships she or he has with others. Ties that are inflexible can snap. Strong ones can be fortified, and new bonds will be formed. Ideally, the ties that persist will form a web of support for the ill person and for all those who are interconnected with her.

Predictable difficulties and opportunities will emerge as people grapple with how to offer and accept help, forgiveness, and good-byes. Fear, guilt, and anger, though uncomfortable, offer chances to be intimate through sharing thoughts and emotions. Problems may be easier to handle if you anticipate and prepare for them. The emphasis in this section is on the very human ways the people who are closest to us can disappoint us, and we them. Such disappointments are also windows for refining our behaviors. Most important of all, serious illness is often the occasion when you discover your and others' capacity to love in unforeseen ways.

Siblings, Friends, Relatives

Though you will likely have support from siblings, friends, and relatives, your illness will also frighten some people. It can remind them of their own mortality, of others who have died whom they miss, and of how they will miss you when you are gone. Those closely related to you might fear that they are more prone to develop cancer as a result of its surfacing in the family. Some might end or reduce their contact with you, driven away unconsciously by their fears. Others may be present but emotionally distant. It is not uncommon that friends and relatives inquire about how you are but resist hearing any more than a superficial answer. They may hide their own feelings, perhaps hiding their lives from you also, in the belief that anything but your illness is inconsequential. They may try to cheer you when you would prefer to talk about serious matters. A few may resent that you need, or receive, a great deal of attention from others and may be harboring anger that confuses you.

Such reactions are typical. Keep in mind that people's behavior reflects who they are, so though some may leave you, either literally or emotionally, their behavior is not about you. They may even profoundly care about you, but their own fears can overwhelm them. You could try talking with them about the distance you feel, and you can always hope a change will occur. It may be less hurtful, though, to accept that certain behaviors will not change. You may find yourself wanting more than they are able to give. Though it may be far from ideal, consider that given their limitations they are doing the best they can. It also may be hard for you in the midst of crisis to remember that as much as they may have deep affection for you, their lives are ongoing, and they need to continue to be joyful about what nurtures their lives.

Parents

If your parents are alive, they may have great difficulty seeing that your health is possibly worse than their own, and the thought that you might precede them in death could cause them great sorrow. They may harbor guilt, to the point of defensiveness, that they are responsible for your illness, either because of heredity or because they fear something in your upbringing may have caused your cancer. For at least two reasons neither they nor you need to concern yourself with such blame. First, the causes of breast cancer are not conclusively known. Even if you did inherit a genetic predisposition, your parents could not have known they harbored the gene, and the only way to prevent such a gene from being passed along would have been for them not to have given birth to you. Second, a hereditary predisposition most often is only one factor in the development of breast cancer and likely not the most important one. In terms of the other factors, if they or you knew you were doing something that would cause the disease, you likely would have avoided it.

For your part, you may find yourself angry with a parent for long-standing or ongoing reasons. The intensity of a life-threatening illness may offer you an opportunity to be liberated from this hostility, perhaps by working with a counselor to productively express or otherwise resolve it. You may also find yourself concerned for your parents. You may have imagined at some point that you would be taking care of them, or perhaps already are, and worry about the stresses on them and who will assist them in the future. You can do your best to prepare for their future care, but what happens is not fully in anyone's hands. For now, you can help them feel less helpless. To forge a more loving connection let a parent know something small that she or he could do for you within his or her physical limitations. Perhaps you can let them know how lucky you are to have their care and their love in ushering you into, and possibly out of, life.

Spouse or Significant Other

Your husband, wife, or partner is very likely horribly upset and quite fearful about your illness. The person with whom you share your life must juggle helping you while maintaining work, home, and personal responsibilities. Spouses can be upset because they are powerless to stop what is happening to you and afraid that they cannot live up to your idea of a good partner. They may worry about medical bills, how to take over what you contributed to your life together, how to recover after you are gone, and how to go on living without you. As difficult as it may be to allow your partner to express his or her frustrations and fears, doing so may allow you to empathize and become closer. Hopefully your partner can express angst in a way that does not lay blame on you or your condition. If being honest is difficult, a counselor may be able to help you communicate. The realization of your suffering and death can unearth deep love that previously went unrecognized. However, illness and impending death can also make plain a relationship's flaws. They can be the final straw in a troubled or superficial bond, with you or your partner opting to end it. A few spouses and partners leave in fright, like a child might; if that happens, you may need to call upon others close to you or on professional services for extra support.

Your sexual life with your partner may change, sometimes becoming more tender and profound and sometimes becoming less satisfying because of emotional tensions or changes in your body. Tell your partner honestly your fears about being physically intimate. Let him or her know what you cannot feel and what feels good, and try experimenting with new ways of being physically intimate. A side effect of cancer treatments is often a lowered libido and physical limitations. Your doctor likely will not address sexual issues unless you mention you are experiencing problems. Do not hesitate to ask what can be done to enhance a lagging sexual desire since increasingly more is known about how to remedy this concern.

If you are single, you may be fearful about forging a new romantic relationship. As long as we are alive, however, we are in relationship with others. Let your heart and mind guide you, and be honest with anyone who may become an intimate partner. A relationship's worth and depth are not measured simply by its length.

Children

Adult children will have some of the same concerns as a spouse—for example, how to care for you while continuing to work, how to allot time to other loved ones, and how to have some personal time themselves. They may want to participate by helping you make decisions, though you may need to be mindful not to let them take over if that is not what you would like. Similar to friends and relatives, they may not fulfill your expectations. It may help to be clear with them about what you would and would not like them to do. Telling them repeatedly, however, is likely futile and can cause ill will. If they cannot meet your needs, it is best to look to others.

You may find that what is most difficult about facing the future is knowing that you will not be physically present for your children, particularly if they are young. You can do all you can to prepare for their future, but for now what is most important is that they know you love them. You can show them and tell them many times before you die. You can leave mementos, images, and cards to remind them of your affection and to advise them in years to come. It may help to remember that however their lives unfold, it always was to some significant extent not in your control. At present, realize that they, like you, are going through a traumatic time. Recognize how this may be affecting them, point them to resources, and have confidence in their resilience.

Children, young ones in particular, will be afraid about what will happen to them after you die. Talk with them in simple and concrete ways about what their lives may be like when you are physically gone. Let them know who will care for them and what you will leave for them to remember you by. Record in writing or in images your wishes for their lives. Share your wisdom and what you have found beautiful in the world.

As much as you and others might be thinking about your young children, they can be overlooked during hectic times. Your children probably feel the world is less safe than it was before you became ill, and at this confusing, scary, and needy time, they may feel left out and ignored. Maintain familiar schedules as much as possible, and when necessary, establish new routines that they can count on. Be sure to plan time into the routine for them to be with you and other caring adults. Perhaps make a point to do one small thing together each day. It may help them if you read aloud a book about death directed to their age group and share feelings and thoughts with each other. The Web sites in the following resource box offer ideas and reading lists. Give them a small task to help you that makes them feel important, and let others know in their presence how much they help. Be clear with them about what you are and are not capable of, and reassure them that you love and have faith in them. Children understand more than adults usually realize.

Adolescents, developmentally, are nearly as egocentric as young children. At this stage their concerns are to be accepted by their peers and to become more independent. They may be conflicted about wanting their freedom and knowing that you are in need. They do not want to be overprotected, and at the same time, they may still want you to take care of them and be an adult who is in control. They will have some of the same fears as young children, but they will often cover up their confusion and concerns. They may show their fears indirectly by becoming moody, angry, and depressed. They may withdraw, denying that you are not well. Such behavior does not mean they do not care.

Experts suggest that a parent who is dying of cancer should not expect much extra of adolescents, and they stress that communications be kept open. Teenagers do not want to be different from their peers, so encouraging them to engage in their normal activities is helpful for them. Give them one or two important, but not overly adult, responsibilities to help you out, and praise them for their contribution. Look for times when you can show you have confidence in them. Also, look for opportunities that allow them to be vulnerable and to share their feelings if they choose. Encourage them, too, to talk with a trusted adult or counselor, to read books that have been written for young people in their situation, and to connect with peers who have a parent who has cancer or who is seriously ill.

For all those closest to you, be honest about how you are doing and how you are feeling, including young children, though you will need to talk with them in an especially simple and gentle manner. If you run into rocky times when interrelating with those who matter to you most, a counselor may be able to bring you closer and deepen your ties. Cancer centers and hospice usually have materials and professionals to help you and your loved ones, especially children, deal with your illness. The links below are helpful as well. You can give your loved ones and yourself a great gift if you are able to share your feelings in this tumultuous time and if you can encourage them to live their lives to the fullest now and in your absence.

SUPPORT FOR YOUNG CHILDREN AND ADOLESCENTS

- Kids Konnected: Offers an extensive web site of information for children with a parent who has cancer, including locations of support groups and a newsletter.
  http://www.kidskonnected.org

- KidsCope: Offers a number of publications and links to local support groups and web sites.
  http://www.kidscope.org

- Hurricane Voices: Provides a reading list for children and adolescents.
  http://www.hurricanevoices.org/index.htm

Those Caring For You

Taking care of the seriously ill can be a deeply rewarding way to connect with another person and expand one's humanity. It can be highly demanding as well. If only a few people are involved in the care of someone who is dying, they are likely to be overwhelmed. You can help those who are looking after you by accepting help from a wider circle of caretakers, including friends, relatives, and acquaintances who have offered their assistance, along with accepting professional caretaking. In doing so, those closest to you will have more energy and time to enjoy being with you.

You may want to write out your needs and think about who could help you. Find out what your county's department of social services can do to assist as well. Once you know what aid is available, consider formalizing a support network. Ask someone to take on the role of leader (it could be a rotating role). The leader could contact people and suggest ways they could assist you, and those willing to volunteer could choose their level of support. Based on others' responses, a calendar could be created detailing who is doing what and when. The leader also needs to periodically ask volunteers if they want to change their commitment. It is important that people in the support network feel free to be honest with the leader about their limitations.

To support those helping you, you could encourage them to support one another, perhaps by doing something as simple as calling one another to see how their lives are going. You could show your appreciation for your caregivers by simply thanking them verbally after they do something, by making brief calls, by sending thanks in writing on small cards or over e-mail, or by offering small gifts, perhaps giving them something of yours that you suspect they would like or giving them meaningful bookmarks or refrigerator magnets. Encourage those caring for you to spend time with others and engage in activities that are nurturing to them. Letting them care for you and expressing your desire that they take care of themselves is offering them a double gift. Encourage them to seek professional support as well. Sometimes a social worker can lead them to additional sources of aid for you, and they may find help by going to counseling or support groups specifically for caregivers. Health insurance may cover some of these costs, and some cancer centers offer certain support without charge. The links below lead to further information to help troubleshoot common problems and to find additional help.

SUPPORT FOR CAREGIVERS

- Cancer Caregiving: Offers both emotional and practical tools for the caregiver.
  http://www.cancercaregiving.com

- Cancercare: Provides free professional support services for anyone affected by cancer; includes online, telephone, and in-person counseling; arranges telephone support for teenage caregivers.
  http://www.cancercare.org

(Resources, continued)

- National Family Caregivers Association: Provides information and
  education for caregivers.
    http://www.nfcacares.org

- Mothers Supporting Daughters with Breast Cancer: Offers education about
  how mothers can help daughters who have breast cancer.
    http://www.mothersdaughters.org

- Gilda's Club: Offers information on where to find or start a club in which
  families are offered emotional and social support free of charge.
    http://www.gildasclub.org

- *Share the Care: How to Organize a Group to Care for Someone Who Is
  Seriously Ill*, by Cappy Capossela and Sheila Warnock

At Ease near Life's End

The goal of human life is constructing an architecture of the soul.

—Simone Weil, from *La connaissance surnaturelle*

Near life's end we are usually freer to be who we are without pretensions
and to see more clearly what matters. When death approaches, the reduction of time becomes like a press that squeezes out the less important,
and we carve away the unnecessary, less life-giving excess (7). In this way
death can help you take action on what matters most to you. If possible, it
is time to take the trip you have dreamt about, visit the people you love,
and do what exalts your being. Decide what is meaningful to you and start
with the most significant, knowing that you cannot do everything. Be sure
to plan breaks in your activities to rejuvenate yourself.

Perhaps what matters most to you is to live as normally as possible and
share simple pleasures with people in your life. As your energy subsides,
pick one thing each week, or day, that you do not want to do, and do not
do it, so that you can focus on what you do want to. You may be able to
get help from others if something must be done, or perhaps it is fine if it
goes unattended. More and more you know not to postpone what is vital.
You know that the time ahead may be your only chance to see someone

or to say something valuable to loved ones. Whatever has kept you from doing what will lead you and others to greater joy, let the knowledge of impending death remove your hesitation. You may not have the energy in the future. It is now or possibly never.

Reaching Out to Others for Emotional Support

Metastatic cancer is a heavy emotional burden to shoulder in silence. Do not keep pain, fear, and confusion all to yourself. People who have strong bonds can best weather crises and lead more contented lives. One of the most important actions you can take is reaching out to others for help, particularly if you live alone or need people who can better understand what you are experiencing. A number of people may want to help but may be unsure what to do. You can learn who would like to help by simply keeping in touch with others or by creating a support network as mentioned in the previous section. One way to stay in contact with others is to send out funny or poignant postcards or e-mails that let people know how you are. If you would like more contact, you could include a note that you would be pleased to have people call or stop by. Others will follow your cues, not always knowing what you would like unless you tell them.

What most people need for emotional support is a good listener. Not everyone is able to be one. If someone does not know to be a good listener but is interested in becoming one, you could share with her or him some frequently advocated guidelines. Such recommendations usually can be found in brochures available from cancer clinics and hospice programs or on cancer care Web sites. The guidelines generally advise people to listen without interrupting and without trying to change the other person's feelings or point of view. They recommend listening to the ill person express fears and anger without trying to offer solutions unless called upon for advice. They suggest allowing the ill person to talk about death without imposing one's own ideas unless asked to share them.

Listening is a particularly intimate request, so you may want to ask for other kinds of support as well. Consider what you and others could enjoy together, perhaps offering a number of possibilities and letting them choose. For example, you might request the following:

> To be remembered in people's prayers
> To have poems or inspirational literature read to you
> To be brought a meal

To have someone join you in listening to music or watching a favorite
     movie or television program
To have someone join you in looking over old pictures or family
     movies
To have someone sit with you in silence
To have someone hold your hand or give you a gentle hug

When you are facing a difficulty, such as surgery, or perhaps when you are
losing heart, you could invite over a circle of friends to be part of what
Dr. Rachel Naomi Remen has named "the stone ritual" (8). To conduct this
ritual you need to find a stone or some small meaningful object that is
passed around the circle of friends. While holding the stone, each person
in turn relates a hardship that she or he endured in life. Then each names
his or her source of strength at that troublesome time, such as patience,
faith, or courage, and says how he or she called upon it from within or
found it elsewhere. As they tell their stories, people imbue the stone with
the source of their strength so that it will be there in spirit for you. When
you need to, hold this stone to be reminded of your connection to all suffering beings and to their strength in times of adversity.

Emotional support is particularly wonderful when it is mutual. You
might feel lonely at times because people are not sharing what is happening in their lives. They can keep you connected to other loved ones,
to your workplace, and most importantly, to themselves if you make a
point to ask about their lives and feelings. Listening to others may keep
you from focusing obsessively on your own situation and console you that
life is ongoing. As much as possible, give them the gift of your attention.
Ask people to share their joys, disappointments, and plans for the future.
Everyone can use a good listener, and you may be in a position to offer
more time than many others. It is especially meaningful for both listener
and speaker if you do not feel the need to put on a false front or to judge
one another's lives.

You may discover a different level of empathy when communicating
with others who have metastatic breast cancer. You can find support
groups, and sometimes a cancer "buddy," through a number of sources
such as the American Cancer Society, your health-care practitioners, and
breast cancer organizations, which you can access using the links in the
next resource box. Women with late-stage breast cancer frequently have
different concerns than those in early stages, so links leading to the online
groups in the following box are primarily for those with metastatic breast

cancer. When first entering a group, get a feel for its character. Some support groups are professionally led and others are highly informal. Some delve deeply into personal feelings; others disseminate information about cancer. Simply being in a group will not necessarily help you thrive, so trust your intuition in deciding whether to stay involved. You can always return to a group, and in the meantime you can acquaint yourself with other groups or means of emotional support.

ONLINE BREAST CANCER COMMUNITIES AND EMOTIONAL SUPPORT

- CLUB-METS-BC
  http://www.acor.org/club-mets-bc.html

- Breast Cancer Support: Look for the virtual meeting place for those with recurrence.
  http://bcsupport.org

- Inflammatory Breast Cancer Mailing List
  http://www.ibcsupport.org

- Sisters Network, a National African-American Breast Cancer Survivorship Organization: Offers support and information specific to African-American women, including links to affiliate chapters.
  http://www.sistersnetworkinc.org

- breastcancer.org: Provides discussion boards and chat rooms.
  http://www.breastcancer.org

- Network of Strength: Provides messages boards.
  http://www.networkofstrength.org

- The Wellness Community: Offers free support of many kinds, including ways to enhance life and reduce isolation.
  http://www.thewellnesscommunity.org/corporate

Putting Regrets to Rest and Reconciling with Others

And forgive us our trespasses, as we forgive those who have trespassed against us.

—The Lord's Prayer

It is not unusual when one's life is coming to its end to be plagued with thoughts that certain choices we made harmed others and ourselves. Over the span of a lifetime disappointments and regrets are inescapable. Some people let go of them quickly, but many cover them over. Dying breaks down these defenses. You may find that as you review your life, past actions, or inactions, come back to haunt you. The acknowledgment of a wrongdoing can be difficult, especially if you hold the unrealistic notion that you should be nearly perfect. Many people discover that speaking about their wrongdoing aloud to a friend who can keep confidences, or to a clergy member, or a counselor, can be liberating. This type of cleansing is similar to the confessional practiced in some faiths. Having another person sit with you as you express your regret can keep you from getting stuck unproductively in guilt and self-hatred. When you face your transgression, allow yourself to experience remorse. Remorse frees people to get outside of themselves and realize their humanity. Such sorrow can enable you to move on, now wiser. You are free to take responsibility, stopping the behavior and/or making amends of some kind.

It may be appropriate and necessary to do something to make up for your wrongdoing. Before making direct amends, consider the consequences carefully and possibly seek counsel. Some amends are hurtful to the person who is contacted. She or he might not want to be reminded of what happened or never realized your offense. You do not have make amends to someone directly; for example, if you betrayed a friend who never realized your transgression, you could make a point to speak well of her to others. If you were cruel or neglectful to an animal, you could donate money to an animal shelter. It is never too late to do something within your physical and financial means. If the person or people you harmed are not alive, you could pass along some loving act, knowing in your heart that you are doing it for the person you wronged. For example, you could bring flowers to an elderly person who is alone in a nursing home if you felt you should have done more for your parents.

If it is appropriate for you to make a direct amend, consider the best way to do so. You may want to apologize in person or less directly in writing. Perhaps go over what you plan to say with someone whose judgment you trust before you approach the other person. It is easy to get into unnecessary explanations that may sound to the other person like you are not accepting responsibility. Keep it simple. The best approach may be to say nothing more than that you are sorry and to ask for forgiveness. Perhaps a gesture of some kind, or a small gift, is appropriate. Realize the wronged person may not be ready to forgive you, but know that your amends will have positive effects if done sincerely. Making an amend takes courage. If one is called for, be sure to gather that courage before it is too late.

Saying Good-Bye

We need, in love, to practice only this: letting each other go.

For holding on comes easily; we do not need to learn it.

—Rainer Maria Rilke, "Requiem for a Friend"

Good-byes are difficult, but they can put your heart at ease, as well as the hearts of those who love you. Good-byes need not be formal and final. Your farewell to others could take various forms, from a meaningful talk, to a kiss on the cheek, to a last laugh. Most important is an acknowledgment of your and another person's caring for each other. Many people feel bad about not having had a chance to say good-bye to a loved one, and many long to hear the words "I love you," perhaps for the first time, perhaps as the last words they hear from someone. Once again, people will often look to you for a cue that it is time for good-byes. While you have energy, make it a point to see people who matter to you, either individually or as a group. Doing this does not mean you are going to die right away, but you want to be sure you can enjoy their company when possible.

If you are feeling up to being social and like bringing people together, have a celebratory gathering at which you and those to whom you want to say good-bye tell one another what you mean to each other or what you learned from each other. Another possibility is to ask each person to bring a photo or a memento of a time you spent together, giving each person a chance to tell the story behind the image or object. Perhaps you have something special you would like to say to someone privately. Individually you may want to tell loved ones what they have meant to you, how you enjoyed them, and what you hope for them, or you may want to ask them to think of you when they see, hear, taste, or smell something. You could ask loved ones if they have anything they want to tell you or would like you to know. Perhaps you want to show your affection in a unique manner. You might write a song, make something with your hands, or create a list of readings and/or music that represents your love or insights about life. Be watchful, however, not to get too caught up in creating something to leave since memories of being together are the most precious remembrance. As you become less concerned with worldly matters, you may not want much company. If you are inclined, you could mail good-byes to people. There are also Internet sites that will send your final words after you are deceased. (See "Obituaries, Markers, Epitaphs, Final Good-Byes" in chapter 7.) Possibly, too, your preference is to depart this life without farewells.

Being Present in Life

Each moment is absolute, alive, and significant. The frog leaps, the cricket sings,
a dewdrop glitters on the lotus leaf, a breeze passes through the pine branches and
the moonlight falls on the murmuring stream.

—D. T. Suzuki

The Chinese word for "opportunity" consists of two characters, *huì* and *jī*. The character *huì* means an occasion. The character *jī* means a time when something is beginning to change. The occasion of dying is the most profound change, and realizing that this astounding transformation will occur can be an opportunity. Though to us this change can feel like a crisis, from a wider perspective, from nature's perspective, dying is simply an occasion. Sensing clearly that we, and everything that exists, are impermanent can reveal the inseparable nature of birth and death and can remind us that we are a part of the unending flow of change, one that unites us with all being. Such a perspective can release us from our fears and allow us to appreciate the present.

Life calls out to us until the moment we take our leave. While our body, eyes, ears, nose, mouth, and mind function, we can focus on any sense to experience living. Even bedridden, we can feel the breeze on our arm; we can see the sunlight filtering through the window shade; we can hear distant voices in conversation; we may smell what is cooking down the hall. We can focus on our breath and observe the air moving in and out of our body. We can notice what many often pass by. As we near death, little is required of us, and we become again more like an infant experiencing the immediate. Pleasant or not, it is existence. Living in awareness by focusing on what is happening at any given moment is a way to live completely until one's final breath. We can be simply and truly who and what we are. We can be relaxed and confident that what has ushered us into life, what has composed our life, and what will shepherd our departure is never ceasing.

Further Reading

Books and Films with Personal Accounts of Late-Stage Breast Cancer or Dying

Advanced Breast Cancer: A Guide to Living with Metastatic Disease, 2nd ed., by Musa Mayer. Patient Centered Guides, 1998.

Before I Say Good-bye: Recollections and Observations from One Woman's Final Year, by Ruth Picardie. Owl Books, 2003.

Cancer in Two Voices, by Sandra Butler and Barbara Rosenblum. Spinsters Ink Books, 1991.

The Cancer Journals, by Audre Lorde. Spinsters Ink Books, 1980.

On Death and Dying, by Elisabeth Kubler-Ross. Macmillan, 1969.

The Death of Ivan Ilyich, by Leo Tolstoy (fiction). Bantam Dell, 1981.

Grace and Grit, by Ken Wilber. Shambhala Publications, 1993.

Hollis Sigler's Breast Cancer Journal, by Hollis Sigler. Hudson Hills Press, 1999.

Intimate Death: How the Dying Teach Us How to Live, by Marie De Hennezel. Vintage, 1998.

Kitchen Table Wisdom, by Rachel Naomi Remen. Riverhead Hardcover, 1996.

Morrie: In His Own Words, by Morrie Schwartz. Delta, 2000.

The Quiet War: Profiles of Women Facing Advanced Breast Cancer/Resource Guide. Affinityfilms, 2007.

Recovering from Mortality: Essays from a Cancer Limbo Time, by Deborah Cumming. Novello Festival Press, 2005.

Books That Address Concerns of the Dying

Good Days, Bad Days: The Self in Chronic Illness and Time, by Kathy C. Charmaz. Rutgers University Press, 1991.

The Four Things That Matter Most: A Book about Living, by Ira Byock. Free Press/ Simon and Schuster, 2004.

Full Catastrophe Living: Using the Wisdom of Your Body and Mind to Face Stress, Pain, and Illness, by Jon Kabat-Zinn. Delta, 1990.

Here for Now: Living Well with Cancer through Mindfulness, by Elana Rosenbaum. Satya House Publications, 2007.

No Regrets: A Ten-Step Program for Living in the Present and Leaving the Past Behind, by Hamilton Beazley. Wiley, 2004.

Books That Offer Wisdom in Facing Death

Handbook for Mortals: Guidance for People Facing Serious Illness, by Joanne Lynn. Oxford University Press, 1999.

Lessons from the Dying, by Rodney Smith. Wisdom Publications, 1998.

No Death, No Fear, by Thich Nhat Hanh. Riverhead Trade, 2003.

Reflections on Death

At some instinctual level all living creatures avoid death. Human beings are no different. Even so, some have been graced with, or have developed, the capacity to live well when highly conscious of their mortality. When you are feeling anxious about ceasing to be in this life, the following quotes, taken from both Eastern and Western traditions, may comfort you.

What is life? It is the flash of a firefly in the night. It is the breath of a buffalo in the wintertime. It is the little shadow which runs across the grass and loses itself in the sunset.
— Crowfoot

Death belongs to life as birth does. The walk is in the raising of the foot as in the laying of it down.
— Tagore, *Stray Birds*, CCLXVII

Accustom yourself to the belief that death is of no concern to us, since all good and evil lie in sensation and sensation ends with death. Therefore the rightful belief that death is nothing to us makes a mortal life happy, not by adding to it an infinite time, but by taking away the desire for immortality. Death is therefore of no concern to us; for while we exist death is not present, and when death is present we no longer exist. . . . People sometimes flee death as the greatest of evils, sometimes long for it as a relief from the evils of life. The wise neither renounce life nor fear its end; for living does not offend them nor do they suppose that not to live is in any way evil. As they do not choose the food that is most in quantity but that which is most pleasant, so they do not seek the enjoyment of the longest life but of the happiest.
— Epicurus in a letter to Menoeceus

There is good hope that death is a blessing for it is one of two things: either the dead are nothing and have no perception of anything, or it is, as we are told, a change and a relocating for the soul from here to another place. If it is complete lack of perception, like a dreamless sleep, then death would be a great advantage. For I think if one had to pick out that night during which a person slept soundly and did not dream, put beside it the other nights and days of life, and then see how many days and nights had been better and more pleasant than that night, not only a private person but the great king would find them easy to count compared with the other days and nights. If death is like this I say it is an advantage, for all eternity would then seem to be no more than a single night. If, on the other hand, death is a change from here to another place, and what we are told is true and all who have died are there, what greater blessing could there be?
—Socrates from Plato's *Apology*

That which dies in a person is only the five senses. That which continues to exist beyond the senses is immense, unimaginable, sublime.
—Anton Chekhov, *Notebook*, 1904

Perhaps the best cure for the fear of death is to reflect that life has a beginning as well as an end. There was a time when you were not; that gives us no concern. Why then should it trouble us that a time will come when we shall cease to be? To die is only to be as we were before we were born.
—William Hazlitt, *Table Talk*, 1821

It is the most supremely interesting moment in life, . . . and I count it as the greatest good fortune to have these few months so full of interest and instruction in the knowledge of my approaching death. It is so simple to one's own person as any fact of nature, the fall of a leaf or the blooming of a rose, and I have a delicious consciousness, ever present, of wide spaces close at hand, and whisperings of release in the air.
—Alice James, in a letter to her brother, 1891

I have always believed that the moment of death is the norm and goal of life.
—Simone Weil, in one of her last letters

For myself, as it happens, almost the only thing I have never doubted is that our sojourn here on earth is part of a larger process.
—Malcolm Muggeridge, *Half in Love with Death*, 1970

The soul, no longer having any great commerce with the body, burgeons and comes into full flower.
—Seneca

What the caterpillar calls the end of the world, the rest of the world calls a butterfly.
—Richard Bach

Is death the last sleep? No, it is the last and final awakening.
—Sir Walter Scott

Look upon death as a going home.
—Chinese proverb

This must be my birthday there in paradise.
—Joseki's death poem

Nothing is ever really lost, or can be lost,
No birth, identity, form—no object of the world.
Nor life, nor force, nor any visible thing;
Appearance must not foil, nor shifted sphere confuse thy brain.
Ample are time and space—ample the field of Nature.
—Walt Whitman, *Leaves of Grass*, 1884

For what is it to die but to stand naked in the wind and to melt into the sun?
And what is it to cease breathing, but to feel the breath from its restless tides, that it may rise and expand and see God unencumbered?
Only when you drink from the river of silence shall you indeed sing.
And when you have reached the mountain top, then you shall begin to climb.
And when the earth shall claim your limbs, then shall you truly dance.
—Kahlil Gibran, *The Prophet*, #68

Would you know a simile for life and death?
Compare them then to water and ice.
Water binds together to become ice;
Ice melts and turns back to water.
What has died must live again,
What has been born shall return to death.
Water and ice do no harm to each other;
Life and death are both of them good.

—Han-shan, *Cold Mountain*

Absolute and Relative Risk

In order to understand results of clinical trials that describe what can reduce your risk of recurrence or disease progression (also called increased disease-free survival time), it is helpful to understand two statistical concepts — *relative risk reduction/relative benefit* (reverse but basically synonymous notions) and *absolute risk reduction/absolute benefit* (reverse but also basically synonymous notions). Relative risk reduction/relative benefit is sometimes called a *hazard ratio* in clinical trial reports. Often these statistics are expressed as fractions rather than percentages (for example 0.5 instead of 50 percent).

For an example of relative risk reduction/relative benefit, hypothetically assume that a study concluded that 6 out of 100 people taking experimental Drug X had a recurrence. In contrast, 10 out of 100 people in the control group who did not take Drug X had a recurrence. The risk of reduction is calculated by dividing the number of patients with a recurrence taking the drug by the number of patients with a recurrence not taking the drug, so relative risk is 6/10 = 0.6 or 60 percent. The relative risk reduction/relative benefit is calculated by subtracting the risk of reduction from 1 (1 − 0.6 = 0.4) or 40 percent. Similarly, if in a different study with a different group of patients, 3 out of 1,000 people had a recurrence while they were taking Drug Y while 5 out of 1,000 people not taking Drug Y had a recurrence, this would also yield a 60 percent risk of reduction and the same relative risk reduction/relative benefit of 40 percent, despite the fact that the number of people affected is much smaller. This is shown in table 5.

Table 5 also shows the calculation for the absolute risk reduction/absolute benefit of these two hypothetical studies. The absolute risk reduction/absolute benefit is calculated by taking the percentage (event rate) of recurrence for those in the group taking the drug, then subtracting the percentage (event rate) of recurrence for those in the group not taking the drug. So for study 1, taking the drug decreased participants' chances of having a recurrence by 4 percent over those who did not take the drug

Table 5. Relative and absolute benefit. This table illustrates how a relative benefit of 60 percent may be obtained in two very different situations, based on the number of people at risk for disease. With a lower number of people at risk, the absolute benefit is correspondingly lower.

	Recurrence taking drug	Recurrence not taking drug	Relative benefit from taking drug	Absolute benefit from taking drug
Study 1, Drug X	6 of 100 people, or 6%	10 of 100 people, or 10%	6/10 = 0.6 1 − 0.6 = 0.4 or 40%	6/100 − 10/100 = 4/100 = −.04 or 4%
Study 2, Drug Y	3 of 1,000 people, or 0.3%	5 of 1,000 people, or 0.5%	3/5 = 0.6 1 − 0.6 = 0.4 or 40%	3/1000 − 5/1000 = 2/1000 = −.002 or 0.2%

Table 6. Variation of absolute benefit based on initial risk of recurrence.

Initial risk for recurrence	Relative benefit of a therapy	Absolute benefit from therapy	Risk of recurrence after therapy
20%	40%	0.2 × 0.4 = 0.08 8%	0.2 − 0.08 = 0.12 12%
40%	40%	0.4 × 0.4 = 0.16 16%	0.4 − 0.16 = 0.24 24%
60%	40%	0.6 × 0.4 = 0.24 24%	0.6 − 0.24 = 0.36 36%

(6/100 −10/100 = −4/100 or −.04) or in other words taking the drug affords an absolute benefit of 4 percent in reducing recurrence. You can see that drug Y, though it had the same relative benefit as drug X, has a lower absolute benefit. This table illustrates how a relative benefit of 60 percent may be obtained in two very different situations, based on the number of people at risk for disease. With a lower number of people at risk, the absolute benefit is correspondingly lower.

Keep in mind another consideration; the true absolute risk reduction/ absolute benefit for an individual depends upon the person's initial risk for recurrence. In clinical trial reports the absolute risk reduction/absolute benefit is based on the average of initial risk for recurrence for all who are participating in the trial. If your risk for recurrence is higher than the average of those in the trial, your corresponding benefit will be higher. Table 6 gives some examples of how absolute benefit can change based on initial risk of recurrence, while the relative benefit remains the same.

In short, when you hear that a drug or therapy reduces your chances for having a breast cancer recurrence by some percentage, if possible, get the percentage in terms of absolute risk reduction/absolute benefit, and further, take into consideration your initial risk of recurrence or disease progression. Most medications have problematic side effects. If you learn that a drug reduces recurrences by 40 percent, you may want to take this drug. If you know, however, that the absolute risk reduction/absolute benefit of this drug is 4 4percent, you may or may not be willing to take the treatment, depending on the side effects. Unfortunately, clear estimates of an individual person's risk of progression with metastatic disease are difficult to determine, so oncologists rely on the relative benefits reported in studies combining a diverse population of tumors.

ABSOLUTE RISK AND BENEFIT

- breastcancer.org: Provides an additional explanation of relative and absolute risk.
  http://www.breastcancer.org/risk/understanding.jsp

resources

Diet and Breast Cancer

Learning how just one substance interacts with cancer is challenging; imagine the difficulty in learning how various foods and cancer interrelate. Variables such as when in someone's lifespan something is eaten, what other food and drink are consumed at the same time, and how one's body metabolizes a food component all make for an incalculable number of variables and complex interactions. Even so, nutritionists have some helpful advice. While no diet has been shown to affect the course of cancer when it recurs, numerous studies have shown that diet can affect initial breast cancer risk and risk of recurrence.

The following is a distillation of standard diet recommendations from authoritative sources, including research studies focused on hormonal and breast cancer prevention. This dietary advice is based largely on statistical studies investigating the relationship of diet to those who do and do not develop various cancers worldwide. Unlike supplementation, which can interfere with treatment or possibly cause harm, the recommendations below are considered relatively safe. If your current diet is far different from these recommendations, you may want to seek outside support to help you more closely adhere to these suggestions. Most cancer centers have nutritionists and dieticians who can offer you aid (1).

Eat Plenty of Plants

A recent study showed that eating five to seven servings of fruits and vegetables a day decreased the risk of developing a breast cancer by 36 percent in a subset of patients (2). There is no substitute for filling your plate with colorful fruits and vegetables at every meal. Food components thought to prevent cancer that have been synthesized into pills (3) have so far not lived up to the cancer-prevention capabilities of the foods themselves (4).

Serving examples:

1 cup of raw leafy vegetable

½ cup of other vegetables (cooked or chopped raw)

¾ cup of vegetable or fruit juice

1 medium piece of fruit

½ cup of fruit (chopped, cooked, frozen, canned)

2 tablespoons dried fruit

Vary your choices, avoiding highly processed starchy vegetables like French fries. Increase your intake of cruciferous vegetables, the kind with a stalk in the middle, such as broccoli, cabbage, cauliflower, brussels sprouts, and kale. These cruciferous vegetables contain beneficial chemicals like I3C (indole-3-carbinol), which have anti-cancer and cancer-preventive actions. These vegetables also contain sulforaphane, which stimulates the production of your own detoxifying enzymes. Berries, such as strawberries, blueberries, and raspberries, are particularly rich sources of plant nutrients. Mushrooms, often overlooked in our diet, also contain numerous compounds that fight cancer in Petri dish studies. There are many edible varieties, including the shitake, crimini, oyster, enoki, portabella, and white button.

In general look for food that is organic, unspoiled, and most recently picked off the tree or vine. Barring these choices, look for frozen, dried, or canned foods, generally in that order. Select food that is the least processed. Eating unprocessed foods will reasonably assure that your diet is high in fiber and low in animal fat, sugar, and salt.

Increase Your Fiber Intake

Eat crunchy, tasty whole grains, beans, roots, and tubers, as well as a variety of nuts in moderation. Choose brown, full-bodied bread, cereals, and rice over white, hulled, and flattened grains. Choose food with more heft and texture that has longer cooking times. For example, cook oat groats or steel cut oats instead of rolled oats or instant oatmeal. Choose whole foods over those with ingredients that have been through manufacturing processes. Spend more time in the fresh food and frozen food aisle rather than the snack, cereal, and baked goods aisles. The more a food has been processed, the more likely it has lost its nutrients and fiber.

Fiber has a number of health benefits, due in part to its fermentation in the colon to short-chain fatty acids, but it may also influence circulating estrogen levels. The recent Women's Cohort Study in the United Kingdom concluded that a diet rich in fiber from cereals reduces breast cancer risk by 52 percent in premenopausal, but not postmenopausal, women (5). Dr. David Rose of the American Health Foundation in New York found a 20 percent drop in estrogen levels of women who ate 30 grams of fiber, 15 grams of which were wheat bran (6). It is also well appreciated that Finnish women have about half the rate of breast cancer as American women; that may be associated with their average daily intake of 30 grams of fiber (compared to 14 grams per day for American women). Aiming for 30 grams of fiber daily is easy if you eat five servings of fruit and vegetables along with other unprocessed foods. For example:

> **5 grams:** ½ cup cooked or dried beans, peas, or lentils or 1 cup high-fiber wheat bran cereal
>
> **2 grams:** a medium-sized piece of fruit or slice of whole wheat bread

Try Organic Produce

Organic foods are those grown without added pesticides, antibiotics, or growth hormones. Many pesticides have been shown to be endocrine disruptors—chemicals that may increase the incidence of hormone-related cancers. Not all food needs to be organic, as produce in particular varies in the amount of pesticide residue on its edible portion. You can learn more about the levels of pesticides and organic foods using the links in the next resource box.

The most contaminated foods (and those worth paying more for organic versions) are the following:

Peaches	Pears
Apples	Grapes (imported)
Sweet bell peppers	Spinach
Celery	Lettuce
Nectarines	Potatoes
Strawberries	Carrots
Cherries	

In addition, a body of research is beginning to demonstrate that organically grown produce contains more of the phytochemicals thought to provide health benefits, probably as a result of the plant's working harder to fight pests and infections.

ORGANIC FOOD

- Environmental Working Group: Lists what foods have the most and least pesticides.
    http://www.ewg.org

- Environmental Working Group: Offers a shopper's guide for buying organic produce.
    http://www.foodnews.org/walletguide.php

Decrease Your Meat Consumption

A study of South American women showed that the possibility of developing breast cancer rose with the amount of meat a woman ate, particularly red or fried meat. Women who ate the most meat had three to four times the risk of the low meat eaters (7, 8).

Limit your consumption of meat to 3 ounces or less per meal, preferably lean poultry. Cooking red meat can produce heterocyclic amines, a group of cancer-causing substances (9). Slow roast or microwave meat or fish rather than frying or boiling it to well done. Avoid meat that is charred, smoked, salted, or nitrate cured. In general, cattle and pigs that are pasture-raised without added growth hormones are healthier for you and the environment. Similarly, poultry that has been organically raised without added antibiotics and growth hormones is healthier.

Watch Your Fat Intake

As mentioned in chapter 1 under "Reducing Your Chances of Recurrence," the Women's Intervention Nutrition Study (WINS) concluded that women with breast cancer who ate a low-fat diet (approximately 20 percent of their calories were from fat) had a reduced risk of recurrence. This diet was particularly advantageous for women with ER-negative disease. It could be that those who followed the low-fat diet had fewer recurrences because they lost more weight. Weight loss reduces body fat, which reduces circulating estradiol. Reducing estradiol is helpful in warding off a recurrence. It is less certain whether or not a low-fat diet reduces the initial risk of getting breast cancer. However, low-fat diets are beneficial in helping many people maintain a healthy weight. Being overweight is a risk factor for getting breast cancer in post-menopausal women.

In choosing fats, opt for plant- rather than animal-derived fats. Mediterranean women who had more than one serving of olive oil daily were less likely to develop breast cancer than those who did not (11). Substitute unrefined (extra virgin) olive oil for other fats where possible. For example, instead of butter, try flavoring your bread with olive oil and using olive oil to flavor popcorn or sauté vegetables. A tablespoon of olive oil has nearly 14 grams of fat and 120 calories. If you use other oils, pick cold-pressed, unrefined oil, preferably canola oil, which, unlike olive oil, can withstand heat. Avoid refined oils (corn oil), saturated fats (butter/cream), and hydrogenated oils (found in many margarines).

It may be that certain fats are detrimental and others not. One of the investigators of the Women's Health Initiative study, Dr. Marcia Stefanick, suggests that it may be more important to reduce saturated and trans-fats as opposed to maintaining an overall low-fat diet. The use of some fats in cooking can be beneficial, as some plant chemicals that have cancer-fighting properties (such as lycopene) are better absorbed by the human body when combined with fat.

Add Dairy Products to Your Diet

Multiple studies have shown a decreased risk of breast cancer in women who consume two or more servings of dairy products daily. It is postulated that the calcium and vitamin D in dairy products may account for some of the observed effect. It is unknown whether diary product consumption alters recurrence or progression risk. Choose low-fat dairy options, such as 1 percent or fat-free milk and yogurt. To avoid exposure to food additives, such as antibiotics and bovine growth hormone, you may want to consider organic versions of dairy products when possible.

Make Sure That Your Diet Is Nutritionally Complete

Nutritionists agree that the best way to ingest vitamins and minerals is in foods rather than in pills. Still, to provide the body with the complete spectrum of vitamins and minerals many nutritionists recommend supplementing your diet. Be certain to get enough vitamins and minerals, but be cautious about ingesting harmfully large quantities.

The "Daily Value" listed on most vitamin and mineral supplements is actually an outdated term that is increasingly being replaced by new terminology. The Institute of Medicine of the U.S. National Academy of Sciences has published a series of guidelines called the Dietary Reference Intakes (DRI), which you can access using the link in the next resource box. DRIs include the Estimated Average Requirement (EAR), Recommended Dietary Allowance (RDA), Adequate Intake (AI), and Tolerable Upper Intake Level (UL). While these may seem complicated, the new methodology takes into account the varying needs for vitamins and minerals as a function of age and gender. To simplify, the RDA or AI refer loosely to what is now called the Daily Value, while the UL is the upper limit for safe intake (or the "don't exceed" level). Unfortunately, the continued use of "Daily Value" by supplement makers does not always correspond with the RDA or AI established by this new system, but look for DRI terminology to be phased in over the next few years. Sample DRIs are shown in table 7.

DIETARY GUIDELINES

- U.S. Department of Agriculture: Offers extensive dietary guidelines, including DRI tables and reports.
    http://fnic.nal.usda.gov/nal_display/index.php?info_center=4&tax_
        level=2&tax_subject=256&topic_id=1342

Uncertain Territory

A number of foods, especially those with possible estrogenic activity, have a complex and/or uncertain relationship with breast cancer recurrence.

Table 7. Sample Dietary Reference Intakes (DRIs) for women aged 19–70

	Daily RDA or AI	UL (Don't Exceed)
Vitamin A*	700 mcg (2,333 IU)	3,000 mcg (10,000 IU)
Folate	400 mcg	1,000 mcg
Vitamin B6	1.3–1.5 mg	100 mg
Vitamin B12	2.4 mcg	Not determined
Vitamin C	75 mg	2,000 mg
Vitamin D	5–15 mcg (200–600 IU)	50 mcg (2,000 IU)
Vitamin E	15 mg	1,000 mg
Calcium	1,000–1,200 mg	2,500 mg
Iron	8–18 mg	45 mg
Selenium	55 mg	400 mg
Zinc	8 mg	40 mg

*Vitamin A recommendations have grown complicated since preformed vitamin A is often mixed with vitamin A precursors (or building blocks) that each have different potencies for producing the vitamin. The microgram listing refers to "retinol activity equivalents" (RAE), where 1 RAE = 1 mcg retinol, 12 mcg beta-carotene, 24 mcg alpha-carotene, or 24 mcg beta-cryptoxanthin. The older term, international units (iu), is provided for comparison.

Source: Food and Nutrition Board, Institute of Medicine, National Academies

Soy and Other Foods High in Isoflavones

Soybeans, or soy, contain isoflavones, a type of plant estrogen. Though plant and animal estrogens differ, ample evidence suggests that some plant estrogens inhibit the estrogen-binding sites on human breast cancer cells by keeping the human estrogen, estradiol, from having a tumor-promoting effect. Therefore, some plant estrogens may prevent breast cancer in women who have not previously had the disease (12). Females from Asian countries, whose diets are often rich in soy substances such as tofu, end up with an increased incidence of breast cancer if they relocate to the United States, leading some to speculate that a decrease in soy once they came to the United States led to the increase in breast cancer (13). Though some studies have pointed to soy's possible protective effect, it may be that this effect occurs when soy is eaten during adolescence (14, 15).

However, once breast cancer is diagnosed, particularly estrogen-receptor-positive breast cancer, high doses of plant estrogens are not recommended. Hormonal drugs that block estradiol from stimulating breast cancer cells, or block estradiol synthesis, are used in treating breast cancer and for preventing recurrence. Hence, plant estrogens may interfere with the beneficial effects of anti-estrogen drugs, such as tamoxifen and aromatase inhibitors. A study in mice showed that a soy isoflavone, genistein, interfered with tamoxifen in reducing the growth of estrogen-receptor-positive breast tumors (16).

Most nutritionists who have studied soy effects are of the opinion that it is reasonable for those who have been diagnosed with breast cancer to eat soy foods when not under treatment, but there is no evidence that it enhances survival. Further, they advise those with breast cancer against taking soy supplements and soy milk since these concentrate the active chemicals to levels far greater than in foods. If you cannot drink cow's milk, or are concerned about its consumption, experiment with almond or rice milk as a substitute. To further confuse matters, it appears that the form in which soy is consumed (fermented soy versus soy protein isolate) may determine whether soy has a positive or negative effect on breast cancer (17). For now it is known that soy consumed throughout life may prevent breast cancer, but breast cancer patients should not expect that soy will favorably affect the outcome of their disease.

Flaxseed

Compounds in flaxseed are thought to have a mild estrogenic effect, which raises questions as to whether this supplement may enhance the growth of estrogen-receptor-positive breast cancer. Current thinking is that flaxseed compounds may compete with estradiol to produce a lower net growth stimulatory effect. In addition, flaxseed's alpha-linolenic acid (ALA) is converted in the body, albeit inefficiently, into omega-3 fatty acids known as DHA and EPA. These are the same omega-3 fatty acids found in fish oil that in one study were associated with slower growth and spread of breast cancer. The relationship of these oils to the prevention or development of breast cancer is currently inconclusive, although a collective examination of previous studies (called a "meta-analysis") is suggestive that omega-3 fatty acids may have some breast cancer–preventative activity (18). Animal studies have shown that flaxseed given as 5 percent or 10 percent of a diet can decrease breast cancer growth and increase the benefit of tamoxifen. These studies have been primarily performed by Dr. Lilian Thompson's group at the University of Toronto. Human studies have not yet been

performed confirming these findings. This remains an active area of investigation. Until more is known, it is safest to avoid flaxseed when taking
hormonal drugs or undergoing radiation treatment. Instead, fish oil may
be a better and safer source of DHA, EPA, and other omega-3 fatty acids.

Nutrition during Cancer Treatment

While the above recommendations are the ideal, many women find it difficult to eat well during chemotherapy or radiation treatment. Chemotherapy may cause nausea, taste changes, constipation, diarrhea, or
mouth sores, all of which may affect food intake and/or nutritional status.
Radiation may cause stomach or esophageal pain or nausea, depending
on the site radiated. Often women experience a lack of appetite due to
disease progression. Some may experience a lack of appetite because liver
or abdominal involvement physically restricts stomach space. Others may
experience a lack of appetite from hormones secreted by the cancer. Still
others may have nausea due to brain metastases or nausea from supportive medications.

The American Cancer Society has extensive recommendations for dealing with each of the above problems, with specific links to each topic in
the resource box below.

EATING WHILE UNDERGOING TREATMENT

American Cancer Society: Offers recommendations for dealing with each of
the following eating problems, which may arise during treatment.

* Changes in Taste and Smell
    http://www.cancer.org/docroot/MBC/content/MBC_6_2X_When_
        Things_Arent_Tasting_Right.asp?sitearea=MBC

* Constipation
    http://www.cancer.org/docroot/MBC/content/MBC_6_2X_
        Constipation_bowel_movement_problems.asp?sitearea=MBC

* Sore or Irritated Mouth or Throat
    http://www.cancer.org/docroot/MBC/content/MBC_6_2x_Sore_or_
        Irritated_Mouth_or_Throat.asp?sitearea=MBC

resources

resources

(Resources, continued)

- Dry Mouth or Thick Saliva

    http://www.cancer.org/docroot/MBC/content/MBC_6_2X_Dry_Mouth_
       or_Thick_Saliva.asp?sitearea=MBC

- Poor Appetite

    http://www.cancer.org/docroot/MBC/content/MBC_6_2X_Poor_
       Appetite.asp?sitearea=MBC

- Diarrhea

    http://www.cancer.org/docroot/MBC/content/MBC_6_2X_Diarrhea
       .asp?sitearea=MBC

- Nausea and Vomiting

    http://www.cancer.org/docroot/MBC/content/MBC_6_2X_When_
       Youre_Feeling_Queasy.asp?sitearea=MBC

- Trouble Swallowing

    http://www.cancer.org/docroot/MBC/content/MBC_6_2X_Difficulty_
       with_Swallowing.asp?sitearea=MBC

- Fatigue

    http://www.cancer.org/docroot/MBC/content/MBC_6_2X_Fatigue
       .asp?sitearea=MBC

Further Reading

Eating Well through Cancer: Easy Recipes and Recommendations during and after Treatment, by Holly Clegg and Gerald Miletello. Favorite Recipes Press, 2006.

CAM Centers

What follows is sampling of CAM centers to make you aware of the many places offering varying kinds of CAM care. Some are exclusively for cancer patients, but all have personnel who have background in addressing the needs of cancer patients. This list is not exhaustive and is not meant as an endorsement of any physician or center. It is important that you use the resources in Chapter 5 to investigate specific doctors or centers more thoroughly.

Integrative Cancer Centers

These are centers that focus on standard cancer treatment but also incorporate complementary modalities.

Duke Integrative Medicine
3475 Erwin Road
Durham, NC 27705
Phone: 866-313-0959
http://www.dukeintegrativemedicine.org

Block Center for Integrative Cancer Care
1800 Sherman Avenue, Suite 515
Evanston, IL 60201
Phone: 847-492-3040
http://www.blockmd.com

Dana Farber Cancer Institute
Leonard P. Zakim Center for Integrative Therapies
44 Binney Street
Shields Warren Building, #G560

Boston, MA 02115
Phone: 617-632-3322
Fax: 617-632-3988
E-mail: anne_doherty@dfci.harvard.edu

Mayo Clinic
Complementary and Integrative Medicine Program
200 First Street, SW
Rochester, MN 55905
Phone: 507-284-8913
Fax: 507-284-5370
E-mail: cimprogram@mayo.edu

M. D. Anderson Cancer Center
Integrative Medicine Clinic
(Requires referral from an M. D. Anderson physician)
1515 Holcombe Blvd., Unit 8
Houston, TX 77030-4009
Phone: 713-792-6072
Fax: 713-794-4700

Memorial Sloan-Kettering Cancer Center
Integrative Medicine Service
Bendheim Integrative Medicine Center
1429 First Avenue
New York, NY 10021
Inpatient hospital services
1275 York Avenue
New York, NY 10065
Phone: 646-888-0800

San Diego Cancer Center
Integrative Oncology Program
910 Sycamore Avenue, Suite 102
Vista, CA 92081
Phone: 760-598-1700
1200 Garden View Road, Suite 200
Encinitas, CA 92024
Phone: 760-634-6661

University of California at Los Angeles
Simms/Mann-UCLA Center for Integrative Oncology
200 UCLA Medical Plaza, Suite 502
Los Angeles, CA 90095-6934
Phone: 310-794-6644
Fax: 310-794-9615
E-mail: SimmsMannCenter@mednet.ucla.edu

Complementary Care Centers

The following list of centers and programs does not imply our endorsement; rather we provide them to give you a sampling of the range of complementary support available in various settings.

Commonweal Cancer Help Program
Founded in 1985, this center was among the first of its kind; it offers six-week-long retreats.
PO Box 316
Bolinas, CA 94924
Phone: 415-868-0970
http://www.commonweal.org

Smith Farm Center for the Healing Arts
Smith Farm Cancer Help Program
1632 U Street, NW
Washington, D.C. 20009
Phone: 202-483-8600
http://www.smithfarm.com

Harmony Hill Cancer Retreats
E. 7362 Hwy 106
Union, WA 98592
360-898-2363
http://www.harmonyhill.org

The Light Center
1542 Woodson Road
Baldwin, KS 66066
Phone: 785-255-4583
ltcenter@grapevine.net

Sunstone Cancer Support Foundation
2545 North Woodland Drive
Tucson, AZ 85749
Phone: 520-749-1928
http://www.sunstonehealing.net

Simonton Cancer Center
New Patient Program
PO Box 890
Pacific Palisades, CA 90272
Phone: 310-459-4434
http://www.simontoncenter.com/index.html

Callanish Healing Retreats
2902 West Broadway, #314
Vancouver, BC, Canada V6K 2G8
Phone: 604-732-0633
http://www.callanish.org

Tapestry Retreat
Department of Psychosocial Resources
Tom Baker Cancer Centre
1331 29th Street, NW
Calgary, AB, Canada T2N 4N2
Phone: 403-670-1767
http://www.cancerboard.ab.ca/tapestry

Bristol Cancer Help Centre
Grove House, Cornwallis Grove
Clifton, Bristol, England BS8 4PG
Phone: 011-44-0272-743216
http://www.bristolcancerhelp.org

Yarra Valley Living Centre/Gawler Foundation
PO Box 77G, Yarra Junction
Victoria, Australia 3797
Phone: 011-61-059-67-730
Fax: 011-61-059-67-1715
http://www.gawler.org

Centers with Unconventional and Unproven Cancer Care

These centers are not recommended but are provided as examples of the
types of sites whose treatments do not meet the standards of evidence-
based medicine.

Livingston Foundation Medical Center
Devised by the late Virginia Livingston, MD, in 1971, the center is
based on her belief that a microbe she called Progenitor Crytocides
caused cancer when the immune system was weakened. It includes
vaccines, one using the patient's bacteria, along with a vegetarian diet
and psychotherapy.
3232 Duke Street
San Diego, CA 92100
Phone: 619-224-3515
The American Cancer Society has a detailed description and evaluation
of the center's approaches:
http://www.cancer.org/docroot/ETO/content/ETO_5_3X_Livingston-
Wheeler_Therapy.asp?sitearea=ETO

Burzynski Clinic
Dr. Stanislaw R. Burzynski reported in the early 1970s that peptides
and amino acid derivatives called antineoplastons could reprogram
cancer cells. The clinic's treatment, lasting nine months or more, is
administered orally or through an IV infusion on an outpatient basis.
http://www.cancermed.com
The NCI has concluded that there is insufficient evidence to support the
use of antineoplastons in cancer because only small patient numbers
have been used in studies to date.
http://www.cancer.gov/cancertopics/factsheet/Therapy/antineoplastons

Immunology Research Center (Immuno-Augmentative Therapy, IAT)

Established in 1988, the center is based on the theory proposed by the late Lawrence Burton, PhD, who believed certain substances in the blood were necessary to prevent cancer development. A patient's blood is tested for protein deficiencies, then a tailored vaccine of cytokines is created to correct imbalances.

Freeport, Grand Bahama Island

Phone: 809-352-7455

A recent study of forty-six cancer patients receiving IAT concluded that there was no evidence for its effectiveness.

Glossary of Medical and Scientific Terms

The definitions used here are provided by the authors or were adapted or copied either directly from the National Cancer Institute's "Dictionary of Cancer Terms" (www.cancer.gov/dictionary) or *Merriam-Webster's Medical Dictionary OnLine* (http://medical.merriam-webster.com/medical).

Ablation: In medicine, the removal or destruction of a body part or tissue or its function. Ablation may be performed by surgery, hormones, drugs, radio-frequency, heat, or other methods.

Adjuvant therapy: Treatment given after surgery to increase the chances of a cure. Adjuvant therapy may include chemotherapy, radiation therapy, hormone therapy, or biological therapy.

Amino acid: One of several molecules that join together to form proteins. There are twenty common amino acids found in proteins.

Angiogenesis: Blood vessel formation. Tumor angiogenesis is the growth of new blood vessels needed for tumors to grow. This is caused by the release of chemicals by the tumor.

Angiogenesis inhibitor: A substance that may prevent the formation of blood vessels. In anti-cancer therapy, an angiogenesis inhibitor prevents the growth of blood vessels from surrounding tissue to a solid tumor. Some naturally occurring inhibitors are thrombospondin, angiostatin, and endostatin.

Anti-angiogenesis: Prevention of the growth of new blood vessels.

Antibody: An antigen-specific receptor, also called an immunoglobulin, made by B-lymphocytes. Antibodies are a critical component of the immune system; they circulate in the blood and bind to foreign antigens and tumor cells, marking them for destruction by immune proteins or other immune cells. Monoclonal antibodies (mAb) are laboratory-produced antibodies that can locate and bind to cancer cells wherever they are in the body. Each one recognizes a different protein on certain cancer cells. They are used in cancer detection or therapy and can be administered alone or used to deliver drugs, toxins, or radioactive material directly to a tumor.

Antioxidant: A substance that protects cells from the damage caused by free radicals (unstable molecules made by the process of oxidation during normal metabolism). Free radicals may play a part in cancer, heart disease, stroke, and other diseases of aging. Antioxidants include beta-carotene; lycopene; vitamins A, C, and E; and other natural and manufactured substances.

Apoptosis: A normal series of events in a cell that lead to its death. Also called cell suicide or programmed cell death.

Aromatase: An enzyme converting androstenedione and testosterone ("male" steroid hormones) to estradiol (a female hormone) in multiple tissues.

Aromatase inhibitor: A class of drugs that inhibits the action of aromatase. Includes anastrozole (Arimidex), letrozole (Femara), and exemestane (Aromasin).

Ascites: Abnormal buildup of fluid in the abdomen that may cause swelling. In late-stage cancer, tumor cells may be found in the fluid in the abdomen. Ascites also occurs in patients with liver disease.

Atypical ductal hyperplasia (ADH): A benign (noncancerous) condition in which ductal cells look abnormal under a microscope and are increased in number.

Axilla: The underarm or armpit.

Axillary lymph node: One of many lymph nodes found in the axilla; the primary nodes that drain the breast.

Basement membrane: A specialized, sheet-like structure of the extracellular matrix that separates cells from the surrounding connective tissue and thereby serves as a boundary of a tissue. The basement membrane must be broken down in order for cancer cells to invade surrounding tissue.

Benign: A swelling or growth that is not cancerous and does not spread from one part of the body to another.

Biological therapy: Treatment to stimulate or restore the ability of the immune system to fight infection and disease. Biological therapy is also used to lessen side effects that may be caused by some cancer treatments. Also known as immunotherapy, biotherapy, or biological response modifier (BRM) therapy.

Biopsy: The removal of cells or tissue for examination by a pathologist. The pathologist may study the tissue under a microscope or perform other tests on the cells or tissue. There are many different types of biopsy procedures. The most common types include (1) incisional biopsy, in which only a sample of tissue is removed; (2) excisional biopsy, in which an entire lump or suspicious area is removed; and (3) needle biopsy, in which a sample of tissue or fluid is removed with a needle. When a wide needle is used, the procedure is called a core biopsy. When a thin needle is used, the procedure is called a fine-needle aspiration biopsy.

Brachial plexopathy: A condition marked by numbness, tingling, pain, weakness, or limited movement in the arm or hand. It is caused by an impairment of the brachial plexus, a network of nerves that affect the arm and hand. In breast cancer, the most common causes are recurrence in the axilla and radiation damage. If not treated promptly, the damage could become permanent.

BRCA1: A gene on chromosome 17 that normally helps to suppress cell growth. A person who inherits a mutated (changed) BRCA1 gene has a higher risk of getting breast, ovarian, or prostate cancer.

BRCA2: A gene on chromosome 13 that normally helps to suppress cell growth. A person who inherits a mutated (changed) BRCA2 gene has a higher risk of getting breast, ovarian, or prostate cancer. Other cancers have been linked to mutations in this gene as well.

Bronchoscopy: A procedure that uses a bronchoscope to examine the inside of the trachea, bronchi (air passages that lead to the lungs), and lungs. A bronchoscope is a thin, tube-like instrument with a light and a lens for viewing. It may also have a tool to remove tissue to be checked under a microscope for signs of disease. The bronchoscope is inserted through the nose or mouth. Bronchoscopy may be used to detect cancer or to perform some treatment procedures.

Cell: The individual unit that makes up the tissues of the body. All living things are made up of one or more cells.

Cell cycle: The sequence of events by which a cell enlarges, duplicates its DNA, and divides. The cell cycle consists of four successive phases (G1, S, G2, and M) and involves many genes, including cyclins and cyclin-dependent kinases (CDKs). Access to growth factors, adhesion to extracellular matrix, and cell cycle checkpoints are some of the many factors that regulate the cell cycle. Disregulation of the cell cycle can lead to the uncontrolled growth characteristic of cancer cells.

Cell division: The process by which two daughter cells are produced from one parent cell.

Cerebrospinal fluid (CSF): The fluid that surrounds the brain and spinal cord; also called spinal fluid.

Cervical lymph node: One of numerous lymph nodes found in the neck.

Chemoprevention: The use of drugs, vitamins, or other agents to try to reduce the risk of or delay the development or recurrence of cancer.

Chemotherapy: Treatment with drugs that kills cancer cells.

Chromosome: A long, tightly packaged DNA molecule that contains the genetic instructions essential for the life of a cell and allows the transmission of genetic information from generation to generation.

Clavicle: Collarbone.

Clinical trial: A type of research study that tests how well new medical treatments or other interventions work in people. Each study is designed to test new methods of screening, prevention, diagnosis, or treatment of a disease.

Complete response: The disappearance of all signs of cancer in response to treatment. This does not always mean the cancer has been cured. Also called complete remission.

Concurrent therapy: A treatment that is given at the same time as another.

Contralateral: Having to do with the opposite side of the body.

Cowden syndrome: An inherited syndrome that results most commonly (80 percent of the time) from a mutation in the PTEN gene on chromosome 10. Patients with the syndrome have an increased risk of breast, endometrial, and thyroid cancer.

Cytoplasm: The fluid inside a cell but outside the cell's nucleus. Most chemical reactions in a cell take place in the cytoplasm.

Cytotoxic: Cell-killing.

Dendritic cell(s): A special type of antigen-presenting cell (APC) that activates T lymphocytes. These cells exist in many tissues, including the skin and mucous membranes and can travel to lymph nodes or spleen to interact with other immune cells. In a sense, dendritic cells are the sentinels that alert other immune cells of an attack.

Disease-free survival (DFS): The length of time after treatment for a specific disease during which a patient survives with no sign of the disease. Disease-free survival may be used in a clinical study or trial to help measure how well a new treatment works.

Disease progression: Cancer that continues to grow or spread.

DNA (deoxyribonucleic acid): The molecules inside cells that carry genetic information and pass it from one generation to the next.

DNA methylation: A type of epigenetic mark. Changes in methylation affect gene expression; the more methylated a stretch of DNA, the less likely it is to be transcribed to RNA.

DNA repair: The process through which mutations in DNA are repaired. The basic DNA repair mechanism involves nucleases (which cut out the damaged area of DNA), polymerases (which fill in the gap with the correct nucleotides), and ligases (which seal the nick between the new segment of DNA and the original DNA strand).

DNA replication: The copying or duplication of a DNA molecule. DNA in a cell is replicated in preparation for cell division so that the two daughter cells will each receive a complete copy of the DNA of the parent cell. While this process is extremely accurate, errors do occur. The cell has proofreading and DNA repair mechanisms to fix these mistakes.

Double blind: A clinical trial in which the method for analyzing data has been specified in the protocol before the study has begun; the patients have been randomly assigned to receive either the study drug or alternative treatment, and neither the patient nor the physician(s) conducting the study know which treatment is being given to a patient.

Duct: The tube through which milk passes from the lobules to the nipple.

Ductal carcinoma *in situ* (DCIS): A noninvasive condition in which abnormal cells are found in the lining of a breast duct. The abnormal cells have not spread outside the duct to other tissues in the breast. In some cases, ductal carcinoma *in situ* may become invasive cancer and spread to other tissues, although it is not known at this time how to predict which lesions will become invasive. Also called intraductal carcinoma.

EGFR (epidermal growth-factor receptor): The protein found on the surface of some cells and to which epidermal growth factor binds, causing the cells to divide. It is found at abnormally high levels on the surface of many types of cancer cells, so these cells may divide excessively in the presence of epidermal growth factor. Also known as ErbB1 or HER1.

Eligibility criteria: In clinical trials, requirements that must be met for an individual to be included in a study. These requirements help make sure that patients in a trial are similar to each other in terms of specific factors such as age, type and stage of cancer, general health, and previous treatment. When all participants meet the same eligibility criteria, it gives researchers greater confidence that results of the study are caused by the intervention being tested and not by other factors.

Endpoint: In clinical trials, an event or outcome that can be measured objectively to determine whether the intervention being studied is beneficial. The endpoints of a clinical trial are usually included in the study objectives. Some examples of endpoints are survival, improvements in quality of life, relief of symptoms, and disappearance of a tumor.

Epidemiology: The study of the incidence, distribution, causes, and control of disease in a population.

Epigenetic: Having to do with the chemical attachments to DNA or the histone proteins around which it coils. Epigenetic marks change the pattern of genes expressed in a given cell or tissue by amplifying or muting the effect of a gene, but they do not alter the actual DNA sequence. Unlike mutations to DNA sequence, epigenetic modifications are typically reversible. Epigenetic markers include acetyl groups, methyl groups, phosphate groups, and the peptide ubiquitin. Tumor cells often contain epigenetic abnormalities.

Estrogen receptor (ER): A protein found inside the cells of the female reproductive tissue, some other types of tissue, and some cancer cells. The hormone estrogen will bind to the receptors inside the cells and may cause the cells to grow. Cancer cells that are ER-positive need estrogen to grow and may stop growing when treated with hormones that block estrogen from binding.

Extracellular: Outside of the cell.

Fine needle aspiration (FNA): The removal of tissue or fluid with a thin needle for examination under a microscope. Also called FNA biopsy.

Fluorescent *in situ* hybridization (FISH): A technique used to look at chromosomes (the parts of a cell that contain genetic information in the form of DNA) or genes (specific regions of DNA in chromosomes that make RNA and proteins). Pieces of DNA containing a fluorescent dye are made in the laboratory and added to cells on a glass slide. When viewed under a microscope with a special light source, parts of chromosomes or genes that bind the pieces of DNA show up as colored.

Gamma Knife therapy: A treatment using gamma rays, a type of high-energy radiation that can be tightly focused on small tumors or other lesions in the head or neck, so that very little normal tissue receives radiation. The gamma rays are aimed at the tumor from many different angles at once and deliver a large dose of radiation exactly to the tumor in one treatment session. This procedure is a type of stereotactic radiosurgery. Gamma Knife therapy is not a knife and is not surgery. Gamma Knife is a registered trademark of Elekta Instruments.

Gene: The functional and physical unit of heredity passed from parent to offspring. Genes are segments of DNA, and most genes contain the information for making a specific protein. The DNA sequence of a gene determines the amino acid sequence of a protein.

HER2 (human epidermal growth-factor receptor 2): A protein involved in normal cell growth. It is found in high levels on some breast cancer cells. Also called HER2/neu and ErbB2.

HER2 overexpression: A genetic alteration in the HER2 gene that produces an increased amount of the growth-factor receptor protein on the tumor cell surface, causing cells to divide, multiply, and grow more rapidly than normal. Women whose tumors overexpress the HER2 protein are likely to have a more aggressive type of breast cancer with a poorer prognosis, shorter time to disease progression, increased relapse rate, shortened survival, and disease that is not as responsive to standard therapies, including certain chemotherapy regimens.

Histologic grade: Describes how closely tumor cells look like normal cells of the same tissue type. Also sometimes called differentiation. Cells that look more like normal breast cells are called well differentiated. Cells that look least like normal breast cells are called poorly differentiated.

Hyperplasia: An abnormal increase in the normal cells of the breast.

Hyperthermia therapy: A type of treatment in which body tissue is exposed to high temperatures to damage and kill cancer cells or to make cancer cells more sensitive to the effects of radiation and certain anti-cancer drugs.

Inflammatory breast cancer: A type of breast cancer in which the breast looks red and swollen and feels warm. The skin of the breast may also show the pitted appearance called peau d'orange (like the skin of an orange). The redness and warmth occur because the cancer cells block the lymph vessels in the skin.

Intensity-modulated radiation therapy (IMRT): A type of three-dimensional radiation therapy that uses computer-generated images to show the size and shape of the tumor. Thin beams of radiation of different intensities are aimed at the tumor from many angles. This type of radiation therapy reduces the damage to healthy tissue near the tumor.

Internal mammary lymph node: One of a number of lymph nodes that lie on both sides of the sternum (breast bone). Less than 5 percent of breast lymph drains to the internal mammary lymph nodes.

Intracellular: Inside of a cell.

Intrathecal chemotherapy: Treatment in which anti-cancer drugs are injected into the fluid-filled space between the thin layers of tissue that cover the brain and spinal cord.

Invasive (or infiltrating) ductal carcinoma: The most common type of invasive breast cancer. It starts in the cells that line the milk ducts in the breast, grows outside the ducts, and often spreads to the lymph nodes. May also be called adenocarcinoma, ductal type.

Invasive lobular carcinoma: Cancer that begins in the lobules (the glands that make milk) of the breast and has spread into the surrounding breast tissues. May also be called adenocarcinoma, lobular type.

Leptomeningeal carcinomatosis (also carcinomatous meningitis): Cancer involvement of the meninges (covering of the brain).

Li-Fraumeni syndrome: A rare, inherited familial cancer syndrome characterized by tumors at multiple sites. A mutation of the p53 tumor suppressor gene predisposes family members who inherit it to develop multiple cancers.

Ligand: A linking or binding molecule that binds to a specific complementary site on (forms a complex with) another molecule. For example, a growth factor is a ligand for its growth-factor receptor.

Lobular carcinoma *in situ* (LCIS): A condition in which abnormal cells are found in the lobules of the breast. LCIS seldom becomes invasive cancer; however, having lobular carcinoma *in situ* in one breast increases the risk of developing breast cancer in either breast.

Lobule: A milk-forming glandular structure of the breast.

Lymph node: A rounded mass of lymphatic tissue that is surrounded by a capsule of connective tissue. Lymph nodes filter lymph (lymphatic fluid), and they store lymphocytes (white blood cells). They are located along lymphatic vessels.

Lymphedema: A swelling of the arm from lymph fluid, a condition that about 18 percent of breast cancer patients develop after having lymph nodes removed.

Lytic bone metastasis: Destruction of an area of bone due to cancer.

Meninges: The membranous coverings of the brain and spinal cord.

Metastasis (pl. metastases): The spread of cancer from one part of the body to another. A tumor formed by cells that have spread is called a "metastatic tumor" or a "metastasis." The metastatic tumor contains cells that are like those in the original (primary) tumor.

Microtubules: Cellular structures that help move chromosomes during mitosis.

Mitosis: The process by which a single parent cell divides to make two daughter cells. Each daughter cell receives a complete set of chromosomes from the parent cell. This process allows the body to grow and replace cells.

Mutation: Any change in the DNA sequence of a cell. Mutations may be caused by mistakes during cell division or by exposure to DNA-damaging agents in the environment. Mutations can be harmful, beneficial, or have no effect. If they occur in cells that make eggs or sperm, they can be inherited; if mutations occur in other types of cells, they are not inherited. Certain mutations may lead to cancer or other diseases.

Neoadjuvant: Treatment given before surgery. Types of neoadjuvant therapy may include chemotherapy, radiation therapy, and hormone therapy.

Nuclear grade: An evaluation of the size and shape of the nucleus in tumor cells and the percentage of tumor cells that are in the process of dividing or growing. Cancers with low nuclear grade grow and spread less quickly than cancers with high nuclear grade.

Nucleotides: The building blocks of nucleic acids (DNA and RNA). The four nucleotide bases are guanine (G), cytosine (C), adenine (A) and thymine (T).

Nucleus: The part of the cell that contains the chromosomes; it is bounded by its own nuclear membrane.

Ommaya reservoir: A device surgically placed under the scalp and used to deliver anti-cancer drugs to the fluid surrounding the brain and spinal cord.

Oncogene: A gene that normally directs cell growth. If altered, an oncogene can promote or allow the uncontrolled growth of cancer. Alterations can be inherited or caused by an environmental exposure to carcinogens. Myc, as, and erb are examples of oncogenes. The normal allele (alternative form of a gene) is called a proto-oncogene.

Overall survival: The percentage of people in a study or treatment group who are alive for a given period of time after diagnosis or treatment. It is often measured five years after diagnosis or treatment and called the five-year survival rate. Also called survival rate.

Palliative care: Activities that ease the symptoms of a disease or the side effects of treatment for a disease. Palliative care does not cure the disease. It is aimed at improving quality of life, and it addresses the psychological, social, and spiritual needs of patients and their families. Also called palliative therapy, comfort care, supportive care, and symptom management.

Paracentesis: A procedure involving numbing the skin and inserting a needle into the abdomen to remove fluid from the peritoneal cavity (the space within the abdomen that contains the intestines, the stomach, and the liver); it may be either diagnostic (to determine the cause of the fluid) or therapeutic (to remove as much fluid as possible).

Parenchyma: The essential or functional elements of an organ.

Partial response: A decrease in the size of a tumor, or the regression by more than 50 percent but less than 100 percent of the extent of cancer in the body.

Pathologic staging: A method used to determine the stage of cancer. Tissue samples are removed during surgery or a biopsy. The stage is determined based on how the cells in the samples look under a microscope.

Peau d'orange: A dimpled condition of the skin of the breast, resembling the skin of an orange, sometimes found in inflammatory breast cancer.

Pericardial effusion: An abnormal collection of fluid inside the sac that covers the heart.

Photodynamic therapy: Treatment with drugs that become active when exposed to light. These drugs kill cancer cells. May be used to treat chest wall recurrences.

Pleura: Thin layers of tissue covering the lungs and lining the interior wall of the chest cavity. The pleura protect and cushion the lungs. This tissue secretes a small amount of fluid that acts as a lubricant, allowing the lungs to move smoothly in the chest cavity while breathing.

Pleural effusion: An abnormal collection of fluid between the thin layers of tissue (pleura) lining the lungs and the wall of the chest cavity.

Pleurodesis: A medical procedure that uses chemicals or drugs to cause inflammation and adhesion between the layers of the pleura. This procedure prevents the buildup of fluid in the pleural cavity. It is used as a treatment for severe pleural effusion.

Port-a-cath: An implanted device through which blood may be withdrawn and drugs may be infused without repeated needle sticks. Also called a port.

Progesterone receptor (PR): A protein found inside the cells of the female reproductive tissue, some other types of tissue, and some cancer cells. The hormone progesterone will bind to the receptors inside the cells and may cause the cells to grow. Cancer cells that are PR-positive need progesterone to grow and will usually stop growing when treated with hormones that block progesterone from binding.

Progression-free survival: The length of time during and after treatment in which a patient is living with a disease that does not get worse. Progression-free survival may be used in a clinical study or trial to help find out how well a new treatment works.

Progressive disease: Cancer that is growing, spreading, or getting worse.

Protein: A molecule made up of amino acids that are needed for the body to function properly. Proteins are the basis of body structures such as skin and hair and of substances such as enzymes, cytokines, and antibodies.

Proto-oncogene: A gene that promotes normal cell growth and differentiation.

Quality of life: The overall enjoyment of life. Many clinical trials measure aspects of an individual's sense of well-being and ability to perform various tasks to assess the effects of cancer and its treatment.

Radiation therapy: The use of high-energy radiation from x-rays, gamma rays, neutrons, protons, and other sources to kill cancer cells and shrink tumors. Radiation may come from a machine outside the body (external-beam radiation therapy), or it may come from radioactive material placed in the body near cancer cells (internal radiation therapy). Systemic radiation therapy uses a radioactive substance, such as a radiolabeled monoclonal antibody, that travels in the blood to tissues throughout the body. Also called radiotherapy and irradiation.

Radiosurgery: A type of external radiation therapy that uses special equipment to position the patient and precisely give a single large dose of radiation to a tumor. It is used to treat brain tumors and other brain disorders that cannot be treated by regular surgery. It also is being studied in the treatment of other types of cancer. Also called stereotaxic radiosurgery, stereotactic radiosurgery, and radiation surgery.

Receptor: A molecule inside or on the surface of a cell that binds to a specific substance and causes a specific physiologic effect in the cell.

RECIST criteria: The standard criteria used for performance measurement in solid tumor clinical trials. The response criteria for evaluation include complete response (CR), partial response (PR), progressive disease (PD), and stable disease (SD).

Recurrence: The return of cancer at the same site as the original (primary) tumor or in another location after the original tumor had disappeared.

    Local: The cancer returns in the same place as the original cancer or is very close to it.

    Regional: The cancer returns in lymph nodes or tissues near the place of the original cancer.

    Distant: The cancer has spread (metastasized) to organs or tissues far from the place of the original cancer.

Refractory: Cancer that has not responded to treatment.

Relapse: The return of signs and symptoms of cancer after a period of improvement.

Response rate: The percentage of patients whose cancer shrinks more than 50 percent following treatment.

Selective estrogen-receptor modulator (SERM): A drug that acts like estrogen on some tissues but blocks the effect of estrogen on other tissues. Tamoxifen and raloxifene are selective estrogen-receptor modulators.

Signal transduction: Usually refers to the series of steps that occurs in the cell cytoplasm after a receptor has bound its ligand to communicate/transduce the signal to the cell nucleus. The "signal" of an activated receptor is carried through the cells by various intracellular messengers and cascades of enzymes. Often the signal will be sent to the nucleus, where genes are turned on and/or off to change the function of the cell. Sometimes referred to as downstream signaling.

Stable disease: A tumor may shrink but not enough to be categorized as a partial response (that is, tumor reduction greater than 50 percent). Or a tumor may increase in size but not enough to be considered progressive disease (that is, tumor growth greater than 20 percent). Such tumors, in which there is no significant change in size, are classified as stable disease.

Stage: The extent of a cancer, especially whether the disease has spread from the original site to other parts of the body. The stages of cancer vary for each cancer type and staging system used. Generally, cancers can be classified as follows:

    Stage 0: The cancer is still confined to the tissue in which it started. Also called carcinoma *in situ*.

    Stage I: The tumor is larger than in Stage 0 and has invaded the surrounding basement membrane, but it remains localized.

    Stage II: The tumor is larger, and cancer cells may be present in nearby lymph nodes.

    Stage III: Cancer has spread to nearby lymph nodes and/or tissue.

    Stage IV: Cancer has spread to distant lymph nodes and/or organs.

Standard treatment: A currently accepted and widely used treatment for a certain type of cancer, based on the results of past research. Also known as standard therapy.

T-cells or T-lymphocytes: White blood cells responsible for generating cell-mediated immune responses. Some T-cells (helper T-cells) enhance the response of other effector cells, including B cells, macrophages, and NK cells, by secreting cytokines. Others (cytotoxic T-cells) can directly kill virus-infected cells and tumor cells. T-cells are antigen-specific, but unlike antibodies they recognize their antigen only when it is cut into tiny pieces that are loaded into MHC molecules and displayed on the surface of a cell.

Targeted therapy: A type of treatment that uses drugs or other substances to identify and attack specific cancer cells while limiting the effect on normal cells.

Thoracentesis: A procedure involving numbing the skin, inserting a needle into the pleural cavity around the outside of the lung, and withdrawing fluid; it may be either diagnostic (to determine the cause of the fluid) or therapeutic (to remove as much fluid as possible).

Toxicity: Harmful side effects from an agent being tested.

Transcription: The synthesis of a single-stranded, complementary RNA molecule from a DNA template in the cell nucleus. When a gene is transcribed, it is said to be expressed. Not all genes are expressed in all cells.

Translation: The synthesis of a polypeptide chain (protein) from its mRNA template.

Translational research: Research that bridges the gap between laboratory research and its application to the clinic. This type of research, which often involves teams of scientists, conveys new ideas and discoveries between the lab and clinic, both to increase our understanding of cancer and to advance the diagnosis, treatment, and prevention of cancer.

Tumor-suppressor gene: A gene that normally inhibits excessive cell proliferation. Mutations that permanently disable tumor-suppressor genes can cause a cell to grow uncontrollably, leading to tumor development. Examples of tumor suppressors are pRB and p53. pRB (retinoblastoma protein) regulates the cell cycle at cell cycle checkpoints; p53 regulates the activity of certain molecules involved in the cell cycle, and it also prevents DNA replication and cell division in normal cells with damaged DNA.

Tyrosine kinases: A large group of enzymes important in cell growth, differentiation, and development.

Vaccine: A substance or group of substances meant to cause the immune system to respond to a tumor or to microorganisms, such as bacteria or viruses.

VEGF (vascular endothelial growth factor): A protein that is secreted by oxygen-deprived cells, such as cancerous cells. VEGF stimulates new blood vessel formation, or angiogenesis, by binding to specific receptors on nearby blood vessels, encouraging new blood vessels to form.

White blood cells: A variety of cells that fight invading germs, infection, and allergy-causing agents. Also called leukocytes.

References

Introduction

1. M. Garcia, A. Jemal, E. M. Ward et al., *Global Cancer Facts and Figures 2007* (Atlanta, Ga.: American Cancer Society, 2007).

2. B. Jonsson and N. Wilking, "Market Uptake of New Oncology Drugs," *Annals of Oncology* 18, Suppl. 3 (2007): iii31–iii48.

3. D. M. Parkin, F. Bray, J. Ferlay, and P. Pisani, "Global Cancer Statistics, 2002," *CA Cancer Journal for Clinicians* 55 (2005): 74–108.

4. American Cancer Society, *Breast Cancer Facts and Figures 2007–2008* (Atlanta, Ga.: American Cancer Society).

Chapter 1. Local and Distant Recurrence

1. L. A. G. Ries, D. Melbert, M. Krapcho et al., "SEER Cancer Statistics Review, 1975–2005," 2008. Available at http://seer.cancer.gov/csr/1975_2005/. Based on November 2007 SEER data submission, posted to the SEER Web site, 2008.

2. L. A. Carey, E. C. Dees, L. Sawyer et al., "The Triple Negative Paradox: Primary Tumor Chemosensitivity of Breast Cancer Subtypes." *Clinical Cancer Research* 13, no. 8 (2007): 2329–34.

3. S. Paik, G. Tang, S. Shak et al., "Gene Expression and Benefit of Chemotherapy in Women with Node-Negative, Estrogen Receptor-Positive Breast Cancer," *Journal of Clinical Oncology* 24, no. 23 (2006): 3726–34.

4. M. Buyse, S. Loi, L. van't Veer et al., "Validation and Clinical Utility of a 70-Gene Prognostic Signature for Women with Node-Negative Breast Cancer," *Journal of the National Cancer Institute* 98, no. 17 (2006): 1183–92.

5. T. Saphner, D. C. Tormey, and R. Gray, "Annual Hazard Rates of Recurrence for Breast Cancer after Primary Therapy," *Journal of Clinical Oncology* 14, no. 10 (1996): 2738–46.

6. C. L. Rock and W. Demark-Wahnefried, "Nutrition and Survival after the Diagnosis of Breast Cancer: A Review of the Evidence," *Journal of Clinical Oncology* 20, no. 15 (2002): 3302–16.

7. M. D. Holmes, W. Y. Chen, D. Feskanich, C. H. Kroenke, and G. A. Colditz, "Physical Activity and Survival after Breast Cancer Diagnosis," *Journal of the American Medical Association* 293, no. 20 (2005): 2479–86.

8. C. H. Kroenke, W. Y. Chen, B. Rosner, and M. D. Holmes, "Weight, Weight Gain, and Survival after Breast Cancer Diagnosis," *Journal of Clinical Oncology* 23, no. 7 (2005): 1370–78.

9. J. P. Pierce, M. L. Stefanick, S. W. Flatt et al., "Greater Survival after Breast Cancer in Physically Active Women with High Vegetable-Fruit Intake Regardless of Obesity," *Journal of Clinical Oncology* 25, no. 17 (2007): 2345–51.

10. R. T. Chlebowski, G. L. Blackburn, C. A. Thomson et al., "Dietary Fat Reduction and Breast Cancer Outcome: Interim Efficacy Results from the Women's Intervention Nutrition Study," *Journal of the National Cancer Institute* 98, no. 24 (2006): 1767–76.

11. L. Holmberg and H. Anderson, "HABITS (Hormonal Replacement Therapy after Breast Cancer—Is It Safe?), a Randomised Comparison: Trial Stopped," *Lancet* 363, no. 9407 (2004): 453–55.

12. E. von Schoultz and L. E. Rutqvist, "Menopausal Hormone Therapy after Breast Cancer: The Stockholm Randomized Trial," *Journal of the National Cancer Institute* 97, no. 7 (2005): 533–35.

13. V. G. Vogel, J. P. Costantino, D. L. Wickerham et al., "Effects of Tamoxifen vs. Raloxifene on the Risk of Developing Invasive Breast Cancer and Other Disease Outcomes: The NSABP Study of Tamoxifen and Raloxifene (STAR) P-2 Trial," *Journal of the American Medical Association* 295, no. 23 (2006): 2727–41.

14. M. Baum, A. U. Budzar, J. Cuzick et al., "Anastrozole Alone or in Combination with Tamoxifen versus Tamoxifen Alone for Adjuvant Treatment of Postmenopausal Women with Early Breast Cancer: First Results of the ATAC Randomised Trial," *Lancet* 359, no. 9324 (2002): 2131–39.

15. A. Howell, J. Cuzick, M. Baum et al., "Results of the ATAC (Arimidex, Tamoxifen, Alone or in Combination) Trial after Completion of 5 Years' Adjuvant Treatment for Breast Cancer," *Lancet* 365, no. 9453 (2005): 60–62.

16. P. E. Goss, J. N. Ingle, S. Martino et al., "A Randomized Trial of Letrozole in Postmenopausal Women after Five Years of Tamoxifen Therapy for Early-Stage Breast Cancer," *New England Journal of Medicine* 349, no. 19 (2003): 1793–1802.

17. P. E. Goss, J. N. Ingle, S. Martino et al., "Randomized Trial of Letrozole Following Tamoxifen as Extended Adjuvant Therapy in Receptor-Positive Breast Cancer: Updated Findings from NCIC CTG MA.17," *Journal of the National Cancer Institute* 97, no. 17 (2005): 1262–71.

18. R. C. Coombes, E. Hall, L. J. Gibson et al., "A Randomized Trial of Exemestane after Two to Three Years of Tamoxifen Therapy in Postmenopausal Women with Primary Breast Cancer," *New England Journal of Medicine* 350, no. 11 (2004): 1081–92.

19. R. Jakesz, W. Jonat, M. Gnant et al., "Switching of Postmenopausal Women with Endocrine-Responsive Early Breast Cancer to Anastrozole after 2 Years' Adjuvant Tamoxifen: Combined Results of ABCSG Trial 8 and ARNO 95 Trial," *Lancet* 366, no. 9484 (2005): 455–62.

20. B. Thurlimann, A. Keshaviah, A. S. Coates et al., "A Comparison of Letrozole and Tamoxifen in Postmenopausal Women with Early Breast Cancer," *New England Journal of Medicine* 353, no. 26 (2005): 2747–57.

21. M. Gnant, B. Mlineritsch, W. Schippinger et al., "Endocrine Therapy Plus Zoledronic Acid in Premenopausal Breast Cancer," *New England Journal of Medicine* 360, no. 7 (2009): 679–91.

22. M. P. Longnecker, P. A. Newcomb, R. Mittendorf et al., "Risk of Breast Cancer in Relation to Lifetime Alcohol Consumption," *Journal of the National Cancer Institute* 87, no. 12 (1995): 923–29.

23. C. A. Swanson, R. J. Coates, K. E. Malone et al., "Alcohol Consumption and Breast Cancer Risk among Women under Age 45 Years," *Epidemiology* 8, no. 3 (1997): 231–37.

24. S. M. Zhang, I. M. Lee, J. E. Manson, N. R. Cook, W. C. Willett, and J. E. Buring, "Alcohol Consumption and Breast Cancer Risk in the Women's Health Study," *American Journal of Epidemiology* 165, no. 6 (2007): 667–76.

25. K. W. Singletary and S. M. Gapstur, "Alcohol and Breast Cancer: Review of Epidemiologic and Experimental Evidence and Potential Mechanisms," *Journal of the American Medical Association* 286, no. 17 (2001): 2143–51.

26. P. Reynolds, S. Hurley, D. E. Goldberg et al., "Active Smoking, Household Passive Smoking, and Breast Cancer: Evidence from the California Teachers Study," *Journal of the National Cancer Institute* 96, no. 1 (2004): 29–37.

27. E. R. Bertone-Johnson, "Vitamin D and Breast Cancer," *Annals of Epidemiology* 19, no. 7 (July 2009): 462–67.

28. P. A. Bryant, J. Trinder, and N. Curtis, "Sick and Tired: Does Sleep Have a Vital Role in the Immune System?" *National Review of Immunology* 4, no. 6 (2004): 457–67.

29. M. L. Chen, J. S. Chen, C. L. Tang, and I. F. Mao, "The Internal Exposure of Taiwanese to Phthalate — An Evidence of Intensive Use of Plastic Materials," *Environment International* 34, no. 1 (2008): 79–85.

30. P. D. Darbre and P. W. Harvey, "Paraben Esters: Review of Recent Studies of Endocrine Toxicity, Absorption, Esterase and Human Exposure, and Discussion of Potential Human Health Risks," *Journal of Applied Toxicology* 28, no. 5 (2008): 561–78.

31. M. Feychting and U. Forssen, "Electromagnetic Fields and Female Breast Cancer," *Cancer Causes Control* 17, no. 4 (2006): 553–58.

32. C. Doyle, L. H. Kushi, T. Byers et al., "Nutrition and Physical Activity during and after Cancer Treatment: An American Cancer Society Guide for Informed Choices," *CA Cancer Journal for Clinicians* 56, no. 6 (2006): 323–53.

33. E. D. Pisano, C. Gatsonis, E. Hendrick et al., "Diagnostic Performance of Digital versus Film Mammography for Breast-Cancer Screening," *New England Journal of Medicine* 353, no. 17 (2005): 1773–83.

34. D. Saslow, C. Boetes, W. Burke et al., "American Cancer Society Guidelines for Breast Screening with MRI as an Adjunct to Mammography," CA *Cancer Journal for Clinicians* 57, no. 2 (2007): 75–89.

35. T. Kuukasjarvi, J. Kononen, H. Helin, K. Holli, and J. Isola, "Loss of Estrogen Receptor in Recurrent Breast Cancer Is Associated with Poor Response to Endocrine Therapy," *Journal of Clinical Oncology* 14, no. 9 (1996): 2584–89.

36. R. Allison, T. Mang, G. Hewson, W. Snider, and D. Dougherty, "Photodynamic Therapy for Chest Wall Progression from Breast Carcinoma Is an Underutilized Treatment Modality," *Cancer* 91, no. 1 (2001): 1–8.

37. T. Yau, C. Swanton, S. Chua et al., "Incidence, Pattern and Timing of Brain Metastases among Patients with Advanced Breast Cancer Treated with Trastuzumab," *Acta Oncologica* 45, no. 2 (2006): 196–201.

38. G. M. Clark, G. W. Sledge Jr., C. K. Osborne, and W. L. McGuire, "Survival from First Recurrence: Relative Importance of Prognostic Factors in 1,015 Breast Cancer Patients," *Journal of Clinical Oncology* 5, no. 1 (1987): 55–61.

39. P. Shie, R. Cardarelli, D. Brandon, W. Erdman, and N. Abdulrahim, "Meta-analysis: Comparison of F-18 Fluorodeoxyglucose-Positron Emission Tomography and Bone Scintigraphy in the Detection of Bone Metastases in Patients with Breast Cancer," *Clinical Nuclear Medicine* 33, no. 2 (2008): 97–101.

40. P. Glare, K. Virik, M. Jones et al., "A Systematic Review of Physicians' Survival Predictions in Terminally Ill Cancer Patients," *British Medical Journal* 327, no. 7408 (2003): 195–98.

41. S. K. Chia, C. H. Speers, Y. D'Yachkova et al., "The Impact of New Chemotherapeutic and Hormone Agents on Survival in a Population-Based Cohort of Women with Metastatic Breast Cancer," *Cancer* 110, no. 5 (2007): 973–79.

42. S. H. Giordano, A. U. Buzdar, T. L. Smith, S. W. Kau, Y. Yang, and G. N. Hortobagyi, "Is Breast Cancer Survival Improving?" *Cancer* 100, no. 1 (2004): 44–52.

Chapter 2. Immediate Concerns and Best Care

1. S. DeSanto-Madeya, S. Bauer-Wu, and A. Gross, "Activities of Daily Living in Women with Advanced Breast Cancer," *Oncology Nursing Forum* 34, no. 4 (2007): 841–46.

2. K. L. Kahn, "On Referral Patterns for Patients with Breast Cancer," *Journal of Clinical Oncology* 25, no. 3 (2007): 244–46.

3. J. Z. Ayanian and E. Guadagnoli, "Variations in Breast Cancer Treatment by

Patient and Provider Characteristics," *Breast Cancer Research and Treatment* 40, no. 1 (1996): 65–74.

4. C. R. Gillis and D. J. Hole, "Survival Outcome of Care by Specialist Surgeons in Breast Cancer: A Study of 3,786 Patients in the West of Scotland," *British Medical Journal* 312, no. 7024 (1996): 145–48.

5. M. A. Gilligan, J. Neuner, X. Zhang, R. Sparapani, P. W. Laud, and A. B. Nattinger, "Relationship between Number of Breast Cancer Operations Performed and 5-Year Survival after Treatment for Early-Stage Breast Cancer," *American Journal of Public Health* 97, no. 3 (2007): 539–44.

6. P. J. Roohan, N. A. Bickell, M. S. Baptiste et al., "Hospital Volume Differences and Five-Year Survival from Breast Cancer," *American Journal of Public Health* 88, no. 3 (1998): 454–57.

7. C. R. Gillis and D. J. Hole, "Survival Outcome of Care by Specialist Surgeons in Breast Cancer: A Study of 3,786 Patients in the West of Scotland," *British Medical Journal* 312, no. 7024 (1996): 145–48.

8. N. Hebert-Croteau, J. Brisson, J. Lemaire, J. Latreille, and R. Pineault, "Investigating the Correlation between Hospital of Primary Treatment and the Survival of Women with Breast Cancer," *Cancer* 104, no. 7 (2005): 1343–48.

9. B. E. Hillner, T. J. Smith, and C. E. Desch, "Hospital and Physician Volume or Specialization and Outcomes in Cancer Treatment: Importance in Quality of Cancer Care," *Journal of Clinical Oncology* 18, no. 11 (2000): 2327–40.

10. J. Groopman, *How Doctors Think* (Boston: Houghton Mifflin, 2007).

11. Institute of Medicine, *To Err Is Human: Building a Safer Health System* (Washington: National Academies Press, 2000).

12. L. A. Siminoff, P. Ravdin, N. Colabianchi, and C. M. Sturm, "Doctor–Patient Communication Patterns in Breast Cancer Adjuvant Therapy Discussions," *Health Expect* 3, no. 1 (2000): 26–36.

13. B. Booth, R. Glassman, and P. Ma, "Oncology's Trials," *Nature Reviews* 2, no. 8 (2003): 609–10.

14. B. G. Ryder, *The Alpha Book on Cancer and Living* (Alameda, Calif.: Alpha Institute, 1993).

Chapter 3. Medical Treatments

1. T. Kuukasjarvi, J. Kononen, H. Helin, K. Holli, and J. Isola, "Loss of Estrogen Receptor in Recurrent Breast Cancer Is Associated with Poor Response to Endocrine Therapy," *Journal of Clinical Oncology* 14, no. 9 (1996): 2584–89.

2. J. Zidan, I. Dashkovsky, C. Stayerman, W. Basher, C. Cozacov, and A. Hadary, "Comparison of HER-2 Overexpression in Primary Breast Cancer and Metastatic Sites and Its Effect on Biological Targeting Therapy of Metastatic Disease," *British Journal of Cancer* 93, no. 5 (2005): 552–56.

3. G. M. Clark, G. W. Sledge Jr., C. K. Osborne, and W. L. McGuire, "Survival from First Recurrence: Relative Importance of Prognostic Factors in 1,015 Breast Cancer Patients," *Journal of Clinical Oncology* 5, no. 1 (1987): 55–61.

4. W. Boogerd, A. A. Hart, and I. S. Tjahja, "Treatment and Outcome of Brain Metastasis as First Site of Distant Metastasis from Breast Cancer," *Journal of Neurooncology* 35, no. 2 (1997): 161–67.

5. G. Friedel, U. Pastorino, R. J. Ginsberg et al., "Results of Lung Metastasectomy from Breast Cancer: Prognostic Criteria on the Basis of 467 Cases of the International Registry of Lung Metastases," *European Journal of Cardiothoracic Surgery* 22, no. 3 (2002): 335–44.

6. C. Ludwig, E. Stoelben, and J. Hasse, "Disease-Free Survival after Resection of Lung Metastases in Patients with Breast Cancer," *European Journal of Surgical Oncology* 29, no. 6 (2003): 532–35.

7. G. Vlastos, D. L. Smith, S. E. Singletary et al., "Long-Term Survival after an Aggressive Surgical Approach in Patients with Breast Cancer Hepatic Metastases," *Annals of Surgical Oncology* 11, no. 9 (2004): 869–74.

8. M. G. Mack, R. Straub, K. Eichler, O. Sollner, T. Lehnert, and T. J. Vogl, "Breast Cancer Metastases in Liver: Laser-Induced Interstitial Thermotherapy— Local Tumor Control Rate and Survival Data," *Radiology* 233, no. 2 (2004): 400–409.

9. M. Selzner, M. A. Morse, J. J. Vredenburgh, W. C. Meyers, and P. A. Clavien, "Liver Metastases from Breast Cancer: Long-Term Survival after Curative Resection," *Surgery* 127, no. 4 (2000): 383–89.

10. J. Bines, D. M. Oleske, and M. A. Cobleigh, "Ovarian Function in Premenopausal Women Treated with Adjuvant Chemotherapy for Breast Cancer," *Journal of Clinical Oncology* 14, no. 5 (1996): 1718–29.

11. D. J. Slamon, B. Leyland-Jones, S. Shak et al., "Use of Chemotherapy Plus a Monoclonal Antibody against HER2 for Metastatic Breast Cancer That Overexpresses HER2," *New England Journal of Medicine* 344, no. 11 (2001): 783–92.

12. C. E. Geyer, J. Forster, D. Lindquist et al., "Lapatinib Plus Capecitabine for HER2-Positive Advanced Breast Cancer," *New England Journal of Medicine* 355, no. 26 (2006): 2733–43.

13. H. A. Burris 3rd, H. I. Hurwitz, E. C. Dees et al., "Phase I Safety, Pharmacokinetics, and Clinical Activity Study of Lapatinib (GW572016), a Reversible Dual Inhibitor of Epidermal Growth Factor Receptor Tyrosine Kinases, in Heavily Pretreated Patients with Metastatic Carcinomas," *Journal of Clinical Oncology* 23, no. 23 (2005): 5305–13.

14. K. Miller, M. Wang, J. Gralow et al., "Paclitaxel Plus Bevacizumab versus Paclitaxel Alone for Metastatic Breast Cancer," *New England Journal of Medicine* 357, no. 26 (2007): 2666–76.

15. J. C. Weeks, E. F. Cook, S. J. O'Day et al., "Relationship between Cancer

Patients' Predictions of Prognosis and Their Treatment Preferences," *Journal of the American Medical Association* 279, no. 21 (1998): 1709–14.

Chapter 4. Understanding Cancer Development, Treatment, and Emerging Therapies

1. J. M. Hall, M. K. Lee, B. Newman et al., "Linkage of Early-Onset Familial Breast Cancer to Chromosome 17q21," *Science* 250, no. 4988 (1990): 1684–89.
2. Y. Miki, J. Swensen, D. Shattuck-Eidens et al., "A Strong Candidate for the Breast and Ovarian Cancer Susceptibility Gene BRCA1," *Science* 266, no. 5182 (1994): 66–71.
3. R. Wooster, S. L. Neuhausen, J. Mangion et al., "Localization of a Breast Cancer Susceptibility Gene, BRCA2, to Chromosome 13q12-13," *Science* 265, no. 5181 (1994): 2088–90.
4. H. Meijers-Heijboer, A. van den Ouweland, J. Klijn et al., "Low-Penetrance Susceptibility to Breast Cancer due to CHEK2(*)1100delC in Noncarriers of BRCA1 or BRCA2 Mutations," *Nature Genetics* 31, no. 1 (2002): 55–59.
5. C. I. Li, B. O. Anderson, J. R. Daling, and R. E. Moe, "Trends in Incidence Rates of Invasive Lobular and Ductal Breast Carcinoma," *Journal of the American Medical Association* 289, no. 11 (2003): 1421–24.
6. M. M. Tilanus-Linthorst, M. Kriege, C. Boetes et al., "Hereditary Breast Cancer Growth Rates and Its Impact on Screening Policy," *European Journal of Cancer* 41, no. 11 (2005): 1610–17.
7. D. A. Berry, K. A. Cronin, S. K. Plevritis et al., "Effect of Screening and Adjuvant Therapy on Mortality from Breast Cancer," *New England Journal of Medicine* 353, no. 17 (2005): 1784–92.
8. C. E. Geyer, J. Forster, D. Lindquist et al., "Lapatinib Plus Capecitabine for HER2-Positive Advanced Breast Cancer," *New England Journal of Medicine* 355, no. 26 (2006): 2733–43.
9. G. J. Clark and C. J. Der, "Aberrant Function of the Ras Signal Transduction Pathway in Human Breast Cancer," *Breast Cancer Research and Treatment* 35, no. 1 (1995): 133–44.
10. M. Olivier, A. Langerod, P. Carrieri et al., "The Clinical Value of Somatic TP53 Gene Mutations in 1,794 Patients with Breast Cancer," *Clinical Cancer Research* 12, no. 4 (2006): 1157–67.
11. M. Cristofanilli, S. Krishnamurthy, L. Guerra et al., "A Nonreplicating Adenoviral Vector That Contains the Wild-Type p53 Transgene Combined with Chemotherapy for Primary Breast Cancer: Safety, Efficacy, and Biologic Activity of a Novel Gene-Therapy Approach," *Cancer* 107, no. 5 (2006): 935–44.

12. G. C. Alghisi and C. Ruegg, "Vascular Integrins in Tumor Angiogenesis: Mediators and Therapeutic Targets," *Endothelium* 13, no. 2 (2006): 113–35.

13. K. Miller, M. Wang, J. Gralow et al., "Paclitaxel Plus Bevacizumab versus Paclitaxel Alone for Metastatic Breast Cancer," *New England Journal of Medicine* 357, no. 26 (2007): 2666–76.

14. W. J. Gradishar, S. Tjulandin, N. Davidson et al., "Phase III Trial of Nanoparticle Albumin-Bound Paclitaxel Compared with Polyethylated Castor Oil-Based Paclitaxel in Women with Breast Cancer," *Journal of Clinical Oncology* 23, no. 31 (2005): 7794–803.

15. M. Cristofanilli, D. F. Hayes, G. T. Budd et al., "Circulating Tumor Cells: A Novel Prognostic Factor for Newly Diagnosed Metastatic Breast Cancer," *Journal of Clinical Oncology* 23, no. 7 (2005): 1420–30.

Chapter 5. Complementary, Alternative, and Integrative Care

1. W. A. Weiger, M. Smith, H. Boon, M. A. Richardson, T. J. Kaptchuk, and D. M. Eisenberg, "Advising Patients Who Seek Complementary and Alternative Medical Therapies for Cancer," *Annals of Internal Medicine* 137, no. 11 (2002): 889–903.

2. J. A. Astin, "Why Patients Use Alternative Medicine: Results of a National Study," *Journal of the American Medical Association* 279, no. 19 (1998): 1548–53.

3. P. J. Mansky and D. B. Wallerstedt, "Complementary Medicine in Palliative Care and Cancer Symptom Management," *Cancer Journal* 12, no. 5 (2006): 425–31.

4. M. Angell and J. P. Kassirer, "Alternative Medicine: The Risks of Untested and Unregulated Remedies," *New England Journal of Medicine* 339, no. 12 (1998): 839–41.

5. D. J. Newman and G. M. Cragg, "Natural Products as Sources of New Drugs over the Last 25 Years," *Journal of Natural Products* 70, no. 3 (2007): 461–77.

6. F. Arcamone, G. Cassinelli, G. Fantini et al., "Adriamycin, 14-Hydroxydaunomycin, a New Antitumor Antibiotic from S. peucetius var. caesius," *Biotechnology and Bioengineering* 11, no. 6 (1969): 1101–10.

7. F. Arcamone, G. Franceschi, S. Penco, and A. Selva, "Adriamycin (14-Hydroxydaunomycin), a Novel Antitumor Antibiotic," *Tetrahedron Letters* 13 (1969): 1007–10.

8. M. C. Wani, H. L. Taylor, M. E. Wall, P. Coggon, and A. T. McPhail, "Plant Antitumor Agents: VI. The Isolation and Structure of Taxol, a Novel Antileukemic and Antitumor Agent from Taxus brevifolia," *Journal of the American Chemical Society* 93, no. 9 (1971): 2325–27.

9. G. M. Cragg, S. A. Schepartz, M. Suffness, and M. R. Grever, "The Taxol Supply Crisis: New NCI Policies for Handling the Large-Scale Production of

Novel Natural Product Anticancer and Anti-HIV Agents," *Journal of Natural Products* 56, no. 10 (1993): 1657–68.

10. M. E. Wall and M. C. Wani, "Camptothecin and Taxol: Discovery to Clinic — Thirteenth Bruce F. Cain Memorial Award Lecture," *Cancer Research* 55, no. 4 (1995): 753–60.

11. F. Gueritte-Voegelein, D. Guenard, F. Lavelle, M. T. Le Goff, L. Mangatal, and P. Potier, "Relationships between the Structure of Taxol Analogs and Their Antimitotic Activity," *Journal of Medicinal Chemistry* 34, no. 3 (1991): 992–98.

12. A. Cirla and J. Mann, "Combretastatins: From Natural Products to Drug Discovery," *Natural Product Reports* 20, no. 6 (2003): 558–64.

13. B. Halliwell, "Reactive Species and Antioxidants: Redox Biology Is a Fundamental Theme of Aerobic Life," *Plant Physiology* 141, no. 2 (2006): 312–22.

14. H. E. Seifried, D. E. Anderson, E. I. Fisher, and J. A. Milner, "A Review of the Interaction among Dietary Antioxidants and Reactive Oxygen Species," *Journal of Nutritional Biochemistry* 18, no. 9 (2007): 567–79.

15. H. E. Seifried, S. S. McDonald, D. E. Anderson, P. Greenwald, and J. A. Milner, "The Antioxidant Conundrum in Cancer," *Cancer Research* 63, no. 15 (2003): 4295–98.

16. S. J. Korsmeyer, X. M. Yin, Z. N. Oltvai, D. J. Veis-Novack, and G. P. Linette, "Reactive Oxygen Species and the Regulation of Cell Death by the Bcl-2 Gene Family," *Biochimica et Biophysica Acta* 1271, no. 1 (1995): 63–66.

17. K. A. Conklin, "Dietary Antioxidants during Cancer Chemotherapy: Impact on Chemotherapeutic Effectiveness and Development of Side Effects," *Nutrition and Cancer* 37, no. 1 (2000): 1–18.

18. R. Chinery, J. A. Brockman, M. O. Peeler, Y. Shyr, R. D. Beauchamp, and R. J. Coffey, "Antioxidants Enhance the Cytotoxicity of Chemotherapeutic Agents in Colorectal Cancer: A p53-Independent Induction of p21WAF1/CIP1 via C/EBPbeta," *Nature Medicine* 3, no. 11 (1997): 1233–41.

19. C. Chen and A. N. Kong, "Dietary Cancer-Chemopreventive Compounds: From Signaling and Gene Expression to Pharmacological Effects," *Trends in Pharmacological Sciences* 26, no. 6 (2005): 318–26.

20. E. R. Bertone-Johnson, "Vitamin D and Breast Cancer," *Annals of Epidemiology* 19, no. 7 (2009): 462–67.

21. S. M. Zhang, W. C. Willett, J. Selhub et al., "Plasma Folate, Vitamin B6, Vitamin B12, Homocysteine, and Risk of Breast Cancer," *Journal of the National Cancer Institute* 95, no. 5 (2003): 373–80.

22. Y. Cui, J. M. Shikany, S. Liu, Y. Shagufta, and T. E. Rohan, "Selected Antioxidants and Risk of Hormone Receptor-Defined Invasive Breast Cancers among Postmenopausal Women in the Women's Health Initiative Observational Study," *American Journal of Clinical Nutrition* 87, no. 4 (2008): 1009–18.

23. T. Byers and G. Perry, "Dietary Carotenes, Vitamin C, and Vitamin E as Protective Antioxidants in Human Cancers," *Annual Review of Nutrition* 12 (1992): 139–59.

24. G. S. Omenn, G. E. Goodman, and M. D. Thornquist, "Risk Factors for Lung Cancer and for Intervention Effects in CARET, the Beta-Carotene and Retinol Efficacy Trial," *Journal of the National Cancer Institute* 88, no. 21 (1996): 1550–59.

25. I. M. Lee, N. R. Cook, J. M. Gaziano et al., "Vitamin E in the Primary Prevention of Cardiovascular Disease and Cancer: The Women's Health Study: A Randomized Controlled Trial," *Journal of the American Medical Association* 294, no. 1 (2005): 56–65.

26. G. Bjelakovic, D. Nikolova, L. L. Gluud, R. G. Simonetti, and C. Gluud, "Antioxidant Supplements for Prevention of Mortality in Healthy Participants and Patients with Various Diseases," *Cochrane Database of Systematic Reviews* (Online), no. 2 (2008): CD007176.

27. H. Zeng and G. F. Combs Jr., "Selenium as an Anticancer Nutrient: Roles in Cell Proliferation and Tumor Cell Invasion," *Journal of Nutritional Biochemistry* 19, no. 1 (January 2008): 1–7.

28. D. De Grandis, "Acetyl-L-Carnitine for the Treatment of Chemotherapy-Induced Peripheral Neuropathy: A Short Review," *CNS Drugs* 21, suppl. 1 (2007): 39–43, discussion 5–6.

29. P. Jolliet, N. Simon, J. Barre et al., "Plasma Coenzyme Q10 Concentrations in Breast Cancer: Prognosis and Therapeutic Consequences," *International Journal of Clinical Pharmacology Therapy and Toxicology* 36, no. 9 (1998): 506–9.

30. K. A. Conklin, "Coenzyme Q10 for Prevention of Anthracycline-Induced Cardiotoxicity," *Integrative Cancer Therapies* 4, no. 2 (2005): 110–30.

31. B. L. Pfeifer and W. B. Jonas, "Clinical Evaluation of 'Immunoaugmentative Therapy (IAT)': An Unconventional Cancer Treatment," *Integrative Cancer Therapies* 2, no. 2 (2003): 112–19.

32. S. Bonnet, S. L. Archer, J. Allalunis-Turner et al., "A Mitochondria-K+ Channel Axis Is Suppressed in Cancer and Its Normalization Promotes Apoptosis and Inhibits Cancer Growth," *Cancer Cell* 11, no. 1 (2007): 37–51.

33. P. Osterlund, T. Ruotsalainen, R. Korpela et al., "Lactobacillus Supplementation for Diarrhoea Related to Chemotherapy of Colorectal Cancer: A Randomised Study," *British Journal of Cancer* 97, no. 8 (2007): 1028–34.

34. A. B. Kunnumakkara, P. Anand, and B. B. Aggarwal, "Curcumin Inhibits Proliferation, Invasion, Angiogenesis and Metastasis of Different Cancers through Interaction with Multiple Cell Signaling Proteins," *Cancer Letters* 269, no. 2 (2008): 199–225.

35. W. Demark-Wahnefried, T. J. Polascik, S. L. George et al., "Flaxseed Supplementation (Not Dietary Fat Restriction) Reduces Prostate Cancer Prolifera-

tion Rates in Men Presurgery," *Cancer Epidemiology Biomarkers and Prevention* 17, no. 12 (2008): 3577–87.

36. Y. Cui, X. O. Shu, Y. T. Gao, H. Cai, M. H. Tao, and W. Zheng, "Association of Ginseng Use with Survival and Quality of Life among Breast Cancer Patients," *American Journal of Epidemiology* 163, no. 7 (2006): 645–53.

37. K. S. Kulp, J. L. Montgomery, D. O. Nelson et al., "Essiac and Flor-Essence Herbal Tonics Stimulate the *in vitro* Growth of Human Breast Cancer Cells," *Breast Cancer Research and Treatment* 98, no. 3 (2006): 249–59.

38. Y. H. Ju, D. R. Doerge, K. F. Allred, C. D. Allred, and W. G. Helferich, "Dietary Genistein Negates the Inhibitory Effect of Tamoxifen on Growth of Estrogen-Dependent Human Breast Cancer (MCF-7) Cells Implanted in Athymic Mice," *Cancer Research* 62, no. 9 (2002): 2474–77.

39. P. A. Johnstone, G. R. Polston, R. C. Niemtzow, and P. J. Martin, "Integration of Acupuncture into the Oncology Clinic," *Palliative Medicine* 16, no. 3 (2002): 235–39.

40. J. M. Ezzo, M. A. Richardson, A. Vickers et al., "Acupuncture-Point Stimulation for Chemotherapy-Induced Nausea or Vomiting," *Cochrane Database of Systematic Reviews* (Online) 2 (2006): CD002285.

41. M. L. McNeely, K. L. Campbell, B. H. Rowe, T. P. Klassen, J. R. Mackey, and K. S. Courneya, "Effects of Exercise on Breast Cancer Patients and Survivors: A Systematic Review and Meta-Analysis," *Canadian Medical Association Journal* 175, no. 1 (2006): 34–41.

42. C. Buettner, C. H. Kroenke, R. S. Phillips, R. B. Davis, D. M. Eisenberg, and M. D. Holmes, "Correlates of Use of Different Types of Complementary and Alternative Medicine by Breast Cancer Survivors in the Nurses' Health Study," *Breast Cancer Research and Treatment* 100, no. 2 (2006): 219–27.

43. J. W. Carson, K. M. Carson, L. S. Porter, F. J. Keefe, H. Shaw, and J. M. Miller, "Yoga for Women with Metastatic Breast Cancer: Results from a Pilot Study," *Journal of Pain and Symptom Management* 33, no. 3 (2007): 331–41.

44. I. Sola, E. Thompson, M. Subirana, C. Lopez, and A. Pascual, "Non-Invasive Interventions for Improving Wellbeing and Quality of Life in Patients with Lung Cancer," *Cochrane Database of Systematic Reviews* (Online) 4 (2004): CD004282.

45. S. F. Duijts, M. P. Zeegers, and B. V. Borne, "The Association between Stressful Life Events and Breast Cancer Risk: A Meta-Analysis," *International Journal of Cancer* 107, no. 6 (2003): 1023–29.

46. L. E. Carlson, M. Speca, K. D. Patel, and E. Goodey, "Mindfulness-Based Stress Reduction in Relation to Quality of Life, Mood, Symptoms of Stress, and Immune Parameters in Breast and Prostate Cancer Outpatients," *Psychosomatic Medicine* 65, no. 4 (2003): 571–81.

47. H. J. Yoo, S. H. Ahn, S. B. Kim, W. K. Kim, and O. S. Han, "Efficacy of Progressive Muscle Relaxation Training and Guided Imagery in Reducing Chemo-

therapy Side Effects in Patients with Breast Cancer and in Improving Their Quality of Life," *Support Care Cancer* 13, no. 10 (2005): 826–33.

48. K. L. Tsang, L. E. Carlson, and K. Olson, "Pilot Crossover Trial of Reiki versus Rest for Treating Cancer-Related Fatigue," *Integrative Cancer Therapies* 6, no. 1 (2007): 25–35.

49. D. Labriola, *Complementary Cancer Therapies: Combining Traditional and Alternative Approaches for the Best Possible Outcome* (Roseville, Calif.: Prima Publishing, 2000).

50. A. Sparreboom, M. C. Cox, M. R. Acharya, and W. D. Figg, "Herbal Remedies in the United States: Potential Adverse Interactions with Anticancer Agents," *Journal of Clinical Oncology* 22, no. 12 (2004): 2489–503.

Chapter 6. Managing Pain and Understanding the Dying Process

1. R. Melzack and P. D. Wall, *The Challenge of Pain* (London: Penguin Books, 1982).

2. National Institutes of Health, "Acupuncture: National Institutes of Health Consensus Development Conference Statement." Bethesda, Md., 1997.

3. G. H. Montgomery, K. N. DuHamel, and W. H. Redd, "A Meta-Analysis of Hypnotically Induced Analgesia: How Effective Is Hypnosis?" *International Journal of Clinical and Experimental Hypnosis* 48, no. 2 (2000): 138–53.

4. M. J. Ott, R. L. Norris, and S. M. Bauer-Wu, "Mindfulness Meditation for Oncology Patients: A Discussion and Critical Review," *Integrative Cancer Therapies* 5, no. 2 (2006): 98–108.

5. R. K. Portenoy, H. T. Thaler, A. B. Kornblith et al., "Symptom Prevalence, Characteristics and Distress in a Cancer Population," *Quality of Life Research* 3, no. 3 (1994): 183–89.

6. Washington v. Glucksberg, 521 U.S. 702, 1997, pp. 736–37.

7. C. K. Daugherty and D. P. Steensma, "Overcoming Obstacles to Hospice Care: An Ethical Examination of Inertia and Inaction," *Journal of Clinical Oncology* 21, no. 9 (2003): 42s–45s.

8. B. Karnes, *Gone from My Sight: The Dying Experience* (Stilwell, Kans.: Barbara Karnes Publishing, 1986).

Chapter 7. Practical Matters

1. National Funeral Directors Association, "Statistics, Funeral Service Facts," 2009.

2. National Funeral Directors Association, "Projections for 2025 Based on Past

Five Years' Average Percentage Change and Cremations-to-Deaths Projections for 2010–2025," 2008.

Chapter 8. Emotional and Spiritual Well-Being

1. D. A. Fishbain, R. Cutler, H. L. Rosomoff, and R. S. Rosomoff, "Chronic Pain-Associated Depression: Antecedent or Consequence of Chronic Pain? A Review," *Clinical Journal of Pain* 13, no. 2 (1997): 116–37.
2. K. Charmaz, *Good Days, Bad Days: The Self in Chronic Illness and Time* (New Brunswick, N.J.: Rutgers University Press, 1991), 2, 12.
3. E. Kosofsky-Sedgwick in *Mamm: Women, Cancer, and Community*, September 2000, 24.
4. "Depression," National Institute of Mental Health. Available at http://www.nimh.nih.gov/publicat/depression.cfm#ptdep7 (accessed June 16, 2006).
5. J. Bukberg, J. D. Penman, and J. C. Holland, "Depression in Hospitalized Cancer Patients," *Psychosomatic Medicine* 46 (1980): 999–1004.
6. S. Sontag, *Illness as Metaphor* (New York: Farrar, 1978), 58.
7. "On Our Own Terms: Moyers On Dying," September 10, 2000. Available at http://www.pbs.org/wnet/onourownterms (accessed January 31, 2008).
8. R. Naomi-Remen, *Kitchen Table Wisdom: Stories That Heal* (New York: Riverhead Books [G. P. Putnam], 1996), 151–53.

Appendix B. Diet and Breast Cancer

1. W. Demark-Wahnefried and C. L. Rock, "Nutrition-Related Issues for the Breast Cancer Survivor," *Seminars in Oncology* 30, no. 6 (2003): 789–98.
2. J. Shen, M. D. Gammon, M. B. Terry et al., "Polymorphisms in XRCC1 Modify the Association between Polycyclic Aromatic Hydrocarbon-DNA Adducts, Cigarette Smoking, Dietary Antioxidants, and Breast Cancer Risk," *Cancer Epidemiology Biomarkers and Prevention* 14, no. 2 (2005): 336–42.
3. A. A. Davies, G. Davey Smith, R. Harbord et al., "Nutritional Interventions and Outcome in Patients with Cancer or Preinvasive Lesions: Systematic Review," *Journal of the National Cancer Institute* 98, no. 14 (2006): 961–73.
4. M. T. Williams, N. G. Hord, "The Role of Dietary Factors in Cancer Prevention: Beyond Fruits and Vegetables," *Nutrition in Clinical Practice* 20, no. 4 (2005): 451–59.
5. J. Cade, V. Burley, and D. Greenwood, "Dietary Fibre and Risk of Breast Cancer in the UK Women's Cohort Study," *International Journal of Epidemiology* 36, no. 2 (2007): 431–38.

6. D. P. Rose, M. Goldman, J. M. Connolly, and L. E. Strong, "High-Fiber Diet Reduces Serum Estrogen Concentrations in Premenopausal Women," *American Journal of Clinical Nutrition* 54, no. 3 (1991): 520–25.

7. A. Ronco, E. De Stefani, M. Mendilaharsu, and H. Deneo-Pellegrini, "Meat, Fat and Risk of Breast Cancer: A Case-Control Study from Uruguay," *International Journal of Cancer* 65, no. 3 (1996): 328–31.

8. A. L. Ronco, E. De Stefani, P. Boffetta, H. Deneo-Pellegrini, G. Acosta, and M. Mendilaharsu, "Food Patterns and Risk of Breast Cancer: A Factor Analysis Study in Uruguay," *International Journal of Cancer* 119, no. 7 (2006): 1672–78.

9. D. W. Layton, K. T. Bogen, M. G. Knize, F. T. Hatch, V. M. Johnson, and J. S. Felton, "Cancer Risk of Heterocyclic Amines in Cooked Foods: An Analysis and Implications for Research," *Carcinogenesis* 16, no. 1 (1995): 39–52.

10. R. T. Chlebowski, G. L. Blackburn, C. A. Thomson et al., "Dietary Fat Reduction and Breast Cancer Outcome: Interim Efficacy Results from the Women's Intervention Nutrition Study," *Journal of the National Cancer Institute* 98, no. 24 (2006): 1767–76.

11. C. la Vecchia, E. Negri, S. Franceschi, A. Decarli, A. Giacosa, and L. Lipworth, "Olive Oil, Other Dietary Fats, and the Risk of Breast Cancer (Italy)," *Cancer Causes Control* 6, no. 6 (1995): 545–50.

12. M. Verheus, C. H. van Gils, L. Keinan-Boker, P. B. Grace, S. A. Bingham, and P. H. Peeters, "Plasma Phytoestrogens and Subsequent Breast Cancer Risk," *Journal of Clinical Oncology* 25, no. 6 (2007): 648–55.

13. R. G. Ziegler, R. N. Hoover, M. C. Pike et al., "Migration Patterns and Breast Cancer Risk in Asian-American Women," *Journal of the National Cancer Institute* 85, no. 22 (1993): 1819–27.

14. C. A. Lamartiniere, "Protection against Breast Cancer with Genistein: A Component of Soy," *American Journal of Clinical Nutrition* 71, no. 6 (2000): 1705s–7s; discussion 8s–9s.

15. H. Adlercreutz, "Phytoestrogens and Breast Cancer," *Journal of Steroid Biochemistry and Molecular Biology* 83, nos. 1–5 (2002): 113–18.

16. Y. H. Ju, D. R. Doerge, K. F. Allred, C. D. Allred, and W. G. Helferich, "Dietary Genistein Negates the Inhibitory Effect of Tamoxifen on Growth of Estrogen-Dependent Human Breast Cancer (MCF-7) Cells Implanted in Athymic Mice," *Cancer Research* 62, no. 9 (2002): 2474–77.

17. C. D. Allred, N. C. Twaddle, K. F. Allred et al., "Soy Processing Affects Metabolism and Disposition of Dietary Isoflavones in Ovariectomized BALB/c Mice," *Journal of Agricultural and Food Chemistry* 53, no. 22 (2005): 8542–50.

18. M. Saadatian-Elahi, T. Norat, J. Goudable, and E. Riboli, "Biomarkers of Dietary Fatty Acid Intake and the Risk of Breast Cancer: A Meta-Analysis," *International Journal of Cancer* 111, no. 4 (2004): 584–91.

Index

The letter *f* following a page number denotes a figure; *g* glossary entry; *t* table.

About the Authors

Barbara Lynn Gordon is an associate professor of English at Elon University in North Carolina, where she teaches writing as well as an upper-level interdisciplinary seminar titled "At Death's Door." Her other publications focus on writing centers, first-year composition, and interdisciplinary studies. She has participated in meditation practice for more than twenty years with Osho Gentei Stewart at the North Carolina Zen Center. In July 1995 she was diagnosed with Stage II breast cancer and two summers later was suspected of having metastases, an experience that instigated this book.

Heather S. Shaw is currently training further in breast cancer prevention at the University of North Carolina, Chapel Hill. From 1999 to 2009, she was a breast oncology clinician and assistant professor of medicine at Duke University Medical Center in the Multidisciplinary Breast Program of the Duke Comprehensive Cancer Center. During that time, her clinical practice and research were devoted exclusively to breast cancer. She has been principal investigator or co-principal investigator on dozens of clinical trials in breast cancer patients and has published numerous articles and book chapters about breast cancer and complementary/ alternative medicine in scholarly journals and textbooks. Her research has been funded by the National Institutes of Health and Susan G. Komen for the Cure. She is board-certified in both Internal Medicine and Medical Oncology and will become board-certified in Preventive Medicine.

David J. Kroll is professor and chair of pharmaceutical sciences at North Carolina Central University; adjunct associate professor of medicine at Duke University; and adjunct associate professor of pharmacology at the University of North Carolina, Chapel Hill. He specializes in the action of anti-cancer drugs derived from natural sources. He has authored, with Steven Bratman, *Clinical Evaluation of Medicinal Herbs and Other Therapeutic Natural Products* (1999). He has edited, with Steven Bratman, *Natural Health Bible: From the Most Trusted Source in Health Information Here Is Your A–Z Guide to over 200 Herbs, Vitamins, and Supplements* (1999). His most recent projects, supported by the National Cancer Institute, have focused on the potential interactions between herbs and chemotherapy and the possible utility of milk thistle extracts in various types of cancer. Dr. Kroll also lectures widely to public and professional audiences on herbal medicines and dietary supplements.

Brooke Ratliff Daniel is a private practice medical oncologist at Chattanooga Oncology and Hematology Associates in Tennessee. She has extensive training and experience in palliative care, the practice of cancer medicine focused on reducing pain and suffering and improving the quality of life of cancer patients. She trained with Dr. Shaw while she was a hematology/oncology fellow at the Duke University Medical Center. Dr. Daniel's scholarly publications include articles on tamoxifen and palliative care.

Library of Congress Cataloging-in-Publication Data
Breast cancer recurrence and advanced disease :
comprehensive expert guidance / Barbara L.
Gordon . . . [et al.].
p. cm.
Includes bibliographical references and index.
ISBN 978-0-8223-4742-2 (cloth : alk. paper)
ISBN 978-0-8223-4763-7 (pbk. : alk. paper)
1. Breast—Cancer—Popular works. 2. Breast—
Cancer—Relapse—Popular works. I. Gordon,
Barbara L., 1952–
RC280.B8B67229 2010
616.99′449—dc22   2009047587